CELL BIOLOGICAL ASPECTS OF DISEASE

BOERHAAVE SERIES
FOR POSTGRADUATE
MEDICAL EDUCATION
Vol. 19

PROCEEDINGS OF BOERHAAVE COURSES
ORGANIZED BY
THE FACULTY OF MEDICINE, UNIVERSITY OF LEIDEN,
THE NETHERLANDS

CELL BIOLOGICAL ASPECTS
OF DISEASE

The plasma membrane
and lysosomes

edited by

W.Th. DAEMS

Laboratory for Electron Microscopy, University of Leiden

E.H. BURGER

Laboratory of Cell Biology and Histology, University of Leiden

B.A. AFZELIUS

Wenner-Gren Institute, Stockholm

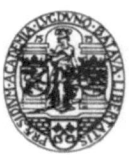

1981

LEIDEN UNIVERSITY PRESS
THE HAGUE / BOSTON / LONDON

Distributors:

for the United States and Canada

Kluwer Boston, Inc.
190 Old Derby Street
Hingham, MA 02043
USA

for all other countries

Kluwer Academic Publishers Group
Distribution Center
P.O. Box 322
3300 AH Dordrecht
The Netherlands

Library of Congress Cataloging in Publication Data   CIP

Main entry under title:

Cell biological aspects of disease.

  (Boerhaave series for postgraduate medical education; v. 19)
  Includes index.
  1. Pathology, Cellular. 2. Plasma membranes. 3. Lysosomes. I. Daems, W.Th.
II. Burger, E.H. III. Afzelius, Björn. IV. Series. [DNLM: I. Disease – Congresses.
2. Pathology – Congresses. 3. Plasma cells – Congresses. 4. Lysosomes – Congresses.
W3 B0672 v. 19/QZ40 C393]
RB25.C33   611′.01815   80-24216

ISBN-13:978-94-009-8614-5   e-ISBN-13:978-94-009-8612-1
DOI: 10.1007/978-94-009-8612-1

Cover design: Paul Burg

CONTENTS

CONTRIBUTORS

Afzelius, B.A., Wenner-Gren Institute, Nortullsgatan 16, S-11345 Stockholm, Sweden

Beek, W.P. van, Division of Cell Biology, Antoni van Leeuwenhoek-Huis, The Netherlands Cancer Institute, Plesmanlaan 121, 1066 CX Amsterdam, The Netherlands

Blitterswijk, W.J. van, Division of Cell Biology, Antoni van Leeuwenhoek-Huis, The Netherlands Cancer Institute, Plesmanlaan 121, 1066 CX Amsterdam, The Netherlands

Bruijn, W.C. de, Laboratory for Electron Microscopy, University of Leiden, Rijnsburgerweg 10, 2333 AA Leiden, The Netherlands

Burger, E.H., Laboratory for Cell Biology and Histology, University of Leiden, Rijnsburgerweg 10, 2333 AA Leiden, The Netherlands

Clarke, J., Clinical Research Centre, Division of Clinical Investigation, Watford Road, Harrow, HA1 3UJ, Middlesex, England

Conzelmann, E., Institut für Organische Chemie und Biochemie der Universität Bonn, Gerhard-Domagkstrasse 1, D-5300 Bonn 1, Federal Republic of Germany

Daems, W.Th., Laboratory for Electron Microscopy, University of Leiden, Wassenaarseweg 62, 2333 AL Leiden, The Netherlands

Damen, J., Laboratory for Physiological Chemistry, University of Groningen, Bloemsingel 10, 9712 KZ Groningen, The Netherlands

D'Arcy Hart, P., National Institute for Medical Research, The Ridgeway, Mill Hill, London NW7 1AA, England

Davis, C., Clinical Research Centre, Division of Clinical Investigation, Watford Road, Harrow, HA1 3UJ, Middlesex, England

Emmelot, P., Division of Cell Biology, Antoni van Leeuwenhoek-Huis, The Netherlands Cancer Institute, Plesmanlaan 121, 1066 CX Amsterdam, The Netherlands

Galjaard, H., Erasmus University, Medical Faculty, Department of Cell Biology and Genetics, P.O. Box 1738, Rotterdam, The Netherlands

Glaumann, H., Department of Pathology, Karolinska Institutet, Huddinge University Hospital, S-14186 Huddinge, Sweden

Gregoriadis, G., Clinical Research Centre, Division of Clinical Investigation, Watford Road, Harrow, HA1 3UJ, Middlesex, England

Groot, P.G. de, B.C.P. Jansen Institute, Laboratory for Biochemistry, Plantage Muidergracht 12, 1018 TV Amsterdam, The Netherlands

Hamers, M.N., Central Laboratory of the Netherlands Red Cross Transfusion Service, Plesmanlaan 125, 1066 CX Amsterdam

Hoekstra, D., Laboratory for Physiological Chemistry, University of Groningen, Bloemsingel 10, 9712 KZ Groningen, The Netherlands

Hoeven, R.P. van, Division of Cell Biology, Antoni van Leeuwenhoek-Huis, The Netherlands Cancer Institute, Plesmanlaan 121, 1066 CX Amsterdam, The Netherlands

Hollemans, M., B.C.P. Jansen Institute, Laboratory for Biochemistry, Plantage Muidergracht 12, 1018 TV Amsterdam, The Netherlands

Jacques, P.J., Department of Biochemical Cytology and Parasitic Diseases, Box CIRMAP 3057, UCL-School of Public Health, Avenue Chapelle aux Champs 30, Brussels, Belgium-1200

Jones, T.C., The New York Hospital – Cornell University Medical Center, Department of Medicine, Division of Infectious Diseases, 525 East 68th Street, New York, N.Y. 10021, U.S.A.

Kalsbeek, R., B.C.P. Jansen Institute, Laboratory for Biochemistry, Plantage Muidergracht 12, 1018 TV Amsterdam, The Netherlands

Kaplan, G., University of Tromsö, Institute of Medical Biology, 9001 Tromsö, Norway

Kapsenberg, M.L., Laboratory of Histology and Cell Biology, Faculty of Medicine, University of Amsterdam, 1e Constantijn Huygensstraat 20, 1054 BW Amsterdam, The Netherlands

Kirby, C., Clinical Research Centre, Division of Clinical Investigation, Watford Road, Harrow, HA1 3UJ, Middlesex, England

Krans, H.M.J., Department of Endocrinology and Metabolic Diseases, University Medical Centre, Rijnsburgerweg 10, 2333 AA Leiden, The Netherlands

Leene, W., Laboratory of Histology and Cell Biology, Faculty of Medicine, University of Amsterdam, 1e Constantijn Huygensstraat 20, 1054 BW Amsterdam, The Netherlands

Manesis, E., Clinical Research Centre, Division of Clinical Investigation, Watford Road, Harrow, HA1 3UJ, Middlesex, England

Marzella, L., Department of Pathology, Karolinska Institutet Huddinge University Hospital, S-14186 Huddinge, Sweden

Mey, J.R. de, Janssen Pharmaceutica Research Laboratories, Laboratory of Oncology, B-2340 Beerse, Belgium

Moolenaar, W.H., Hubrecht Laboratory International Embryological Institute, Uppsalalaan 8, 3584 CT Utrecht, The Netherlands

Neerunjun, D., Clinical Research Centre, Division of Clinical Investigation, Watford Road, Harrow, HA1 3UJ, Middlesex, England

Renswoude, A.J.B.M. van, Laboratory for Physiological Chemistry University of Groningen, Bloemsingel 10, 9712 KZ Groningen, The Netherlands

Roerdink, F.H., Laboratory for Physiological Chemistry, University of Groningen, Bloemsingel 10, 9712 KZ Groningen, The Netherlands

Sanderson, C.J., Transplantation Biology Clinical Research Centre, Watford Road, Harrow HA1 3UJ, England

Sandhoff, K., Institut für Organische Chemie und Biochemie der Universität Bonn, Gerhard-Domagkstrasse 1, D-5300 Bonn 1, Federal Republic of Germany

Scherphof, G.L., Laboratory for Physiological Chemistry, University of Groningen, Bloemsingel 10, 9712 KZ Groningen, The Netherlands

Strijland, A., B.C.P. Jansen Institute, Laboratory for Biochemistry, Plantage Muidergracht 12, 1018 TV Amsterdam, The Netherlands

Tager, J.M., B.C.P. Jansen Institute, Laboratory for Biochemistry, Plantage Muidergracht 12, Amsterdam, The Netherlands

Tegelaers, F.P.W., B.C.P Jansen Institute, Laboratory for Biochemistry, Plantage Muidergracht 12, 1018 TV Amsterdam, The Netherlands

Temmink, J.H.M., Landbouwhogeschool Wageningen, Vakgroep Toxicology, De Dreijen 12, 6703 BC Wageningen, The Netherlands

Thompson, G.R., Lpid Metabolism Unit, Hammersmith Hospital, Du Cane Road, London W 12045, England

Trouet, A., Université Catholique de Louvain, International Institute of Cellular and Molecular Pathology, Avenue Hippocrate 75, B-1200 Brussels, Belgium

Vermeer, B.J., Department of Dermatology, University Medical Centre, Rijnsburgerweg 10, 2333 AA Leiden, The Netherlands

Vroman, L., Research Carier Scientist Interface Laboratory, Veterans Administration Hospital, Brooklyn, N.Y. 11209, New York, U.S.A.

Wieringa, Tj., Department of Endocrinology and Metabolic Diseases, University Medical Centre, Rijnsburgerweg 10, 2333 AA Leiden, The Netherlands

Wohlfarth-Bottermann, K.E., Institut für Cytologie und Mikromorphologie der Universität Bonn, Ulrich-Haberlandstrasse 61a, D-5300 Bonn 1, Federal Republic of Germany

Zwaal, R.F.A., Biomedical Centre, Faculty of Medicine, State University of Limburg, P.O. Box 616, 6200 MD Maastricht, The Netherlands

1. CELL BIOLOGY AND MEDICINE: AN INTRODUCTION

W. TH. DAEMS

This volume contains the papers presented at a Boerhaave Course for Post-graduate Education on *The cell-biological aspects of disease: the plasma membrane and lysosomes*. One of the purposes of this introduction is to explain the reasons for this choice of subject.

The first question which might be asked — why a postgraduate course on the cell biological aspects of disease was considered neccessary — is not difficult to answer: the impact of the basic sciences on medicine is immeasurably strong, and among these sciences cell biology has contributed immensely to the advances made in medicine during recent decades. It has provided clues leading to general insights into etiology and pathogenesis as well as to the development of diagnostic tools and a basis for therapeutic methods. These insights derived mainly from the still-increasing body of knowledge about the architecture of cells.

Initially, this knowledge arose from the notion that cells are either simply bags full of enzymes or complex spongelike structures in which all organelles are permanently interconnected (Fig. 1). Later, this notion was replaced by a highly schematized picture of the cell as an essentially two-compartment structure (Fig. 2) in which cell organelles are discrete units separated from each other by membranes, enabling each organelle to maintain an internal microenvironment with optimal conditions for its specific metabolic processes. In this concept, connections between the compartments and between the cell and its environment can be realized by membrane fusion and fission without disturbing these specific microenvironments [1]. Especially the latter view, together with newly acquired knowledge about the metabolic processes occurring in cells, contributed greatly to the development of concepts on the functioning of normal cells and thus provided a baseline for the understanding of pathological processes. In other words, Virchow's concept of cellular disorders as the basis of diseases [2] was revived and pathology again became a cellular pathology. This cellular pathology was developed further into an organelle pathology and, to some extent, a molecular pathology. As a result, it became increasingly evident that the complex symptomatology of diseases can often be attributed to one well-defined agent, to one malfunctioning organelle, or to one missing enzyme.

The advances made in cell biology and, perhaps even more so, in bio-

2

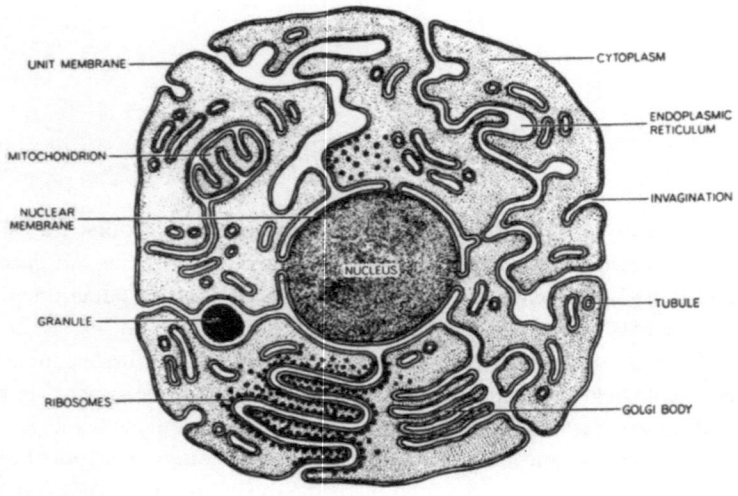

Fig. 1. Schematic drawing of a cell according to Robertson [12].

chemistry and molecular biology, are seen to be revolutionary when we compare the present situation with that of fifty years ago. This progress has been due mainly, if not completely, to the almost simultaneous advances in methodology made in biochemistry, electron microscopy, cytochemistry, automation technology, etc. These methods provided a basis for further research on the complex mechanisms of cell-cell interactions in such situations as morphogenetic and embryonic development, interactions between cells and viruses, microorganisms, or parasites, and defense against tumor cells, as well as in mechanisms underlying neurophysiological processes.

As already mentioned, it is now known that complex symptomatologies often have a single cause. One of the many examples is that of the lysosomal storage diseases, which are caused by a hereditary enzyme deficiency in the lysosomes of all cells of an organism [3]. As a result of this deficiency, certain compoumds normally digested with the help of the missing enzyme will accumulate in the lysosomes. Protracted lysosomal storage usually interferes with the functioning of the cells in which the loaded lysosomes are present. This ultimately disturbs the function of the organ or tissue containing the affected cells and leads to a condition which is usually fatal.

The variety of symptoms shown by patients with a lysosomal storage disease are seemingly unrelated, but can all be explained by the fact that the enzyme deficiency expresses itself when the cells that lack the lysosomal enzyme required for the digestion also contain the compound to be digested. For instance, in Pompe's disease, only organs with cells in which glycogen has to be digested in lysosomes are affected, for instance the liver and the heart;

3

the spleen is unaffected. In Gaucher's disease, the spleen is severely affected, because its macrophages must digest red blood cells but do not have the appropriate enzyme in their lysosomes. The heart is not affected in Gaucher's disease, because although the lysosomes in the muscle cells of the heart lack the same enzyme, these cells do not have to digest red blood cells. There is reason to assume that atherosclerosis is caused by a comparable phenomenon, i.e., a relative deficiency of lysosomal enzymes in the vascular smooth muscle cells, leading to an intralysosomal accumulation of lipoproteins [4].

A similar example of a complex symptomatology based on a single cause is the Kartagener or immotile cilia syndrome in which a dysfunctioning of cilia, caused by a defect in their microtubular structure, results in such seemingly unrelated phenomena as upper respiratory infections, sterility, and situs inversus [5]. Another example concerns white blood cells. Before cell-biological analysis of the functional interactions between plasma membranes and the submembranous contractile proteins became possible, the cause of neutrophil abnormalities was obscure. We now know that disturbances of chemotaxis, phagocytosis, and lysosomal degranulation are due to a disruption of the integrity of the cytoskeleton-membrane organization and that these disturbances explain the failure of bacterial surveillance in, for instance, the Chediak-Higashi syndrome [6].

Cell biology has also had considerable influence on the development of

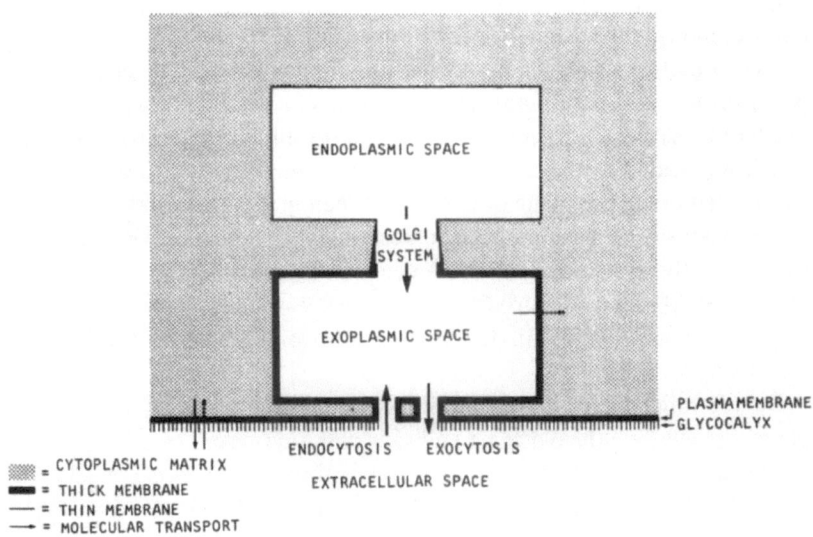

Fig. 2. Schematic drawing of the partition of a cell in an endoplasmic and exoplasmic space. The membranes of the endoplasmic space are relatively thin, whereas those of the exoplasmic space are relatively thick [13].

diagnostic tools such as automatic chromosome analysis and the micro-chemical determination of enzymes in amniotic-fluid cells. Studies on human genetics utilizing cell-biological methods and insights have led to the development of sophisticated approaches in this field.

These and other important contributions to medicine explain why attention is given to cell biology in a postgraduate course like the present one. However, the contributions are so numerous and are spread over so many specialized fields that only a relatively small number of topics can be dealt with in two days. There were two main reasons for limiting the subject matter to the plasma membrane and the lysosomes. In the first place, membranology is one of the areas of cell biology in which knowledge concerning normal function and pathology is now well defined [7]. The fluid mosaic membrane model formulated by Singer and Nicholson [see 8] can be considered one of the major accomplishments in cell biology. Very few concepts have opened such wide perspectives and had such a far-reaching influence [9]. In the second place, any encounter between a cell and its surroundings starts at the cell surface and triggers innumerable processes, many of which involve the plasma membrane [10], in which invagination of the plasma membrane leads to the uptake of part of the *milieu exterieure* into the cell's cytoplasm. This makes endocytosis an important process in the defense of the organism, for instance against microorganisms. Since effective defense means that the material taken up by endocytosis is introduced into the intracellular digestive system, defective fusion between phagosomes and lysosomes will enable microorganisms to escape lysosomal digestion [11]. Detailed knowledge of the lysosomal apparatus opens possibilities for new therapeutic approaches in parasitic diseases that do not respond to conventional treatment.

All of these steps — recognition of the extracellular materials by means of receptors located at the cell surface, the processes involving the motility of these receptors in the plane of the plasma membrane, the uptake of material by endocytosis, the fusion of lysosomes, the relationship between these processes and the systems of microfilaments and microtubuli, and many more — are susceptible to disturbances, and these deviations from normal function have consequences for the normal functioning of cells and hence the organism.

On the other hand, understanding of the normal functioning of cell organelles, including the plasma membrane and its adnexes, can throw light on pathogenetic mechanisms and thus, as mentioned above, open possibilities for the design of appropriate prophylactic or therapeutic measures to replace the trial and error of the empirical approach [3]. This is how modern cell biology can provide contemporary medicine with important improvements in diagnosis and therapy.

It should be emphasized here that collaboration between research scientists and clinicians is not a one-way road: the clinician too has a task, for instance to provide the research worker with pathological material and thus to give him the results of nature's experiments. In addition to experimental studies in animals and model studies, it is the human material, normal and diseased, which must in the end complete the picture. The gap between clinicians and research scientists is, however, still rather wide and at best is not increasing. The collaboration between basic science and medicine is seldom institutionalized, and is usually the result of incidental personal contacts between individuals. The fact that very few medical students are willing to seek a career in basic research and that relatively few of the more than 10,000 clinicians responded to the invitation to attend this Boerhaave course are ominous signs that should not be ignored. There is a challenge here for all of us. Any attempt to change this situation should be based on the notion that basic science, including cell biology, is essential for the progress of medicine.

REFERENCES

1. Duve C de: An integrated view of lysosome function. In: Molecular basis of biological degradative processes. New York, Academic Press, 1978, pp 25–38.
2. Virchow R: Die Cellularpathologie in ihrer Begründung auf physiologische und pathologische Gewebelehre. Berlin, Verlag August Hirschwald, 1862.
3. Tager JM, Hooghwinkel GJM, Daems WTh (eds): Enzyme therapy in lysosomal storage diseases. Amsterdam, Oxford, North-Holland, 1974.
4. Wolinsky H, Fowler S: Participation of lysosomes in atherosclerosis. N Engl J Med 299: 1173–1178, 1978.
5. Afzelius B, Eliasson R, Johnsen Ø, Lindholmer C: Lack of dynein arms in immotile human spermatozoa. J Cell Biol 66: 225–232, 1975.
6. Oliver JM: Cell biology of leucocyte abnormalities. Membrane and cytoskeletal function in normal and defective cells. Am J Pathol 93: 221–259, 1978.
7. Weissman G, Claiburne R (eds): Cell membranes. Biochemistry, cell biology and pathology. New York, HP, 1975.
8. Singer SJ, Nicolson GL: The fluid mosaic model of the structure of cell membranes. Science (NY) 175: 720–731, 1972.
9. Booij HL, Daems WTh (eds): Biomembranen 50 jaar na Gorter en Grendel. Wageningen, Pudoc. 1976.
10. Silverstein SC, Steinman RA, Cohn ZA: Endocytosis. Annu Rev Biochem 46: 669–722, 1977.
11. Jones ThC: Macrophages and intracellular parasitism. J Reticuloendothel Soc 15: 439–450, 1974.
12. Robertson JD: The membrane of the living cell. Sci Am 206: 65–72, 1962.
13. Daems WTh: Functionele morfologie van biomembranen. In: Booij HL, Daems WTh (eds) Biomembranen 50 jaar na Gorter en Grendel. Wageningen, Pudoc, 1976, pp 78–87.

2. RECENT VIEWS ON THE STRUCTURE AND FUNCTION OF THE PLASMA MEMBRANE

R.F.A. ZWAAL

MEMBRANE STRUCTURE

The attainment of an understanding of the molecular structure of biological membranes is a central goal in cell biology, since without this the wide variety of functions which membranes perform cannot be understood. One of the most conspicuous structural features of biological membranes is the bimolecular lipid leaflet, which was first recognized by Gorter and Grendel in 1925 [1]. Their findings initiated some four decades of thought on the molecular architecture, culminating in the fluid mosaic membrane model of Singer and Nicolson in 1972 [2]. The lipid molecules are thought to be arranged in bilayers with polar headgroups directed outward towards the aqueous medium on both sides of the membrane and the hydrocarbon chains pointed towards the centre of the bilayer away from contact with water (Fig. 1). Membrane proteins are bound to the bilayer by both polar and hydrophobic interactions. They are considered to be either peripheral or integral. Peripheral proteins are associated with the membrane predominantly by electrostatic interactions with the polar headgroups of the phospholipids and can in general be detached from the membrane by manipulation of the ionic strength of pH. Integral proteins have a non-polar part of their molecules intercalculated in the lipid bilayer or even span the membrane from one side to the other (Fig. 2). Solubilization of these proteins generally requires the use of detergents [3].

MEMBRANE LIPIDS

The lipid fraction of most mammalian plasma membranes usually accounts for half of the total mass, the remainder being occupied by membrane proteins. The lipids are mainly composed of phospholipids, cholesterol, and, to a smaller extent, of glycolipids (usually gangliosides). Slightly more than half of the phospholipid fraction is composed of the choline-containing phospholipids lecithin and sphingomyelin, the remainder consisting of a wide variety of other phospholipids, of which phosphatidylethanolamine and phosphatidylserine are the most abundant. Due to their amphipathic

8

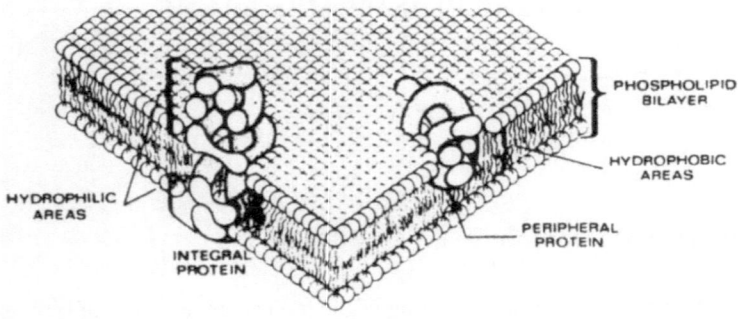

Fig. 1. Fluid mosaic membrane model

nature, phospholipids spontaneously form concentric multilamellar bilayer structures (liposomes) when suspended in an aqueous environment [4] (Fig. 3).

Alternatively, single bilayer vesicles can be prepared in water after sonication of the liposomes [5] or after mixing solutions of lipids in organic solvents with water followed by removal of the solvent [6, 7]. Similar vesicles are also formed after dissolving lipids in the presence of detergents, which are subsequently removed [8, 9]. These techniques have been successfully applied in studies dealing with recombination between lipids and membrane proteins. Judged according to a number of criteria, but especially the result of freeze-fracture electron microscopy, these recombinant structures show a close resemblance to native membranes [9].

Spontaneous formation of closed bilayer structures in aqueous solutions is considered to be a consequence of the unfavourable thermodynamic inter-action of water with the hydrocarbon chains [10] and also requires that these fatty acid chains be in a liquid-crystalline state [11]. The phase transition temperature at which the bilayer changes from a liquid-crystalline to a gel state depends on the length and degree of unsaturation of the apolar side chains and on the nature of the polar headgroup of the phospholipids [12]. The presence of cholesterol in the bilayer exerts a condensing effect on the lipids in the liquid-crystalline state and a liquefying effect on lipids in the gel state, thus bringing about an intermediate condition of the bilayer interior [13]. Moreover, both temperature and enthalpy of the phase transition can be influenced by proteins binding to the bilayer. In bilayers containing mix-tures of phospholipids, such as most biological membranes, a progressive phase change occurs over a broad range of temperatures, which indicates that phase separations into gel and liquid-crystalline areas occur [14]. At physiological temperatures, most naturally occurring lipid mixtures are in the liquid-crystalline state which is accompanied by a rapid molecular motion of the hydrocarbon chains and a great lateral mobility of the phospholipid molecules. This motion is thought to be restricted when lipids are associated with membrane proteins. The lipids in this boundary layer are thought to have more of the characteristics of the gel state below the phase transition temperature. Translocation of phospholipids from one half of the bilayer to the other appear to be a rare event in artificial phospholipid vesicles [15], unless considerable differences in lateral molecular packing are present between the two halves of the bilayer [16]. Also, the introduction of membrane proteins may considerably accelerate this process [17], and half-times of only a few hours have been inferred for translocation (flip-flop) rates of lecithin in red cell membranes [18, 19].

MEMBRANE ASYMMETRY

There is now compelling evidence that both lipids and proteins are asymmetrically distributed between the two halves of the membrane bilayer [20, 21]. The non-random distribution of phospholipids in erythrocyte and platelet plasma membranes in shown schematically in Fig. 4. In both types of membrane phosphatidylserine appears to be almost exclusively located on the cytoplasmic surface, the outer monolayer of the membrane being composed of neutral phospholipids, particularly sphingomyelin [22, 23]. The vectorial arrangement of membrane proteins is more absolute. In general, it appears

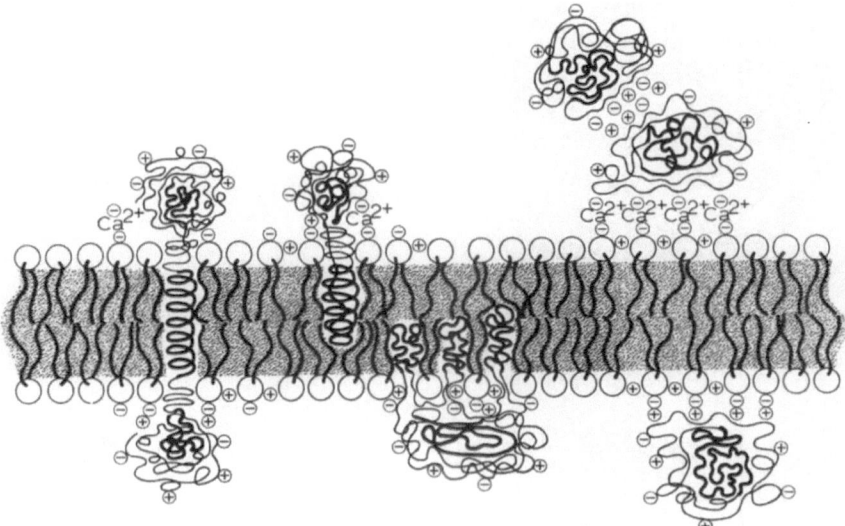

Fig. 2. Schematic representation of proteins interacting with a phospholipid bilayer. The apolar areas of proteins and lipids are represented by heavier lines than those used for the polar areas. Note that hydrophobic domains tend to cluster together away from contact with water.

10

that in most mammalian plasma membranes the majority of the proteins, including the membrane-bound enzymes, are associated with the cytoplasmic side of the membrane, whereas the carbohydrate moieties are almost exclusively found on the exterior surface of the membrane bound either to glycolipids or to glycoproteins extending across the lipid bilayer [3, 24, 25]. An example of such a glycoprotein is the major sialoglycoprotein (glycophorin) of erythrocytes, which has highly localized sites for interaction with the lipid bilayer (Fig. 5). This protein consists of a sincle polypeptide chain of 131 amino acids of known sequence and an average of 16 oligosaccharide chains [26]. The carbohydrates are covalently linked to the N-terminal half of the polypeptide chain and are exposed to the external environment of the cell. The C-terminal part of the molecule, which is rich in proline, extends into the cytoplasm, where it may interact with contractile membrane proteins. The two parts of the molecule are connected by a segment of 23 apolar amino acids, presumably extending across the intramembranous domain and anchoring the membrane-spanning protein by hydrophobic interactions. In model studies this protein exhibits an interaction with lipids, particularly when acidic phospholipids such as phosphatidylserine are present [27]. This has led to the suggestion that a salt bridge between the negatively charged polar headgroup of phosphatidylserine and the positively charged amino

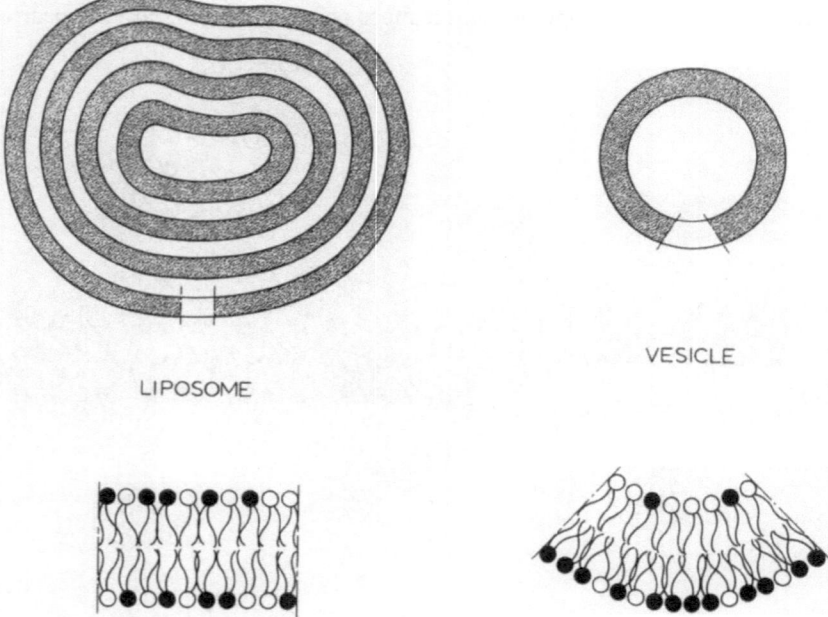

LIPOSOME

VESICLE

Fig. 3. Schematic representation of multilamellar liposomes and unilamellar vesicles obtained after dispersion of lipids in water.

acids on the cytoplasmic side just beyond the hydrophobic region of the protein (-Arg-Arg-Leu-Ile-Lys-Lys-) contributes to the correct orientation of the protein in the membrane.

MEMBRANE FUNCTION

Whereas the lipid bilayer forms the structural framework of the membrane, the proteins mediate most of the biochemical functions that membranes perform. These functional aspects include active and facilitated transport of small molecules through the membrane, enzymatic activities involved in maintaining the status quo of the cell and performing its specific functions, binding of hormones to the cell surface and transduction into chemical signals across the membrane, and many more. It must be emphasized, however, that the majority of these processes occur at lipid-water interfaces. Therefore, a simple distinction between lipids and proteins in terms of structural and functional components of membranes, respectively, cannot always be maintained. Lipids apparently provide the suitable environment, not only for a number of typical membrane processes, but also for related phenomena such as the provision of a catalytic surface for interacting coagulation factors. Nevertheless, with the possible exception of the receptor function of gangliosides for cholera toxin [28], the functional significance of lipids and particularly of lipid asymmetry is much less well understood than that of proteins. Two cases have so far been recognized in which lipid asymmetry may contribute in biological control.

Exocytosis. Recent studies may suggest that in intracellular membranes, phosphatidylserine is almost exclusively present on the outside of the membrane, i.e. on the cytoplasmic surface [29]. From the observation that artificially prepared phospholipid vesicles merge readily in the presence of Ca^{2+} when phosphatidylserine is present at the vesicle surface [30, 31], it can be inferred that the fusion process directly preceding the Ca-induced release of intracellular compounds might be made possible by the presence of phosphatidylserine on the opposing cytoplasmic surfaces of the membranes to be fused [23, 32].

Haemostasis. Recent experiments indicate that procoagulant phospholipids (such as mixtures of negatively charged phosphatidylserine and neutral phospholipids) are absent on the outer surface of blood cells, and are exclusively located on the cytoplasmic surface of the membrane [20, 33]. Moreover, the outer surface of the erythrocyte membrane is devoid of procoagulant activity, whereas strong clot-promoting activity is present on the inner surface. In view

12

of the similar phospholipid asymmetry in erythrocyte and platelet plasma membranes, it has been postulated that the procoagulant effect of platelet phospholipids (platelet factor 3) is present on the inner surface of the membrane [33]. The absence of procoagulant phospholipids on the outer surface of blood cells would avoid a condition of 'permanent' hypercoagulability but requires at the same time that the platelet plasma membrane possess a mechanism which, upon platelet activation, translocates phosphatidylserine through the plasma membrane to provide a catalytic lipid surface for interacting coagulation factors [20].

MEMBRANES AND PATHOLOGY

Finally, the functional role of membrane components can often be inferred from experiments of nature, where structural deviations or alterations in membrane composition are accompanied by certain pathological conditions. In the case of the lipids, alterations in the composition often seem to be a secondary effect, not providing a direct insight into their functional signifi-

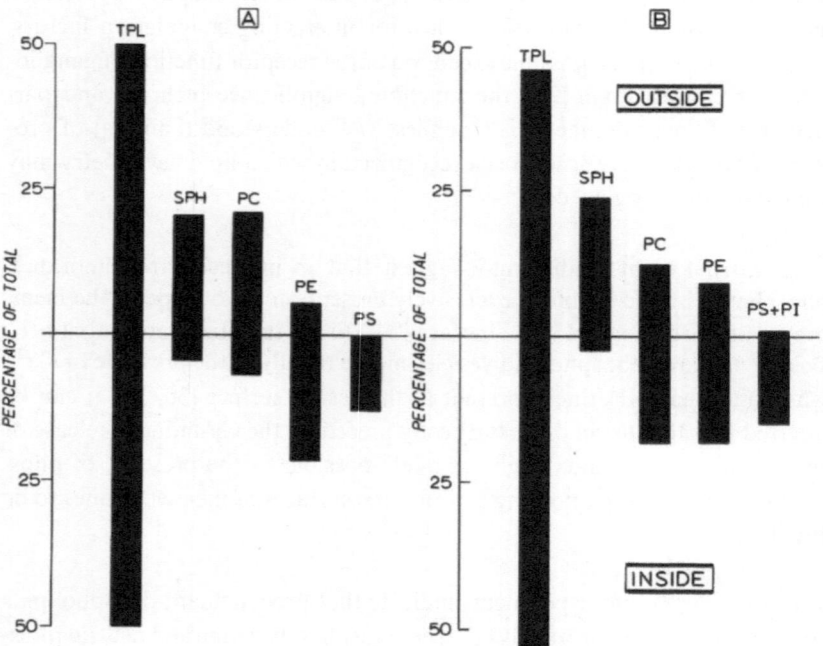

Fig. 4. Asymmetric distribution of phospholipids between inner and outer layers of human red cell membranes (A) and pig platelet membranes (B). TPL, total phospholipid; SPH, sphingomyelin; PC, phosphatidylcholine; PE, phosphatidylethanolamine; PS, phosphatidylserine; PI, phosphatidylinositol.

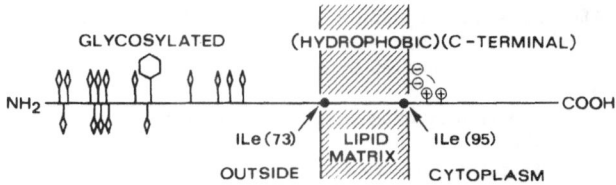

Fig. 5. Schematic representation of the transmembrane orientation of human erythrocyte glycophorin.

cance. For example, the huge increase of cholesterol and lecithin in erythrocytes under the conditions of obstructive and hepatocellular liver disease appears to result from fusion of lipoprotein-X with the red-cell membrane, which leads to target-cell morphology [34]. On the other hand, defects in membrane proteins are often primarily responsible for pathological conditions. Two prominent examples are known for human platelet membranes. Two glycoproteins (presumably similar to erythrocyte glycophorin) are lacking in platelets of patients with Glanzmann's thrombasthenia [35], which is characterized by a defect of platelet aggregation and release induced by ADP or collagen. Platelets of patients with the Bernard-Soulier syndrome lack another membrane glycoprotein [35, 36]. This protein is probably equivalent to the receptor for the Von Willebrand factor, which is necessary for adhesion of platelets to the subendothelium. These platelets also fail to interact with thrombin. In this respect it is remarkable that the complete absence of human erythrocyte glycophorin [En(a-)erythrocytes] is not associated with a pathological condition, presumably because its functions are taken over by band III protein, which appears to be more heavily glycosylated than in normal cells [37].

Twenty-five years ago, the molecular basis of biological membranes was largely unknown. This certainly is no longer the case. Nevertheless, our understanding of the relationships between membrane structure and function is still fragmentary. It is the complexity of the dynamic processes of membranes that has produced far more questions than can at present be answered. That makes this field so interesting — if occasionally frustrating as well.

REFERENCES

1. Gorter E, Grendel F: On bimolecular layers of lipoids on the chromocytes of the blood. J Exp Med 41: 439–443, 1925.
2. Singer SJ, Nicolson GL: The fluid mosaic model of the structure of cell membranes. Science 175: 805–837, 1972.
3. Steck TL: The organization of proteins in the human red blood cell membrane. A review. J Cell Biol 61: 1–20, 1974.

14

4. Bangham AD, Standish MM, Watkins JC: Preparation and use of liposomes as models of biological membranes. J Mol Biol 13: 253–264, 1965.
5. Huan C: Preparation of unilamellar phospholipid vesicles by sonication. Biochemistry 8: 344–351, 1969.
6. Batzri S, Korn ED: Single bilayer liposomes prepared without sonication. Biochim Biophys Acta 298: 1015–1019, 1973.
7. Deamer D, Bangham AD: Large volume liposomes by an ether vaporization method. Biochim Biophys Acta 443: 629–634, 1976.
8. Brunner J, Skrabal P, Hauser H: Single bilayer vesicles without sonication: physicochemical properties. Biochim Biophys Acta 455: 322–331, 1976.
9. Gerritsen WJ, Verkleij AJ, Zwaal RFA, Deenen LLM van: Freeze-fracture appearance and disposition of band 3 protein from the human erythrocyte membrane in lipid vesicles. Eur J Biochem 85: 255–261, 1978.
10. Tanford C: The hydrophobic effect. New York, Wiley, 1973.
11. Gier J de, Mandersloot JG, Deenen LLM van: Lipid composition and permeability of liposomes. Biochim Biophys Acta 150: 666–675, 1968.
12. Dijck PWM van, Kruijff B de, Deenen LLM van, Gier J de, Demel RA: The preference of cholesterol for phosphatidylcholine in mixed phosphatidylcholine-phosphatidylethanolamine bilayers. Biochim Biophys Acta 455: 576–587, 1976.
13. Demel RA, Kruijff B de: The function of sterols in membranes. Biochim Biophys Acta 457: 109–132, 1976.
14. Dijck PWM van, Zoelen EJJ van, Seldenrijk R, Deenen LLM van, Gier J de: Calorimetric behaviour of individual phospholipid classes from human and bovine erythrocyte membranes. Chem Phys Lipids 17: 336–343, 1976.
15. Kornberg RD, McConnel HM: Inside-outside transitions of phospholipids in vesicle membranes. Biochemistry 10: 1111–1120, 1971.
16. Kruijff B de, Wirtz KWA: Induction of a relatively fast transbilayer movement of phosphatidylcholine in vesicles. A ^{13}C NMR study. Biochim Biophys Acta 468: 318–326, 1977.
17. Kruijff B de, Zoelen EJJ van, Deenen LLM van: Glycophorin facilitates the transbilayer movement of phosphatidylcholine in vesicles. Biochim Biophys Acta 509: 537–542, 1978.
18. Renooij W, Golde LMG van, Zwaal RFA, Deenen LLM van: Topological asymmetry of phospholipid metabolism in rat erythrocyte membranes. Evidence for flip-flop of lecithin. Eur J Biochem 61: 53–58, 1976.
19. Bloj B, Zilversmit DB: Asymmetry and transposition rates of phosphatidylcholine in rat erythrocyte ghosts. Biochemistry 15: 1277–1284, 1976.
20. Zwaal RFA: Membrane and lipid involvement in blood coagulation. Biochim Biophys Acta 515: 163–205, 1978.
21. Rothman JE, Lenard J: Membrane asymmetry. Science 195: 743–753, 1977.
22. Zwaal RFA, Roelofsen B, Comfurius P, Deenen LLM van: Organization of phospholipids in human red cell membranes as detected by the action of various purified phospholipases. Biochim Biophys Acta 406: 83–96, 1975.
23. Chap JH, Zwaal RFA, Deenen LLM van: Action of highly purified phospholipases on blood platelets. Evidence for an asymmetric distribution of phospholipids in the surface membrane. Biochim Biophys Acta 467: 146–164, 1977.
24. Zwaal RFA, Roelofsen B, Colley CM: Localization of red cell membrane constituents. Biochem Biophys Acta 360: 159–182, 1973.
25. Bretscher MS: Membrane structure: some general principles. Science 181: 622–629, 1973.
26. Tomita M, Marchesi VT: Amino-acid sequence and oligosaccharide attachment sites of human erythrocyte glycophorin. Proc Natl Acad Sci USA 72: 2964–2968, 1975.
27. Zoelen EJJ van, Zwaal RFA, Reuvens FAM, Demel RA, Deenen LLM van: Evidence for the preferential interaction of glycophorin with negatively charged phospholipids. Biochim Biophys Acta 464: 482–492, 1977.
28. Bennet V, Cuatrecasas P: Mechanism of action of *Vibrio cholerae* enterotoxin. J Membr Biol 22: 1–52, 1975.
29. Nilsson OS, Dallner G: Enzyme and phospholipid asymmetry in liver microsomal membranes. J Cell Biol 72: 568–583, 1977.

30. Papahadjopoulos D, Poste G, Schaeffer DE, Vail WJ: Membrane fusion and molecular segregation in phospholipid vesicles. Biochim Biophys Acta 352: 10–28, 1974.
31. Miller C, Racker E: Fusion of phospholipid vesicles reconstituted with cytochrome C oxidase and mitochondrial hydrophobic protein. J Membr Biol 26: 319–333, 1976.
32. Portis A, Newton C, Pangborn W, Papahadjopoulos D: Studies on the mechanism of membrane fusion: evidence for a intermembrane CA^{2+}-phospholipid complex, synergism with Mg^{2+}, and inhibition by spectrin. Biochemistry 18: 780–790, 1979.
33. Zwaal RFA, Comfurius P, Deenen LLM van: Membrane asymmetry and blood coagulation. Nature 268: 360–362, 1977.
34. Deenen LLM van, Gier J de, Golde LMG van, Nauta ILD, Renooij W, Verkleij AJ, Zwaal RFA: Some topological and dynamic aspects of lipids in the erythrocyte membrane. Nobel Symp 34: 107–118, 1976.
35. Nurden AT, Caen J: Membrane glycoproteins and human platelet function. Br J Haematol 38: 155–160, 1977.
36. Ganguly P: Binding of thrombin to functionally defective platelets: a hypothesis on the nature of the thrombin receptor. Br J Haematol 37: 47–51, 1977.
37. Gahmberg CG, Myllyla G, Leikola J, Pirkola A, Nordling S: Absence of the major sialoglycoprotein in the membrane of human En (a-) erythrocytes and increased glycosylation of band 3. J Biol Chem 251: 6108–6116, 1976.

3. PLASMA MEMBRANE STRUCTURE AS REVEALED WITH FREEZE-FRACTURE METHODS

W. LEENE AND M.L. KAPSENBERG

INTRODUCTION

The ubiquitous trilaminar appearance of cellular membranes as seen in thin-sectioned cells and tissues may reflect some common underlying structural features, which has led to the 'unit membrane' concept [1], but does not contribute essentially to our present insight into membrane structure and function, because too little is known about the chemical mechanism of membrane staining. With the introduction of the freeze-fracture technique (syn.: freeze-cleave, freeze-etch) [2], however, a potent tool became available to analyse the membrane interior and to gather information on the arrangement of various molecules in the membrane.

Since this technique is now widely used in membrane research, it will be useful to provide a guide to the interpretation of freeze-fracture results before discussing some of its interesting applications and perspectives.

INTERPRETING FREEZE-FRACTURE DATA

When a plasma membrane (part of which is presented schematically as a profile in Fig. 1) is freeze fractured, it splits into two leaflets, and external or, according to the nomenclature of Branton et al. [3], extracellular half (E) and an internal or protoplasmic half (P). The fracture proceeds along one plane of the membrane, as can be demonstrated with the complementary replica technique (for an example, see Fig. 8), and is located in the central hydrophobic region between the outer and inner phospholipid layers [4, 5]. As shown in Fig. 2, the external membrane half (E) is partially removed by the fracture process. In this way, two fracture faces can be produced in one membrane region: an external fracture face (EF) and a protoplasmic fracture face (PF) (Fig. 2, PF; Fig. 3, EF and PF).

If replicas of the fracture faces are prepared, internal structures of the membrane can be studied with transmission electron microscopy. Generally,

Abbreviations: EF, external fracture face; FITC, fluorescine isothiocyanate; IMP, intramembranous particles; PHA, phytohemagglutinin; PF, protoplasmic fracture face; sIg, surface immunoglobulin.

W.Th. Daems et al. (eds.), Cell Biological Aspects of Disease, 17–25. All rights reserved.
Copyright © 1981 by Martinus Nijhoff Publishers bv, The Hague/Boston/London.

only one fracture face (external or protoplasmic) is replicated but for the complementary replica technique both fracture faces (the external and proto-plasmic faces of one membrane region) are replicated.

From such studies a general picture of the membrane interior was developed, the smooth areas of the replicas reflecting the pure lipid regions in the membrane, the particles (bumps or intramembranous particles) representing protein macromolecules. Recent observations have, however, made it necessary to regard this generally accepted notion with some caution. In the first place, Verkleij et al. [6] demonstrated that intramembranous particles showing complementary pits can represent inverted micelles of phospholipid molecules (Fig. 3, lipidic particles and complementary pits), indicating that the relative disposition of the intramembranous particles may reflect not only the organization of proteins in the membrane but also the organization of lipids. Secondly, the demonstrability of intramembraneous proteins also depends on their position in the lipid bilayer (integral or peripheral proteins; see Zwaal, this volume, chapter 1), their relation to cytoplasmic proteins, and their susceptibility to the fracture forces employed.

In Fig. 4, the fate of various types of integral membrane proteins in the fracture process is indicated. The transmembrane proteins (T) are pulled out of the external half of the membrane, leaving no complementary pit in that half. The more excentrically located integral proteins (R) do not give rise to intramembrane particle formation in the external fracture face (EF). Peripheral proteins do not give rise to intramembranous-particle formation, and are not indicated in these Figures. Fig. 5 shows how transmembrane proteins firmly anchored to cytoplasmic proteins, e.g., band 3 protein in the erythrocyte plasma membrane [7, 8], may give rise to intramembranous particles in the protoplasmic fracture face (PF). In this case they leave pits in the complementary EF, while other transmembrane proteins are pulled through to the external membrane half. Finally, in the freeze-fracture process transmembrane proteins (e.g., sialoglycoproteins in the erythrocyte plasma membrane) may be cleaved at selected points [8], giving in that case not always rise to the formation of IMP (Fig. 6, broken IMP). It should be concluded from these data (summarized in Fig. 7) that the absence of IMP does not necessarily reflect the absence of proteins in the membrane region studied; on the other hand, although the protein nature of IMP is confirmed for a variety of cells, the mere presence of IMP without additional data does not constitute sufficient proof of the presence of protein molecules in the membrane.

Additional data to identify the structures as proteins must be obtained; how this can be done will be treated in the last section.

Even without knowledge of the true nature of the IMP, much can be learned from the number of particles on the fracture faces and the way in which particles are distributed and redistributed in the membrane. In fact, the

19

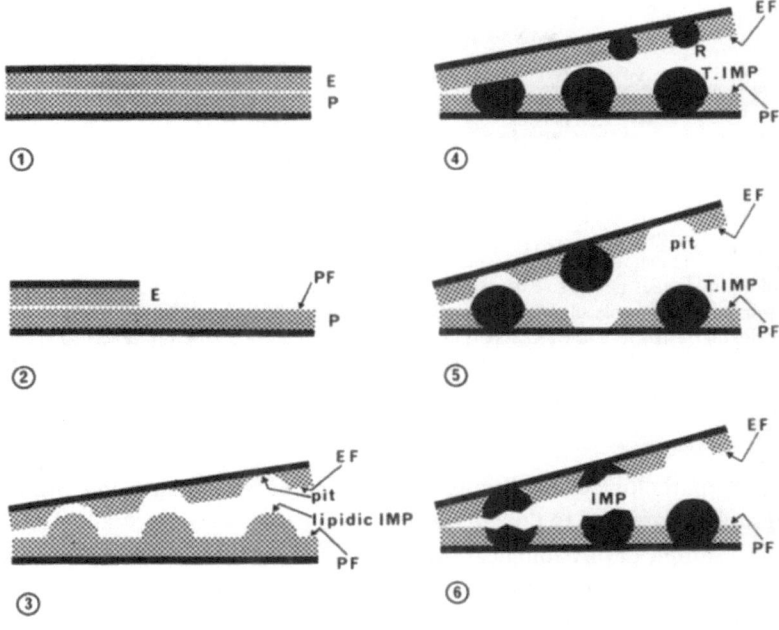

Figs. 1–6. Plasma membrane structures shown by the freeze-fracture technique.

number and distribution of the particles are considered to be characteristic for various types of membranes [9], the extremes being membranes with high metabolic activity, such as the particle-rich erythrocyte plasma membranes, on one hand, and the relatively inert particle-poor plasma membranes of the myelin sheath on the other. The lymphocyte plasma membrane represents an intermediate type with respect to particle density.

It should be noted that these three types of plasma membrane are very similar in structure when studied as membrane profiles in thin sections, which illustrates the discriminating power of the freeze-fracture technique in the investigation of membrane structure.

INTRAMEMBRANOUS PARTICLE AGGREGATION

In the majority of the membranes studied so far the IMP are distributed randomly — the particle density generally being greater in PF than in EF (see Fig. 8) — but under certain physiological conditions (e.g., under the influence of oxytocin [10], vasopressin [11], and antigen-receptor binding

20

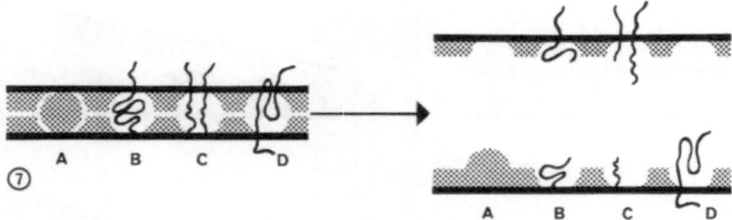

Fig. 7. Plasma membrane components before and after freeze fracturing. A: micelle of phospholipid molecules giving rise to a lipidic IMP in the protoplasmic fracture face; B: a transmembrane protein molecule broken at the level of the hydrophobic layer; no IMP are produced at this site on the fracture faces; C: a partial split transmembrane molecule (or molecular complex) giving a protein IMP in the external fracture face; and D: a protein molecule firmly bound to cytoplasmic structures and therefore adhering to the protoplasmic membrane half, thus contributing to the formation of an IMP in the protoplasmic fracture face.

[12]), or pathological conditions (e.g., malignant transformation [13]), IMP aggregation appears to take place.

An example of physiological IMP aggregation is provided by the results of de Groot's [12] study on the early changes in membrane structure accompanying antigen-receptor aggregation at the cell surface of B-lymphocytes. The earliest sign of antigen-receptor aggregation at the cell surface is the formation of small patches of immunoglobulin molecules (surface immunoglobulins are the antigen-receptors of B-lymphocytes). Freeze-fracture studies on lymphocytes in this condition of sIg aggregation revealed a redistribution of particles in the PF into clusters, apparently accompanying the sIg redistribution at the cell surface. From these findings, it was concluded that the onset of antigen-receptor redistribution at the cell surface – possibly related to cell triggering – is associated with the redistribution of intramembrane structures giving rise to IMP formation.

It should be noted that since the lymphocyte plasma membrane is highly susceptible to artificially induced aggregation phenomena [14], great care must be taken to establish suitable conditions in this type of experiment.

Another example of physiological IMP aggregation is to be found in the formation of intercellular junctions [15], including particle aggregation to form patches in the case of gap junctions. The particles in the gap junctions (i.e., structures constituting the major pathways of intercellular communication) may be arranged in two distinct patterns: a hexagonal array of particles present in the functionally uncoupled state and a more irregular packing of particles in the functionally coupled state [16, 17].

In the study of junctional complexes the freeze fracture technique appears to be indispensable for identification of the nature of the junction. Gap-junction formation between lectin-stimulated lymphocytes was investigated by Kapsenberg [18] and can serve as an example of the dynamics of the plasma membrane in such physiological processes. When rabbit lymphocytes are stimulated with the lectin phytohemagglutinin they agglutinate, and their plasma membranes form broad contact zones between adjacent cells. In the EF of the plasma membranes at the site of the broad contact zones, IMP with a diameter of approximately 11 nm aggregate to clusters and after longer culture periods appear to participate in the formation of gap junctional complexes.

Finally, it should be mentioned that artificially induced IMP aggregation may reflect the underlying microviscosity properties of the membrane. Combined evidence from two different lines of investigation may support this possibility: glycerol-induced particle aggregation in lymphocyte plasma membranes [19] is restricted to the more mature lymphocytes in the thymus [20] (see Fig. 9A and B); and microviscosity measurements of plasma-membrane fractions of subclasses of thymus lymphocytes by Roozemond et al. [21] showed that plasma membrane microviscosity was significantly lower in mature than in immature lymphocytes.

CHARACTERIZATION AND IDENTIFICATION OF INTRAMEMBRANOUS PARTICLES

Characterization of IMP according to size and shape appears to be possible when special rotary shadowing techniques are applied in freeze fracturing [22] or when replicas prepared under less favourable conditions are analysed by a newly developed morphometric method [23]. In general, however, only a few categories of IMP can be distinguished by their characteristic substructure. An example of a distinct category of IMP is represented by the particles with a central pit, first described by McNutt et al. [24] in gap junctions, but also present in a variety of cells and tissues in non-junctional membrane areas [25]; they are thought to correspond to hydrophilic channels in the plasma membrane.

Direct methods to identify molecular structures causing IMP formation are not yet available. However, when intramembrane proteins are accessible from outside the cell, they can be detected by properly labeled antibodies; and coaggregation of the labeled cell-surface structures with intramembrane structures can be taken as evidence for a relationship, if not identity, between cell surface and intramembrane structures.

In this way it has been shown that a number of cell-surface antigens and receptors are related to intramembrane proteins (e.g., the A antigen in the erythrocyte plasma membrane [26]). However, data concerning coaggregation of cell surface and intramembrane structures should be regarded with some caution, especially in the field of lectin receptor research on lymphocytes [27, 28] and erythrocytes [29–31] where the phenomenon of coaggrega-

22

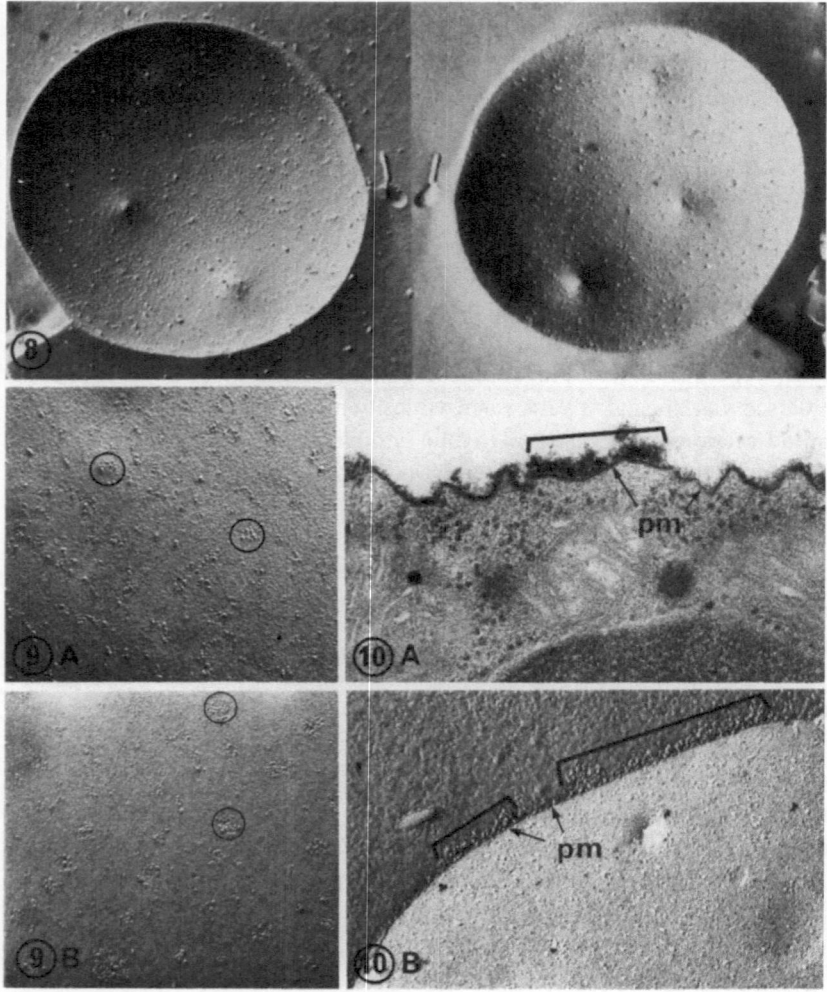

Fig. 8. Complementary replicas of lymphocyte plasma membrane showing uniqueness of the fracture plane through the hydrophobic region of the membrane interior. External fracture face (EF) at the left, protoplasmic fracture face (PF) at the right. Note the difference in particle density between EF and PF.

Fig. 9A and B. Redistribution phenomena in plasma membrane of mature lymphocytes, resulting in small (A, circled) or large (B, circled) clusters of intramembranous particles in the protoplasmic fracture face.

Fig. 10A and B. Double-layer antibody labeling of cell-surface structures visualized in ultrathin sections (A) and in freeze-fracture replicas (B) of lymphocytes. The method for labeling and for demonstrating the label in ultrathin sections was originally described by Roholl [32]. The labeled areas of the plasma membrane (pm) are indicated. Note that in the freeze-fracture replica (B) the relationship between the labeled membrane surface and the underlying structures in the membrane interior (in this case represented by the protoplasmic fracture face) can be investigated. The latter method has been described in detail by Kapsenberg [33].

tion appears to depend on the procedure applied for surface labeling.

To illustrate the essentials of this approach in plasma membrane research, we shall give data about some techniques of cell-surface labeling recently developed in our laboratory. First, a method was developed by Roholl [32] to visualize directly, in ultrathin sections of cells, antibodies directed against cell-surface components, without the use of any special electron-microscopical marker. This method uses a double layer of antibodies (the first comprising antibody directed against the cell-surface antigen, the second antibody directed against the first antibody), which is fixed with a mixture of glutaraldehyde and tannic acid and postfixed and stained in a conventional way. Results with this method are presented in Fig. 10A. Next, Kapsenberg [33], using a comparable method in freeze-fracture experiments, was able to demonstrate the double layer of antibodies in freeze-fracture replicas. This provided a new possibility to study the relationship between cell-surface structures and intramembrane components. The cells shown in Fig. 10A and B were exposed to the lectin phytohemagglutinin (PHA), after which the sites of PHA binding at the cell surface were detected by two-step labeling with antibodies, first with rat antibodies against the lectin and then with goat antibodies against rat immunoglobulins (labeled with FITC for a comparative fluorescence microscopical investigation). No coaggregation of the lectin receptor (PHA-receptor) and underlying membrane components giving rise to IMP formation could be observed in this case.

Although, progress in the characterization and identification of intramembrane structures with the freeze-fracture methodology is rather slow, the perspectives are promising. This approach is the only one available via which plasma-membrane components can be detected, directly visualized, and mapped at the macromolecular level.

REFERENCES

1. Robertson JD: Unit membranes: a review with recent new studies of experimental alterations and a new subunit in synaptic membranes. In: Cell membranes in development. New York, Ronald Press, 1964.
2. Steere RL: Electron microscopy in structural detail in frozen biological specimens. J Biochem Biophys Cytol 3: 45–55, 1957.
3. Branton D, Bullivant S, Gilula NB, Karnovsky MJ, Moor H, Mühlethaler K, Northcote DH, Packer L, Satir B, Satir P, Speth V, Staehelin LA, Steere RL, Weinstein RS: Freeze-etching nomenclature. Science 190: 54–56, 1975.
4. Branton D: Fracture faces of frozen membranes. Proc Natl Acad Sci USA 55: 1048–1056, 1966.
5. Nanninga N: Uniqueness and location of the fracture plane in the plasma membrane of *Bacillus subtilis*. J Cell Biol 49: 564–570, 1971.
6. Verkleij AJ, Mombers C, Leunissen-Bijvelt J, Ververgaert PHJT: Lipidic intramembranous particles. Nature 279: 162–163, 1979.

24

7. Margaritis LH, Yu J, Branton D: Biochemical and structural analysis of intramembrane particles using recombination experiments and rotary shadow freeze-etch microscopy. J Cell Biol 70: 73a, 1976.
8. Edwards HH, Mueller TJ, Morrison M: Distribution of transmembrane polypeptides in freeze fracture. Science 203: 1343–1345, 1979.
9. Branton D: Freeze-etching studies of membrane structure. Philos Trans R Soc Lond [Biol] 261: 133–138, 1971.
10. Chevalier J, Bourguet J, Hugon JS: Membrane associated particles: distribution in frog urinary bladder epithelium at rest and after oxytocin treatment. Cell Tissue Res 152: 129–140, 1974.
11. Kachadorian WA, Wade JB, Di Scala VA: Vasopressin: induced structural change in toad bladder luminar membrane. Science 190: 67–69, 1975.
12. Groot C de, Leene W, Bierman-van Steeg C: Evidence for identity of intramembranous particles with surface-immunoglobulins in rabbit peripheral blood lymphocytes. Ultramicroscopy 2: 127, 1976.
13. Weinstein RS: Changes in plasma membrane structure associated with malignant transformation in human urinary bladder epithelium. Cancer Res 36: 2518–2528, 1976.
14. Groot C de, Leene W: The influence of cryoprotectants, temperature, divalent cations and serum proteins on the structure of the plasma membrane in rabbit peripheral blood lymphocytes. Eur J Cell Biol 19: 19–25, 1979.
15. Staehelin LA: Structure and function of intercellular junctions. Int Rev Cytol 39: 191–283, 1974.
16. Peracchia C, Dulhunty AF: Low resistance junctions in crayfish: structural changes with functional uncoupling. J Cell Biol 70: 419–439, 1976.
17. Peracchia C: Gap junctions. Structural changes after uncoupling procedures. J Cell Biol 72: 628–641, 1977.
18. Kapsenberg ML, Leene W: Formation of B type gap junctions between PHA-stimulated rabbit lymphocytes. Exp Cell Res 120: 211–222, 1979.
19. McIntyre JA, Gilula NB, Karnovsky MJ: Cryoprotectant-induced redistribution of intramembranous particles in mouse lymphocytes. J Cell Biol 60: 192–203, 1974.
20. Leene W, Roholl PJM, Groot C de: Lymphocyte differentiation in the rabbit thymus. Ann Immunol (Paris) 127C: 911–921, 1976.
21. Roozemond RC, Urli DC: Lipid composition and microviscosity of subcellular fractions from rabbit thymocytes. Differences in the microviscosity of plasma membranes from subclasses of thymocytes. Biochim Biophys Acta 556: 17–37, 1979.
22. Margaritis LH, Elgsaeter A, Branton D: Rotary replication for freeze-etching. J Cell Biol 72: 47–56, 1977.
23. Krbecek R, Gebhardt C, Gruler H, Sackman E: Three dimensional microscopic surface profiles of membranes reconstructed from freeze etching electron micrographs. Biochim Biophys Acta 554: 1–22, 1979.
24. McNutt NS, Weinstein RS: The ultrastructure of the nexus. A correlated thin section and freeze cleave study. J Cell Biol 47: 666–688, 1970.
25. Orci L, Perrelet A, Malaisse-Lagae F, Vassalli P: Porelike structures in biological membranes. J Cell Sci 25: 157–161, 1977.
26. Pinto da Silva P, Douglas SD, Branton D: Localization of A antigen sites on human arythocyte ghosts. Nature 232: 194–196, 1971.
27. Loor F: Lymphocyte particle redistribution induced by a mitogenic/capping dose of the phytohemagglutinin of Phaseolus vulgaris. Eur J Immunol 3: 112–116, 1973.
28. Yahara I, Edelman GM: Electron microscopic analysis of the modulation of lymphocyte receptor mobility. Exp Cell Res 91: 125–142, 1975.
29. Pinto da Silva P, Nicolson GL: Freeze-etch localization of concanavalin A receptors to the membrane intercalated particles of human erythrocyte ghost membranes. Biochim Biophys Acta 363: 311–319, 1974.
30. Tillack TW, Scott RE, Marchesi VT: The structure of erythrocyte membranes studied by freeze-etching. II. Localization of receptors for phytohemagglutinin and influenza virus to the intramembranous particles. J Exp Med 135: 1209–1221, 1972.

31. Bächi T, Schnebli HP: Reaction of lectins with human erythrocytes. II. Mapping of Con A receptors by freeze-etching electron microscopy. Exp Cell Res 91: 285–295, 1975.
32. Roholl PJM: A new method for the comparative investigation of fluorochrome labeled cell surface structures on the light- and electron microscopical level. J Immunol Methods (in press).
33. Kapsenberg ML: Mechanism of lymphocyte stimulation: intramembranous particles are not involved in patch and cap formation of PHA-receptors. Exp Cell Res (submitted for publication).

4. FUNCTIONAL ASPECTS OF PLASMA MEMBRANE STUDIES: GROWTH REGULATION BY IONIC FLUXES

W.H. MOOLENAAR

INTRODUCTION

The cell surface plays a crucial role in the regulation of cell metabolism in general and in the regulation of cell proliferation in particular. The plasma membrane receives and transduces growth-stimulatory signals which trigger a cascade of physiological and biochemical events in the cell. Ultimately, these events lead to the initiation of DNA synthesis and cell division. In recent years it has become clear that proliferative signals are mediated by growth-promoting polypeptides or growth factors present in serum and tissues [1, 2]. Serum is the usual source of many as yet unidentified growth factors in cell culture. On the other hand, several growth factors have recently been isolated and purified from a variety of biological sources, including epidermal growth factor from mouse submaxillary glands [3], fibroblastic growth factor from bovine brain [1], and a growth factor from blood platelets [4]. Like all other peptide hormones, growth factors initiate their action by binding to specific receptors on the plasma membrane of their target cells. The first detectable events after growth factor-receptor interaction involve alterations in membrane transport and changes in the levels of cyclic nucleotides. For example, serum stimulation of quiescent fibroblasts or activation of lymphocytes results in a rapid stimulation of the Na^+/K^+ pump [5, 6] and an increase in the rate of uptake of amino acids, sugars, and phosphate into the cell [7, 8]. There is strong evidence that these early membrane events are somehow causally related to the initiation of cell proliferation, but the exact interrelationships are not yet clearly understood.

The intention of this chapter is (a) to identify the immediate ionic membrane changes that occur when cultured neuroblastoma cells are stimulated to grow by the addition of fresh serum to the culture medium, and (b) to elucidate the possible relationship between early changes in ionic fluxes and the initiation of late metabolic events such as protein and DNA synthesis.

NEUROBLASTOMA CELLS AS A MODEL SYSTEM FOR GROWTH-
REGULATION STUDIES

Clonal cell lines derived from the mouse C1300 neuroblastoma, a spontaneous tumor of sympathetic origin, provide a highly convenient model
system for the study of cell growth and differentiation in vitro [9, 10]. Like
most cultured animal cells, neuroblastoma cells require serum for their
growth; after removal of serum from the culture medium they cease growing
but remain viable.

On serum removal, neuroblastoma cells begin to extend neurites and gradually acquire the excitability properties of fully differentiated sympathetic
neurons. On readdition of serum, the neurites retract and, after a lag period of
several hours, DNA replication resumes, followed by cell division. Cells of
some neuroblastoma clones have a great advantage over most other cultured
cells: their size is large enough to permit stable penetration by one or two
intracellular microelectrodes [11].

Generally, continuous intracellular recording of the membrane potential
and membrane resistance from a single cell permits easy detection of rapid
ionic permeability changes induced by membrane ligands such as hormones
and growth factors. Most of the available evidence on early ionic transport
changes after serum stimulation has been obtained with tracer-flux techniques, but the relatively poor time resolution of these methods (of the order
of minutes) has precluded detection of any dynamic membrane changes that
may occur whithin seconds of serum addition. Whenever possible, therefore,
electrophysiological experiments should be performed in addition to ionic
tracer-flux measurements in the study of rapid ionic events after serum
stimulation of cultured cells.

RAPID IONIC EVENTS AFTER GROWTH STIMULATION

Addition of fresh serum to serum-deprived neuroblastoma cells (clone N1E-
115) immediately elicits a sequence of striking ionic events at the plasma
membrane, as inferred from microelectrode and tracer-flux studies [12, 13].
The electrical membrane potential, measured with an intracellular microelectrode, is a direct reflection of (a) the asymmetric distribution of Na^+ and
K^+ across the plasma membrane, and (b) the ratio of Na^+ to K^+ permeability [14]. Low intracellular Na^+ (roughly 10–30 mM) and high intracellular
K^+ (100–150 mM) are maintained by the Na^+/K^+-ATP ase or Na^+/K^+ pump,
a membrane-bound enzyme which continuously carries Na^+ out of the cell
and K^+ into it. Changes in ionic permeabilities manifest themselves as alterations in membrane potential and membrane resistance, whereas changes in

the activity of the Na^+/K^+ pump do not have a direct electrophysiological correlate because Na^+ ions are exchanged for K^+ ions in a virtually electro-neutral way. For that reason, microelectrode studies cannot give a complete picture of growth-factor-induced changes in ionic transport, and unidirectional tracer-flux studies are necessary to characterize ionic transport mediated by the Na^+/K^+ pump.

Electrophysiological observations

Neuroblastoma N1E-115 cells in serum-free medium show resting membrane potentials lying between -30 and -45 mV and a membrane resistance varying from to 10 to 40 M Ω.

As illustrated in Fig. 1, addition of fetal calf serum (FCS, final concentration: 30%) immediately elicits a characteristic triphasic voltage response [12]. The initial phase (I) is a rapid depolarization, reaching maximum peak values between -5 and -15 mV within a few seconds, accompanied by a substantial fall in the membrane resistance. During the next 5–10 s, the membrane repolarizes to a potential value near the original resting level (phase II), whereas the membrane resistance only recovers partially. This hyperpolarizing phase is followed by a new depolarizing phase (III), accompanied by a gradual decrease of the membrane resistance. Phase III reaches a plateau value of about -25 mV at 40–70 s after serum stimulation. Finally both membrane potential and resistance slowly increase again to new steady-state values, which are consistently lower than the prestimulation values. This final recovery usually takes 4–8 min, but occasionally much slower time courses (up to 20 min) are recorded. Peak values of the serum response are dose-dependent, showing saturation at a serum concentration of about 30%. Addition of bovine serum albumin (BSA, final concentration: 25 mg/ml) is without any electrical effect, which indicates that the serum response is not an unspecific protein effect. After washing out the serum-containing medium, the serum response can be elicited again in the same cell. This procedure can be repeated several times before the response eventually becomes 'desensitized.'

The ionic mechanisms underlying the sequential phases are evaluated by measuring the null or reversal potential of the distinct peaks as a function of changes in the external ionic concentration. The null potential of the initial phase I varies between -5 and $+10$ mV and is dependent on the external Na^+ concentration. A threefold reduction of $[Na^+]$ (choline substituted) results in a 20-mV shift of the null potential. A tenfold reduction of external $[Ca^{2+}]$ does not, however, influence the properties of phase I significantly. These results indicate that phase I is mainly caused by an increase in Na^+ permeability. Phase I is not affected by the Na^+-channel blocker tetrodotoxin (10^{-6} g/ml),

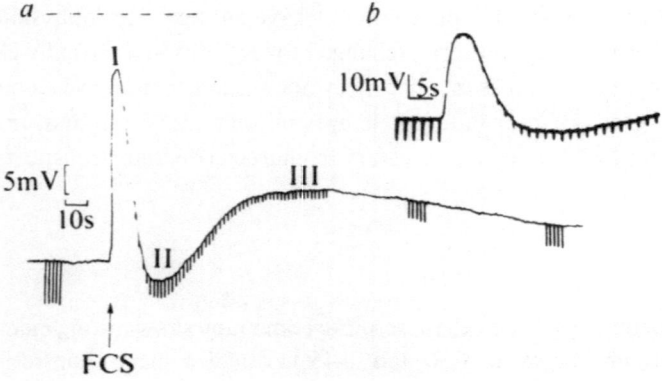

Fig. 1a and b. (a) Intracellular potential recorded from a neuroblastoma cell during addition of fetal calf serum (FCS), showing the characteristic triphasic voltage response. Membrane resistance was monitored as the voltage response to brief hyperpolarizing current pulses. Dashed line represents zero potential level. (b) Oscilloscope recording of the initial phase, clearly showing the changes in membrane resistance. Temperature was $36 \pm 1°C$.

and corresponds to a peak of inward current under voltage-clamp conditions (not illustrated). Thus, it follows that the serum-activated Na^+ conductance is clearly different from the voltage-dependent Na^+ channel underlying the generation of the neuroblastoma action potential [15].

Phase II reaches maximum hyperpolarizing peak values up to -45 mV. In view of the reduced resistance value, this suggests an increase in permeability to K^+, which is the only ion with an equilibrium potential (E_K) more negative than the resting potential ($E_K = -75$ mV; [15]). One component of the K^+ permeability in neuroblastoma cells depends on Ca^{2+} - influx for its activation [16, 17]. Enhancing the driving force for Ca^{2+}-influx by elevating the external $[Ca^{2+}]$ from 1.8 to 10 mM results in a striking shift of the peak value in the hyperpolarizing direction towards E_K, accompanied by a still further decrease of the membrane resistance (Fig. 2). Maximum peak-II values in high $[Ca^2]$ solutions approach -60 mV and are reduced by an increase in external $[K^+]$. The dependence of phase II on both external Ca^{2+} and K^+ indicates that this phase reflects an increase in K^+ permeability accompanied or preceded by a net Ca^{2+} influx into the cytoplasm, presumably via voltage-dependent Ca^{2+} channels. The resulting increase in intracellular $[Ca^{2+}]$ is then thought to underlie the Ca^{2+} -dependent membrane hyperpolarization [16].

The null potential of the slowly depolarizing phase III is about -25 mV and depends on changes in external $[K^+]$ and $[Na^+]$, whereas changes in external $[Ca^{2+}]$ hardly influence phase III. It can be stated, therefore, that phase III reflects an increase in both Na^+ and K^+ permeability.

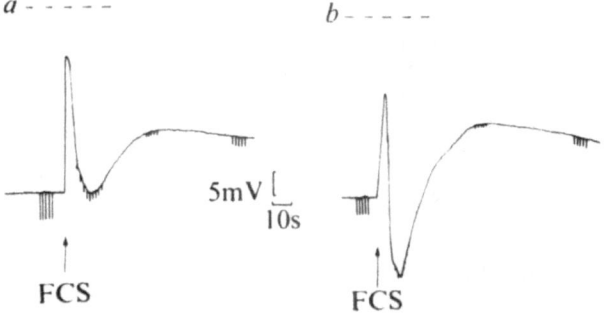

Fig. 2a and b. Effects of external calcium on the serum-induced voltage response. (a) Normal solution (containing 1.8 mM Ca^{2+}); (b) high $[Ca^{2+}]$ solution (containing 10 mM Ca^{2+}). Note the marked enhancement of phase II in a more negative direction, accompanied by a reduction of the membrane resistance. Dashed lines represent zero potential level.

In summary, serum stimulation of mouse neuroblastoma cells elicits a transient membrane potential change due largely to a biphasic increase in Na^+ permeability. As a result, Na^+ ions flow into the cytoplasm while the concomitant rapid change in membrane potential (phase I) triggers the opening of specific Ca^{2+} channels in the membrane, which leads to a transient increase in cytoplasmic free Ca^{2+}.

Which serum factors underly this sequence of ionic permeability changes? Since serum is a complex and undefined mixture of many growth-promoting substances and nutrients, the voltage response may well be induced by more than one single serum factor. Recent experiments [13] have confirmed this idea: peak I is due to a dialyzable FCS factor with molecular weigth of less than 2000, probably not a peptide. Amino acids, neutrotransmitters, steroids, and polyamines have also been excluded as possible candidates. Interestingly, this factor is not detectable in sera of nonfetal origin. The more slowly depolarizing phase III, on the other hand, is due to (a) nondialyzable macromolecular factor(s) present in serum from various sources, including the newborn calf and horse.

Figure 3 shows that growth-depleted serum, which is incapable of supporting growth, fails to induce a significant electrophysiological response. This result is consistent with the view that at least some of the serum constituents underlying the voltage response have growth-promoting activity.

Tracer-flux studies

How are the serum-induced fluxes related to the initiation of subsequent metabolic events preceding DNA synthesis? One of the consequences of the serum-stimulated Na^+ influx will be an increase in intracellular Na^+ concen-

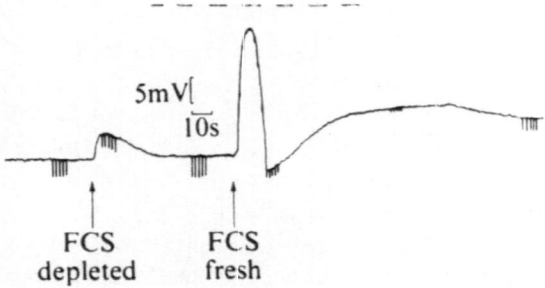

Fig. 3. Effects of growth-depleted and fresh serum on the same cell. Depleted serum was obtained by prolonged exposure of growth medium to a confluent neuroblastoma culture, with daily adjustment of the medium pH.

tration. Intracellular Na^+ and K^+ levels are controlled by the Na^+/K^+ pump and the pump rate is generally proportional to the intracellular Na^+ concentration [18]. As a rule, the pump rate is determined by measuring the ouabain-sensitive influx of labelled K^+ (or Rb^+) into the cells. Figure 4 shows that dialyzed serum gives a roughly twofold stimulation of the Na^+ pump within 10 min. The pump stimulation must be a direct result of the serum-induced Na^+ influx, since in the absence of an inwardly directed Na^+ concentration gradient, serum is incapable of stimulating the pump. Furthermore, the diuretic amiloride, which blocks Na^+ entry into a variety of cells and tissues [19–21], completely inhibits pump stimulation. It is important that amiloride does not affect the basal pump rate level. This strongly suggests that serum opens a specific amiloride-sensitive Na^+ pathway rather than modifying the basal ionic leak permeability. But amiloride acts differently on both phases of increased Na^+ permeability as recorded with microelectrodes. Whereas phase I is completely blocked by amiloride (0.4 mM), phase III is hardly affected. This means that amiloride inhibits Na^+ entry during phase III in an elec-

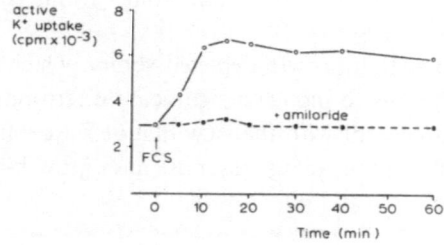

Fig. 4. Stimulation of the Na/K pump, after serum stimulation, as determined from the rate of ouabain-sensitive Rb^+ uptake by neuroblastoma cells deprived of serum for 24 h. Dashed line shows the inhibitory effect of amiloride (0.4 mM). Temperature was 37°C.

trically silent way, the net charge transfer being zero, as during a 1:1 ionic exchange process.

From studies on the mechanism of action of amiloride on epithelial tissues it is clear that the drug blocks passive Na^+ entry in a current-generating way [20]. In mouse skeletal muscle, however, amiloride specifically inhibits an electroneutral Na^+/H^+ exchange process, thus interfering with the recovery of intracellular pH after an acid load [22]. In fertilized sea urchin eggs, too, amiloride has been claimed to block Na^+/H^+ exchange [23], but this finding has been severely questioned [24, 25]. In mouse embryo fibroblasts, amiloride blocks part of a Li^+ uptake mechanism which seems to occur via a Na^+-specific pathway [23]. However, evidence that amiloride blocks Na^+/H^+ exchange in cultured cells is not yet available.

RELATIONSHIP BETWEEN THE EARLY IONIC EVENTS AND THE INITIATION OF DNA SYNTHESIS

An important question that arises now is which, if any, of the rapid ionic effects of the serum growth factors are causally related to the onset of DNA synthesis and cell proliferation? Present evidence points to the increased Na^+ influx during phase III of the electrophysiological response as a necessary requirement for the initiation of DNA synthesis [13]. Inhibition of the early Na^+ influx by amiloride (0.2–0.4 mM) blocks the initiation of DNA synthesis in neuroblastoma cells [13], in fertilized sea urchin eggs [23], and in primary hepatocytes in culture [27]. Furthermore, epidermal growth factor (EGF) rapidly stimulates Na^+ influx in appropriate target cells [26, 27] and evokes a membrane depolarization similar to that induced by dialyzed serum (unpublished results). Conversely, growth-depleted serum devoid of growth-promoting activity fails to induce significant ionic effects.

At present, one can only speculate about the precise mechanisms by which an increase in Na^+ influx triggers subsequent biochemical events that eventually lead to DNA replication. A plausible mechanism seems to be provided by the stimulation of a Na^+/H^+ exchange process. The efflux of protons, coupled in an electroneutral way to Na^+ influx, will result in a rise of intracellular pH, which is a crucial parameter for the rate of numerous intracellular metabolic reactions. In sea urchin eggs a transient rise in intracellular pH occurring shortly after fertilization, appears to be a necessary trigger for the onset of protein synthesis preceding DNA replication [28, 29]. By analogy, a change in intracellular pH, serving as a 'second messenger' for growth-factor-mediated cell proliferation, is here postulated to be a critical parameter in the regulation of animal cell growth.

Serum-stimulated electroneutral Na^+ transport might also include $Na^+/$

34

Ca^{2+} exchange, a process which is intimately involved in the regulation of intracellular free Ca^{2+} levels [30], but there is no evidence that Na$^+$/Ca^{2+} exchange is amiloride sensitive.

For a more detailed interpretation of the mode of action of amiloride on neuroblastoma proliferation, it will be necessary to monitor changes in intracellular Na$^+$ and H$^+$ concentration after serum stimulation.

In addition to H$^+$ and Ca^{2+} fluxes, the transport of several amino acids into the cell is known to be Na$^+$ dependent [31]. Interestingly, hormone-stimulated amino acid transport in cultured hepatocytes is amiloride sensitive [27]. Based on the idea of Na$^+$-dependent changes in H$^+$ fluxes and amino acid transport, the following scheme for the mode of action of serum growth factors shown in Fig. 5 can now be put forward.

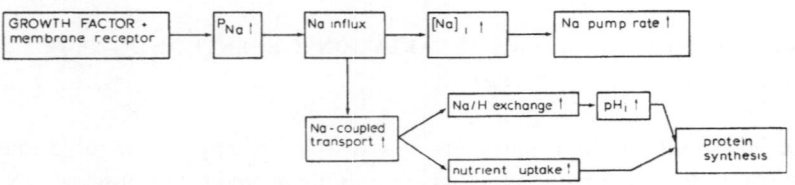

Fig. 5. Flow chart illustrating the mainly hypothetical relations between Na$^+$ permeability change and the late metabolic events such as stimulation of protein synthesis preceding DNA replication.

Although the picture of the mode of action of growth factors in the control of cell proliferation is only just emerging, the cascade of events illustrated in Fig. 5 provides a framework on which future experiments should be based.

Obviously, the sequence of events depicted in Fig. 5 is not in itself sufficient to explain the initiation of DNA synthesis fully. Maximal growth stimulation requires a long-term occupancy of growth-factor receptors; a triggerlike action of mitogenic stimuli, such as the fusion of a sperm with an egg, is usually incapable of initiating proliferation of cultured cells. Furthermore, growth-promoting peptides are rapidly internalized into their target cells, and it might well be that internalized growth factors exert part of their mitogenic activity inside the cell.

The working hypothesis presented here, i.e., that the internal pH is a 'second messenger' of growth factor-receptor interaction, provides an attractive picture of the relationship between early ionic fluxes and late metabolic events of the proliferative response. It is obvious that proof of the validity of this hypothesis must await further experimental work.

Acknowledgement. This work was supported by the Koningin Wilhelmina Fonds.

REFERENCES

1. Gospodarowicz D, Moran JS: Growth factors in mammalian cell culture. Ann Rev Biochem 45: 531–558, 1976.
2. Holley RW: Control of growth of mammalian cells in culture. Nature 258: 487–490, 1975.
3. Savage CR, Cohen S: Epidermal growth factor and a new derivative. J Biol Chem 247: 7609–7611, 1972.
4. Ross R, Vogel A: The platelet-derived growth factor. Cell 14: 203–210, 1978.
5. Rozengurt E, Heppel LA: Serum rapidly stimulates ouabain sensitive Rb influx in quiescent 3T3 cells. Proc Natl Acad Sci USA 72: 4492–4495, 1975.
6. Kaplan JG: Membrane cation transport and the control of proliferation of mammalian cells. Ann Rev Physiol 40: 19–41, 1978.
7. Baserga R: Multiplication and division in mammalian cells. New York, Dekker, 1976.
8. Jimenez de Asua L, Rozengurt E, Dulbecco R: Kinetics of early changes in phosphate and uridine transport and cyclic AMP levels stimulated by serum in density-inhibited 3T3 cells. Proc Natl Acad Sci USA 73: 96–98, 1974.
9. Nelson PG: Nerve and muscle cells in culture. Physiol Rev 55: 1–61, 1975.
10. Prasad KN: Differentiation of neuroblastoma cells in culture. Biol Rev 50: 129–265, 1975.
11. Moolenaar WH, Spector I: Membrane currents examined under voltage clamp in cultured neuroblastoma cells. Science 196: 331–333, 1977.
12. Moolenaar WH, Laat SW de, Saag PT van der: Serum triggers a sequence of rapid ionic conductance changes in quiescent neuroblastoma cells. Nature 279: 721–723, 1979.
13. Moolenaar WH, Mummery CL, Saag PT van der, Laat SW de: Rapid ionic events following serum stimulation of mouse neuroblastoma cells. Cell (in press) 1980.
14. Williams JA: Origin of transmembrane potentials in non-excitable cells. J Theor Biol 28: 287–296, 1970.
15. Moolenaar WH, Spector I: Ionic currents in cultured mouse neuroblastoma cells under voltage-clamp conditions. J Physiol 278: 265–286, 1978.
16. Moolenaar WH, Spector I: The calcium action potential and a prolonged calcium dependent after-hyperpolarization in mouse neuroblastoma cells. J Physiol 292: 297–306, 1979.
17. Moolenaar WH, Spector I: The calcium current and the activation of a slow potassium conductance in voltage-clamped mouse neuroblastoma cells. J Physiol 292: 307–323, 1979.
18. Thomas RC: Electrogenic sodium pump in nerve and muscle cells. Physiol Rev 52: 563–594, 1972.
19. Aceves J, Cereijido M: The effect of amiloride on sodium and potassium fluxes in red cells. J Physiol 229: 709–718, 1973.
20. Bentley PJ: Amiloride: a potent inhibitor of sodium transport across the toad bladder. J Physiol 195: 317–330, 1968.
21. Cuthbert AW: Importance of guanidium groups for blocking sodium channels in epithelia. Mol Pharmacol 12: 945–957, 1976.
22. Aickin CC, Thomas RC: An investigation of the ionic mechanism of intracellular pH regulation in mouse soleus muscle fibres. J Physiol 273: 295–316, 1977.
23. Johnson JD, Epel D, Paul M: Intracellular pH and activation of sea urchin eggs after fertilisation. Nature 262: 661–664, 1976.
24. Cuthbert A, Cuthbert AW: Fertilization acid production in Psammechinus eggs under pH clamp conditions, and the effects of some pyrazine derivatives. Exp Cell Res 114: 409–415, 1978.
25. Shen SS, Steinhardt RA: Intracellular pH and the sodium requirement at fertilization. Nature 282: 87–89, 1979.
26. Smith JB, Rozengurt E: Lithium transport by fibroblastic mouse cells: characterization and stimulation by serum and growth factors in quiescent cultures. J Cell Physiol 97: 441–450, 1978.
27. Koch KS, Leffert HL: Increased sodium ion influx is necessary to initiate rat hepatocyte proliferation. Cell 18: 153–163, 1979.

28. Grainger JL, Winkler MM, Shen SS, Steinhardt RA: Intracellular pH controls protein synthesis rate in the sea urchin egg and early embryo. Dev Biol 68: 396–406, 1979.
29. Epel D: Mechanisms of activation of sperm and egg during fertilization of sea urchin gametes. Curr Top Dev Biol 12: 185–246, 1978.
30. Blaustein MP: The interrelationship between sodium and calium fluxes across cell membranes. Rev Physiol Biochem Pharmacol 70: 34–82, 1974.
31. Guidotti GG, Borghetti AF, Gazzola GC: The regulation of amino acid transport in animal cells. Biochim Biophys Acta 515: 329–366, 1978.

5. SOME STRUCTURAL AND FUNCTIONAL ALTERATIONS IN TUMOR PLASMA MEMBRANES

P. EMMELOT, W.J. VAN BLITTERSWIJK, W.P. VAN BEEK,
AND R.P. VAN HOEVEN

INTRODUCTION: TYPES OF CHANGE IN TUMORS AND THEIR PLASMA MEMBRANES

In the last two decades numerous changes have been described in isolated plasma membranes or the intact surface of tumor cells as compared with homologous normal cells [1–3]. These changes differ widely in character, and concern the various chemical classes of membrane components, their lateral or rotational movements, functional activities related to, for instance, enzymes, antigens, hormone and other receptors, and transport processes, relationships with the cytoskeleton, and intercellular contact mechanisms. The paramount question is therefore which, if any, of these changes are essential to the tumorigencity of cells by being involved in the determination of that potential. Tumorigenicity is defined as the faculty of cells to show neoplasmic behavior in vivo. If growth is restricted to the site of origin or transplantation, the tumor is called benign. Malignant tumor (= cancer) cells, however, proliferate, spread, and grow at secondary sites. Thus, transplantability per se indicates autonomous growth, whereas malignancy is indicated by infiltrative growth, i.e., invasion and metastasis.

Of the recorded membrane changes, none is explicitly known to mediate the tumorigenic cell state directly. If some change were to have such an effect, it would represent the direct expression at the cell surface of (one of) the primary causal events in tumorigenicity. Under causal events we understand those changes brought about by a carcinogenic determinant, very presumably localized in the cell genome, that impose a cell to behave as a tumor cell as defined above. (For the enabling role of antigenic change, see below.)

Changes can also represent secondary expressions associated with or derived (via feedback mechanisms) from the causal events. For instance, the first cell stage operating in hepatocarcinogenesis in the rat, induced by a single carcinogenic event, shows a certain autonomy of growth, while the surface of these cells has lost adenosine triphosphatase and gained γ-glutamyl transpeptidase activity [4, 5]. Liver carcinomas, also in man, may show the same

---

Abbreviations: TSTA, tumor-specific transplantation antigen; CEA, carcinoembryonic antigen; PL, phospholipid; PHA, phytohemagglutinin.

W.Th. Daems et al. (eds.), Cell Biological Aspects of Disease, 37–66. All rights reserved.
Copyright © 1981 by Martinus Nijhoff Publishers bv, The Hague/Boston/London.

enzymatic changes. Yet there is no reason to suppose that these enzymatic changes per se are instrumental in neoplastic growth; rather the opposite is indicated, namely, that these changes are in some way coupled to the more important alteration that confers growth autonomy. Another example is provided by the different activities of the cell-surface enzymes in the various human leukemias: each type of leukemia exhibits a specific profile [6] as compared with lymphocytes. These profiles might reflect the enzymatic activities of intermediary cell stages occurring in the sequential differentiation of the various blood-cell series in which malignant transformation took place. A similar case can be made for other surface expressions, e.g., of the antigenic type, in these malignancies, including the thymus-derived neoplasms.

In view of the increasing awareness that specific chromosomal changes may occur in the various malignant lymphoproliferative disorders in man [7, 8], another interpretation is that the specific enzyme profiles are related to these chromosomal changes. Whatever the case may be, such alterations in enzymatic activities do not seem to be essential for tumorigenicity, but they may serve as 'markers' to identify tumor precursor cell stages, respectively to distinguish between lymphoproliferative disorders.

The cells of many, perhaps all, tumors carry some expression of feto-embryonic gene states detectable by immunological techniques [9–13]. In chemically induced tumors, these 'antigens' are present next to the tumor-specific transplantation antigen (TSTA) [12, 13] (see below). The significance of the embryonic expressions on (and in) tumor cells is not clear. One interpretation is that this phenomenon may represent a secondary phenotypic change associated with the relevant primary change in the genome that confers autonomy of growth, any specificity of the expression being a function of the cell type; mutation in control DNA is another possibility. The above-mentioned capacity to express γ-glutamyl transpeptidase on the cell surface is also a property of embryonic liver cells, as distinct from in vivo liver cells of young and adult rats. The enzyme is also expressed in certain carcinogen-induced lesions whose manifestation depends on a strong growth stimulus; when the stimulus is discontinued, the enzyme expression disappears [5]. Similarly, regenerative growth may in some cases also cause the appearance of certain embryonic expressions. A well-known example of such reexpression of genes normally operating fully only during ontogeny is the presence of carcinoembryonic antigen (CEA), rich in carbohydrates, on the surface of embryonic colon cells as well as on cells of colonic carcinomas, and to various extents in a number of other tumors. Since the carcinoembryonic antigen is readily released by cells and reaches the circulation, it can sometimes be used as a 'marker' to monitor the course of the disease.

Furthermore, from the very randomness of the action of chemical carcinogens [14], purely accidental changes in tumor cell properties may also be expected. In that case different alterations in a given character may occur among separate tumors of the same type. The appearance of TSTA on the cells of chemically induced rat tumors, including hepatomas and sarcomas [12, 13], could be a case in point. Each separate tumor of a given type induced by a given carcinogen exhibits on its cells an individually specific antigen foreign to the host. This heterogeneity can be interpreted in terms of random interaction of carcinogen with target DNA, and thus would represent random mutation. It is conceivable that other random alterations may likewise be induced, and heterogeneity in biochemical reactions among separate tumors of the same type is generally well documented. The very randomness of such alterations may lead one to suppose that, in general, their occurrence does not contribute to the essential changes in the tumor cell phenotype. Descriptively, the essential changes are the loss of — or escape from — growth, positional, and immunological controls, which all in some way or another involve the cell surface or at least have a footing there.

Cancer as one disease is an abstract notion; actually, tumors differing widely in properties are encountered. Also, tumors of the same cell type (origin) may exhibit different grades of malignancy, ranging from well-differentiated and slowly (including locally) growing specimens to anaplastic, rapidly proliferating ones that invade and metastasize, and tumors exhibiting various combinations of these properties also occur. In all of these cases the loss of normal controls appears to differ to various degrees. Thus, whereas the terms benign (exclusively local growth) and malignant (invasive and metastatic growth) are frequently used qualitatively, there is a large spectrum of tumor phenotypes, varying from weakly to highly malignant, in which the underlying differences are quantitative in nature. Accordingly, if tumor cell behavior is mediated by abnormalities in cell-surface processes, there may be quantitative differences in this respect.

In general, then, tumor cell behavior is the outcome (sum effect) of a number of particular phenotypic alterations that show quantitative differences among tumors. But do these alterations also differ qualitatively among tumors? Different mechanisms of change can lead to the same biological end-effect, as exemplified by the escape from immunological control. If this also applied to escape from other controls, the molecular mechanisms by which even identical behavior of separate tumors is expressed could differ. As discussed elsewhere [1], a crucial alteration in the tumor cell surface could involve the lack of some proper configuration acting in normal growth regulation. This lesion might stem from either the absence of or masking by other surface components, or from shedding (by nonlethal autolysis); moreover, the configuration could be present, but the elaboration or transduction of the signal generated by the configuration during its regulatory act might be defective.

Thus, at least four mechanisms could yield the same end-effect. In three of these, the lack of proper configuration would lead to surface heterogeneity among tumor cells [1], and this lack rather than the actual expression present on the tumor surface would be crucial. Now assume that these three mechanisms (and not the fourth) are involved in aberrant growth control. If one could monitor the proper surface configuration without having knowledge of these three mechanisms, one would conclude that the absence of that configuration on tumor cells was the common molecular lesion responsible for the loss of growth control, whereas it was really the end-effect of three mechanisms. Therefore, it is clear that the level of analysis applied determines what one calls a common molecular lesion. To take another example, assume that the transduced signal stemming from the surface configuration after regulatory interaction is compound P. Monitoring of P in tumors would then lead to the conclusion that the common molecular lesion among tumors was the inability to form compound P. Accordingly, if one is unable to distinguish the mechanisms, one would take the molecular effect that is being measured as the common primary change. On this basis the conclusion is not unwarranted that tumorigenicity in separate cases may be governed by lesions in different molecular reactions yielding the same biological or molecular end-effect. However, this is a theoretical, though reasonable, possibility and the conclusion may not necessarily hold for all of the relevant changes in all tumors.

It is in this light that we must view the concept that all tumors share one or more 'qualitatively' identical changes at the molecular level — an attractive but as yet unproven postulate. In that case, all tumors, regardless of species, cell type, mode of growth, carcinogenic determinants, etc., would show the alteration, which would then be a universal marker of tumorigenicity. (However, alternatively, a universal marker does not necessarily represent a causal change.) If the tumor-type specific chromosomal changes referred to above are instrumental in the tumorigenic state, essential phenotypic changes among tumors might be more variable, although common change might still be visualized. In addition, the possibility that the same chromosomal abnormality may be induced independent of the type of carcinogenic determinant (X-irradiation, chemical carcinogen, oncogenic RNA virus) has recently been demonstrated for lymphomas in various mouse strains [15].

In sum, the following types of relevant changes may be distinguished:

1) General changes, which ideally would be causal in tumorigenicity per se;

2) Specific changes, instrumental in the tumorigenicity of a tumor, or a tumor of a given cell type;

3) Selective changes that confer an advantage on tumor cells and intensify an aggressive course, or impose a particular tumor cell behavior (e.g., metastatic target). This category can be subdivided according to whether the change contributes directly or indirectly to a more aggressive course. By

indirect contribution is understood any change that would relieve the cell of the burden of making differentiated products inessential for cell survival. Such changes would be advantageous to the tumor cell, since its metabolic machinery and available metabolites are geared to proliferative processes only. The advantage provided by this type of change consists of the deletion or loss of differentiated function not involved in the normal controls mentioned on page 39. This type of cell simplification or 'dedifferentiation' will not be dealt with further here except to mention that the principle also applies to plasma membranes, e.g., the lack of bile canalicular membranes containing morphological specializations (and enzymes) as part of the plasma membranes of anaplastic but not of differentiated hepatomas [16, 17].

A number of examples of the type of change that contributes more directly to the biological 'success' of the tumor cell at the level of plasma membrane processes will be discussed in the remainder of this paper. The choice of subjects was led by the experience and interest of the authors. In the main, tumors established in vivo will be considered, with special attention to two systems: the rat-hepatoma/liver system (chemically induced tumors maintained as solid tissue or intraperitoneal ascites cells) and the lymphoma/ thymocyte system of the GR/A mouse (tumors [GRSL] arising spontaneously and propagated intraperitoneally as ascites cells). The GRSL, a thymic leukemia or thymoma, will be referred to in the present paper by the term lymphoma. Some related leukemia systems will also be discussed.

We shall end by describing a change in plasma membranes that may qualify as a general marker of cancer cells.

ENZYME TOPOLOGY

Plasma membranes of anaplastic rat hepatomas contain the enzyme hexokinase [18, 19], which catalyzes the first reaction of the glycolytic pathway (glucose $\rightarrow$ glucose-6-phosphate). This enzyme is absent from the plasma membrane of normal liver [17, 18] and well-differentiated mouse [17] and rat hepatomas [20], where its localization is exclusively cytoplasmic. In the anaplastic, rapidly growing tumors with a poor blood supply, the peripheral localization of the enzyme in the cell apparently enables the tumor cells to utilize glucose very efficiently. With the loss of cell contacts between tumor cells, enzymes which otherwise are topologically restricted to a particular part of the plasma membrane may spread along the surface [22]. This could also furnish an advantage to the cells, if the enzyme was involved in transport processes. The latter function is indicated for γ-glutamyltranspeptidase [11]. While the emergence of the latter enzyme appears to be associated with the (neoplastic) growth state of certain cell types, that of hexokinase may repre-

42

sent a separate alteration selected for during tumor progression. The advantage in these examples is conferred by gain of a function that facilitates tumor growth rate rather than causes neoplastic growth. The following sections include examples of advantage conferred on tumor cells by changes, i.e., dysfunction through loss or gain, in processes occurring in normal controls.

STRUCTURAL CONTACT DEVICES

Structural contacts between normal cells in a tissue are maintained mainly by three types of intercellular junction: desmosomes, tight junctions, and gap junctions, each of which has a particular function (Fig. 1). An almost complete loss of gap junctions has been observed in human breast adenocarcinoma [21] and anaplastic rat hepatoma, but not in well-differentiated mouse hepatomas [16, 17, 22]. (At the time of this observation, the gap junctions in the liver/hepatoma system were called tight junctions.) In the breast tumors, tight junctions are almost completely absent, but desmosomes appear normal [21]. Decreases in the number of desmosomes, which apparently function mainly as cell-to-cell anchors (thus acting in positional control), have been

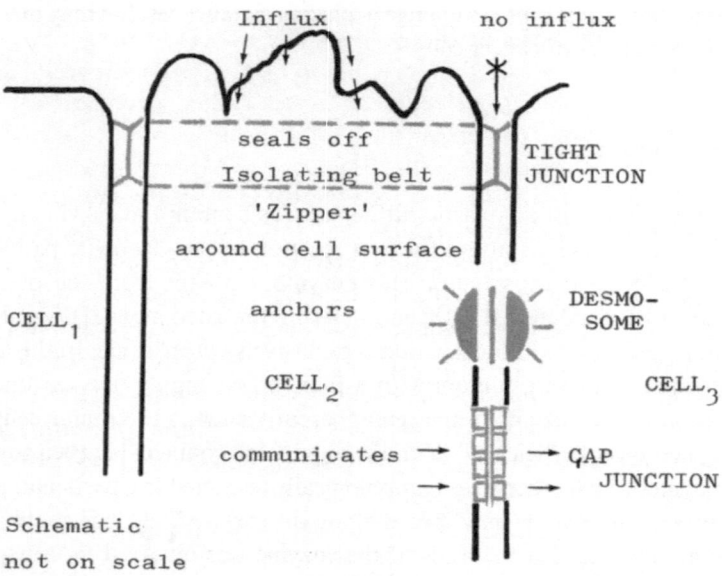

Fig. 1. Schematic representation of junctional complexes.

found to correlate with the invasiveness of human cervix and urinary bladder carcinomas but not in some experimental systems [23, 24]. Regional loss of desmosomes has been observed for invasive cells of chemically induced rat urinary bladder tumors [25]. A numerical deficiency of tight junctions — which have an isolating function by sealing off the cell boundary apically from lumens, and thus govern the direction of inflow of materials into cells, thereby maintaining cell and tissue gradients — will result in cells facing the environment on all sides and to random uptake and disappearance of normal gradients that may also be involved in the local expression of membrane enzymes (alkaline phosphatase [22]). Finally, deficiency in the number or function of gap junctions — which allow intercellular communication [26] because they are permeable to cellular metabolites and metabolic signals (metabolic cooperation) — will lead to the disruption of that process and to cells which are functionally isolated from their neighbors and thus will increase uncoordinated, asocial cell behavior.

In tumors, the plasma membranes of adjacent cells are often separated from each other over much of their surface [23]. This may have an effect on cell proliferation, since the latter process can be modulated by adjacent cells either by cell-to-cell contact or through specific secretory products (compare: loss of gradients). On the other hand, loss of, or decreased apposition of, plasma membranes (and junctions) may also result from growth itself, and these surface phenomena may not be observed, or be less prominent, in slowly growing, well-differentiated tumors. A consistent pattern of change in cell contacts in tumors has not been encountered [22]. This should be viewed in the following context. First, the release of cells from tumor tissue in situ does not (always) seem to be the rate-limiting step in the metastatic process, or necessarily distinguish malignant from benign cells. Secondly, 'statistical' studies in whole tumors may not detect individual changes in a restricted number of cells. Recent results underscore the finding that tumors are composed of heterogeneous cell populations [27–31] that may differ from case to case. Only some of these subpopulations are capable of metastasis and probably also of invasion [32, 33]. Metastatic cells are phenotypic variants of the primary tumor population. Moreover, experience has shown that not all anaplastic tumors do metastasize and that not all well-differentiated tumors lack the capacity of metastasis. Therefore, in studies performed to obtain more insight into the parameters that govern this behavior, the subpopulations should first be isolated by proper selection in vivo and/or in vitro.

METASTASIS

Despite the clonal origin of tumors, cell variants may be present from the start or originate during a tumor's natural history, which can be experimentally prolonged by transplantation. Thus, from tumor cell strains (e.g., melanoma, lymphosarcoma), variant cells can be selected, either biologically or through lectin treatment, that preferentially metastasize to different organs (e.g., the brain, lung, or liver) or show increased metastasis in a particular organ [34–38].

The organ specificity of metastasis by these cell variants is not absolute, but relative. Where lectins have been used for selection, differences in number of metastases or in organ preference are apparently related to differences among the tumor cells as to surface components with affinity for lectin [35, 38]. By an analogous principle of complementary interaction, different affinities of tumor cells to normal cells could lead to differences in the heterotypic association between tumor and normal cells in vivo; selected tumor cells have been shown to agglutinate preferentially with the cells of their preferred normal target tissue [29, 40]. Thus, organ preference as to arrest and colonization may be mediated by adhesive interactions between tumor and normal cells. However, such interaction should not proceed to the stage of contact inhibition of growth imposed by the normal cells on the tumor cells, i.e., heterotypic association should not lead to functional contact resulting in the cessation of DNA synthesis. If it did, the tumor cell would remain dormant.

The formation of multicellular tumor emboli favors lung metastasis, and tumor cells selected for lung memtastasis show enhanced homotypic (= self) association [40]. Other mechanisms may involve nonlethal antibody-induced agglutination of the tumor cells or platelet aggregation at the tumor-cell surface [41]. Clumps of tumor cells or self-adhesion of tumor cells after release from the primary tumor would favor the formation of secondaries if only by their tendency to become stuck in capillaries, as in blood-borne pulmonary metastasis; in addition, tumor-cell clumps can be expected to show decreased contact inhibition by normal cells and less accessibility to immunological attack. Parenthetically, it should be said that cell-surface adhesiveness remains a loose term if not further defined. Thus, adhesiveness in terms of binding to latex particles proved to be inversely related to tumorigenicity in a series of fibroblastoid cell lines [42]; it remains to be established how this relates to homo- and heterotypic cell adhesion.

Since tumor cells capable of metastasis differ from other cells of the (non-selected) parent tumor, metastasis may be effected by subpopulations with particular cell-surface properties [43–45]. For instance, differences in antigenic expression may be especially important, since metastasizing tumor cells are generally not, or only weakly, immunogenic and thus easily escape the immune control of the host. Loss of or deficiency in cell-surface immunogenic components — a dominant factor in metastasis in experimental systems — may be accomplished by various mechanisms (see below). The cellular heterogeneity of tumors with respect to antigenic expression has been clearly demonstrated for a mouse mammary tumor from which five subpopulations were isolated, each differing in the expression of mammary tumor virus antigen [27]; and four antigenic subtypes have been encountered among spontaneous AKR leukemia cells [29].

For DNA synthesis and growth to proceed, normal cells in vitro need a solid substrate to which part of the cell surface is anchored, anchorage being a prerequisite for cell proliferation. Among the various traits of cell transformation, the anchorage independence of growth is the only one that is frequently [46], but not always [47, 48], correlated with the tumorigenicity of cells, i.e., yielding tumors if inoculated in suitable mice. Normal endothelial cells, which are capable of invasion, also show an anchorage-independent growth and produce plasminogen activator [49], another property found among transformed and tumor cells. Since, moreover, anchorage independency alone is not sufficient to enable transformed cells to grow out into tumor on transplantation [50], anchorage-independent growth (and plasminogen activator production) of tumor cells seems to be associated with, or to condition, the infiltrative mode of neoplastic growth rather than autonomous growth per se. Like certain tumor cells, endothelial cells and activated macrophages, the latter two being normal cells with invasive potential, also possess elevated amounts of surface-associated proteolytic enzyme activity [51]. Proteolytic activity by tumor cell — either released extracellularly, including plasminogen activator, or surface-bound — has been found experimentally to be correlated with the infiltrative cell phenotype [51–55]. Proteolysis may not only mediate the penetration of tumor cells through epithelial basal membranes and endothelial linings [55], but in the case of plasmin (the proteolytic component resulting from plasminogen activation) may also inhibit the antibody-induced lysis of tumor cells, as recently demonstrated in human melanoma cells [56]. However, for the formation of collagen or fibrin capsules around certain tumors, which may impede metastasis by acting as a physical barrier or otherwise, see refs. 53, 57, and 58; for a permissive role of fibrin in metastasis, see ref. 41.

In sum, metastasis depends on special properties of both tumor and target-tissue cells ('seed-soil').

GANGLIOSIDES

Changes in the relative amounts of gangliosides (sialic-acid-containing glycosphinglolipids) resulting from enzymatic blocks in glycosylation and accumulation of precursors in transformed and tumor cells and their plasma membranes have been implicated in aberrant growth regulation (reviewed in ref. 59; more than 200 abstracts of research performed in the 1970s have been published recently [60]). However, no consistent pattern of change among tumor cells has been observed [1, 59, 60]. One generalization that can be made, however, is that the glycolipid composition of tumor cells changes little with growth stage. In contrast, the glycolipid composition of normal cells varies with growth state and cell cycle parameters. Hence, the tumor-cell surface is less dynamic and shows a 'frozen' appearance [1] compared with the normal cell surface. (This may be an illustration of a more general phenomenon: the 'uncoupling' in tumors of biochemical reactions from the position of the cell in the cell cycle which otherwise is an enabling or rate-limiting factor for occurrence of the reactions.)

Nonmetastatic rat liver tumors, independent of the degree of differentiation, were recently shown to be characterized by a ganglioside pattern depleted in hematoside (GM_3) and elevated in the products of the monosialoganglioside pathway (GM_1, G_{D1a}). In contrast, metastases from tumors selected from the same parent tumor, whether well or poorly differentiated, exhibited a restoration of the GM_3 level and nearer-normal levels of the monosialogangliosides [61]. From this the conclusion was drawn that ganglioside deletion is not causal in tumorigenicity, but that there are differences between the surface glycolipids of metastatic and nonmetastatic liver tumors. The pattern of these gangliosides in the metastatic material tends to resemble that of another anaplastic rat hepatoma (484a) with metastatic potential [1], whereas that of the nonmetastatic tumors is not unlike that of nonadhesive rat hepatoma ascites cells; the adhesive variant of the latter has GM_3 as major ganglioside [62]. It is not known, however, how such differences are related in terms of cause or effect to the mode of growth (metastatic vs nonmetastatic, adhesive vs nonadhesive; for the differences in glycoprotein aggregation factor and formation of junctional complexes between the ascites hepatomas, see ref. 63). Functionally, however, the exposition of gangliosides at the cell surface might matter more than the amount present in the membrane, these two not necessarlily being related. In this connection it is of interest that antiganglioside antibodies have been reported to inhibit viral transformation [64], but to stimulate thymocyte DNA synthesis [65].

Glycolipids, including gangliosides, may be taken up by cells from serum and function as 'acquired receptors' on the cell surface [66]. According to several observations, serum ganglioside levels are markedly increased in tumor-bearing animals and cancer patients (see abstracts 38, 46, and 58 in ref. 60). If certain of these compounds — which can serve as receptors for hormones or other physiological agonists — were acquired by other cells of the tumor-bearing host, the latter's metabolism would be affected. This would represent an as yet unnoticed type of systemic effect of a tumor on the host.

CHOLESTEROL CONTENT OF MEMBRANES

A rather general phenomenon that has been firmly established for hepatomas and leukemias, in man as well as in animals, is the lack of an inhibitory effect of exogenous cholesterol on the de novo biosynthesis of cholesterol in the tumor cells either in vivo or in vitro; an efficient inhibition occurs in the corresponding normal cells [67] (for a review, see ref. 68).

Compared with normal liver, plasma membranes and intracellular membranes of hepatomas show an increased cholesterol content [69–71] (Table 1); the serum cholesterol in hepatoma-bearing rats is also increased [72]. In our experience [69], the increased cholesterol content is not related to the degree of tumor differentiation (anaplastic rat vs differentiated mouse hepatoma) or the mode of growth (solid vs ascites rat hepatomas), but see ref. 71.

In contrast, lymphoma and leukemia cells and their plasma membranes contain only half as much cholesterol on a phospholipid basis as do normal thymocytes/lymphocytes and their plasma membranes (Table 2); serum cholesterol level is also markedly lower (for GRSL cells, see ref. 73; for Moloney virus-induced mouse lymphoma and human leukemic cells, see ref. 74, a review with pertinent references).

The findings in the hepatoma system are consistent with an 'overproduction' of cholesterol. This does not seem to be the case for the lymphoma/leukemia systems. Apart from a possible parameter involved in the low

Table 1. Plasma membranes: liver/hepatoma system.

System	'Rigidity' (P) pm; total lipid[a]	Cholesterol/ phospholipid	Unsaturation[b] of phospholipids
RAT			
Liver	0.300[c]	0.65	273
Hepatoma-484A, solid	0.337; 0.330	0.89	152
Novikoff hepatoma, ascites	0.350; 0.345	1.09	162
MOUSE			
Liver	0.326; 0.325	0.80	250
Hepatoma-147042	0.307; 0.304	1.00	239
Hepatoma-143066	0.308; 0.296	1.08	263

[a] Total lipid extracted and measured as liposomes; $P =$ fluorescence polarisation, DPH at 25°; pm, plasma membranes.
[b] Number of double bonds in fatty acyls per 100 molec. of total phospholipids (Emmelot P, Van Hoeven RP, *Chem Phys Lipids* 14: 236, 1976).
[c] See ref. 75; this value is calculated (observed P value 0.322 and for the corresponding liposomes: 0.317; $P = 0.311$ and 0.288 for plasma membranes isolated from single cells prepared from intact and regenerating rat liver, respectively). Bile canalicular membranes and junctional complexes are abundant in isolated liver plasma membranes, but depleted or absent in the isolated and in situ plasma membranes of rat hepatomas. However, in situ or isolated plasma membranes of mouse hepatomas (solid) closely resemble mouse liver plasma membranes in these respects.

Table 2. Plasma membranes: thymocyte/lymphoma system of the GR mouse.

Cells	'Rigidity' *(P)*	Cholesterol/ phospholipid
Thymocytes	0.306	0.79
GRSL, well established	0.261	0.32

cholesterol content of these cells mentioned below (p. 51), a systemic effect of the disease affecting the cholesterol-carrying serum lipoproteins might be operative. Moreover, in the case of the GRSL lymphoma the proliferation of the cells may be so rapid that even the 'unrepressed' cholesterol synthesis in these cells and the available serum cholesterol supply may not siffice to provide a higher cholesterol content than the one that is actually reached.

However that may be, the difference in cholesterol content may have different consequences for the plasma membranes of the two tumor systems.

FLUIDITY OF MEMBRANES

Cholesterol confers a more rigid consistency on the unsaturated fatty acyls of the phospholipid bilayer of the membrane via a physicochemical interaction impeding their free motion, whereas interaction with saturated acyls imposes a more fluid condition on the latter. In plasma membranes the former effect apparently predominates, because removal of cholesterol always leads to a more fluid membrane. This is supported by the finding that the increased cholesterol content of the rat hepatoma plasma membranes (solid and ascites tumors), compared with liver membranes, is accompanied by an increased rigidity (decreased fluidity) as measured by fluorescence polarization [75] (Table 1). The use of the spin labeling technique has shown that the microsomal membrane lipid of rat hepatoma is also more rigid than the corresponding normal material [76]. However, the rigidizing effect should not be attributed to, or solely to, cholesterol, since the more saturated nature of the fatty acyl chains of the rat hepatoma phospholipids [77] may determine the effect. This is suggested by the finding that mouse hepatoma plasma membranes showed a somewhat decreased rigidity but the same fatty acyl unsaturation [77] as did liver membranes, although the cholesterol content [69] of these hepatoma membranes was higher than that of the liver membranes. As a result, rat hepatomas possess stronger (plasma) membranes than do liver cells; Novikoff ascites hepatoma cells are notable for their resistance to mechanical disruption.

In contrast, the decreased cholesterol content in plasma membranes of the GRSL (and other leukemia) cells, compared with the thymocyte (lymphocyte) plasma membranes, is accompanied by an increased fluidity [73–75] (Table 2). Hence these membranes are rather fragile and easy to disrupt, as shown by the death of many of these cells on intraperitoneal injection, the debris being rapidly cleared.

Differences in fluidity among tumors may conceivably affect antineoplastic drug entry [78] and other permeability processes.

EFFECT OF TRANSPLANTATION OF SPONTANEOUS GRSL CELLS ON PLASMA-MEMBRANE CHOLESTEROL AND FLUIDITY

The above results were obtained with well-established strains of GRSL cells growing as ascites cells in vivo. However, when cells and plasma membranes from primary, spontaneous GRSL cells or very early transplant generations — the latter growing as ascites cells and in a more solid form in mesenterial lymph nodes and spleen — were studied, their rigidity and cholesterol/PL ratio were not decreased, remaining equal to the corresponding values of thymocyte membranes [79, 80] (Fig. 2). Usually after two to four and occasionally seven transplant generations — when cells grew mainly in the ascites form — these values dropped to the lower ones previously mentioned. This suggests that during transplantation, a particular population of ascites cells is selected (heterogeneity in fluidity among GRSL cells is indicated by Fig. 1 of ref. 79). Furthermore, the emergence of fragile cells may suggest that the selection was aimed against cells with a surface mark that was more detrimental than cell fragility to cell survival in vivo.

Intraperitoneal inoculation of primary GRSL cells and their following transplant generations into immune-deficient, syngeneic mice (400 rads whole-body irradiation) then showed that the rigidity and the cholesterol content of the plasma membranes of these cells hardly changed, if at all, during at least ten transplant generations [79, 80]. However, when these cells were inoculated into normal mice, the low cholesterol and high fluidity of the membranes were again demonstrable.

Before it was concluded that an immune reaction was instrumental in the selection, the possible involvement of another systemic effect of irradiation was investigated. One such effect could have been an increase in serum cholesterol after irradiation, cholesterol then being taken up by the plasma membranes of the GRSL cells. However, when GRSL cells of transplant generations > 10 maintained in nonirradiated mice and with membranes exhibiting the high fluidity and low cholesterol content were transferred to irradiated mice and grew there as ascites cells, these parameters did not normalize. Hence it may be concluded that the selection occurring during transplantation was irreversible for cells in the ascites form, and that the suggested

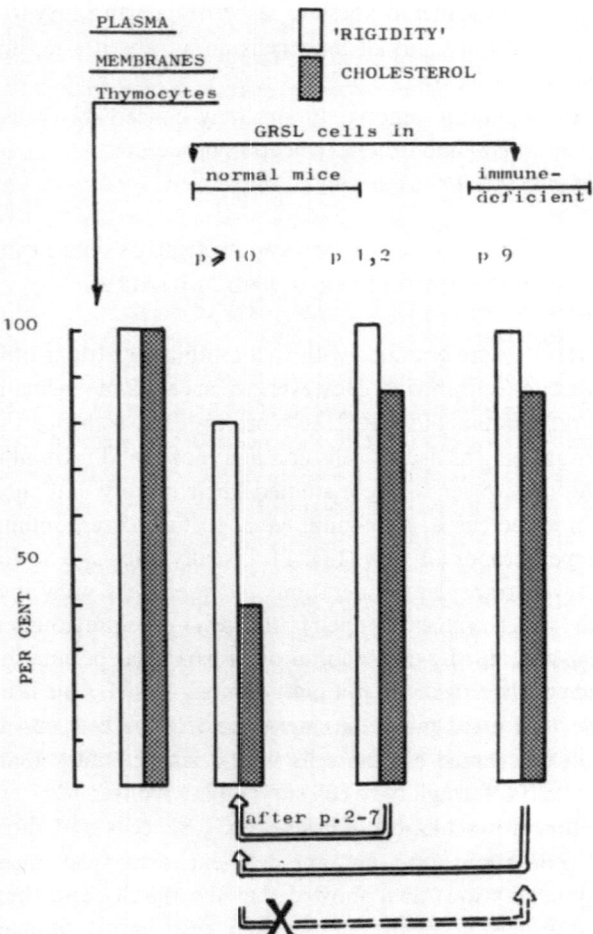

Fig. 2. Cholesterol content and 'rigidity' of GRSL plasma membranes as a function of transplant generation (p) in normal and immune-deficient mice.

systemic effect was apparently not involved. However, the mode of growth was of paramount influence, as suggested by the further finding that whenever established ascites cells happened to grow in a more solid form, normalization of fluidity and cholesterol content did occur.

The conditions for immune selection in this system are as follows. GRSL cells carry the mammary tumor viral antigen, *MLr* [81], and antibody production in these mice occurs within four days after inoculation of the GRSL cells. The early death of fragile GRSL cells upon transplantation may result in a boostering of the immune response in animals that are normally (nontumor bearers) exposed to a low level of endogenous virus. Moreover, heterogeneity in expression of the same antigen among cells of another tumor has been demonstrated [27]. However, the GR/A seems to be deficient in complement. Since selection resulted in fluid cells, the question can be posed as to whether the measure of viral antigen expression at the cell surface (immunogenicity) is inversely related to the fluidity of the membrane. According to some reports [82–84], membrane proteins may be vertically displaced upon change in membrane lipid fluidity — i.e., 'squeezed out' if the membrane becomes more rigid — and this displacement could modulate the antigens themselves or the immune reactions in which the antigens are involved. As to humoral and cellular immune reactions, there are indications both *pro* and *contra* a single or direct relationship between antigen expression or immune reactivity and membrane rigidity [82–95]. On this basis it cannot be decided whether GRSL cells with more rigid membranes would be preferentially disposed of immunologically; but the apparent result of selection is that they are. In this connection, it is of interest that not only did fluidity increase and the cholesterol content of the membranes of the GRSL cells decrease on transplantation, but that these transplanted cells also exhibited a much lower ability to form caps with antibodies against various cell-surface antigens, including the viral one [79]. Thus, a significant change in the distribution potential of cell-surface antigens occurs during the early transplantations.

Compared with lymphocytes, human leukemic cells show the same increase in membrane fluidity and descrease in membrane and serum cholesterol contents [74]. Thus, if the animal model bears some resemblance to the human disease, the possibility should be considered that a similar type of selection might operate in man during the long period required for the clinical manifestation of the disease.

FORMATION OF SATELLITE VESICLES

GRSL cells with more fluid membranes, resulting from selection during early transplantation, still carry viral antigen. However, living GRSL cells in vivo exfoliate part of their plasma membrane components in a concentrated form including the viral antigen, as small membraneous vesicles (Fig. 3) called extracellular membranes or satellite vesicles, which are essentially free of ribosomes but contain microfilament fragments [73, 80, 81, 96, 97]. Noteworthy is the high rigidity of these membranes, which corresponds with their high cholesterol and sphingomyelin (another parameter of rigidity) contents compared with the plasma membranes proper (Table 3). Now the problem may be rephrased in the following terms: Does transplantation select for cells capable of extracellular vesicle formation? Does a low membrane fluidity

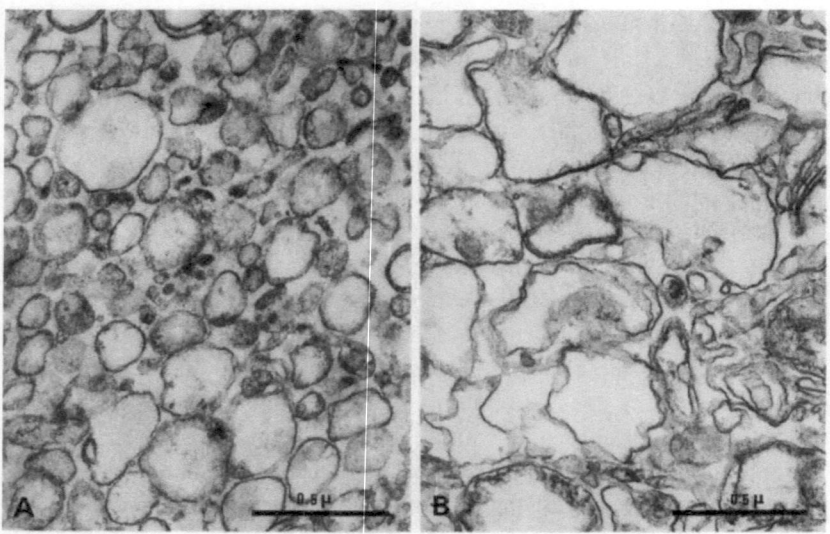

Fig. 3A and B. (A) Extracellular membrane vesicles isolated from the ascites fluid bathing GRSL cells(× 37,500). (B) Plasma membranes isolated from GRSL cells (× 37,500). Bar indicates 0.5 μ (Courtesy Dr. C.A. Feltkamp, The Netherlands Cancer Institute.)

Table 3. Properties of isolated plasma membranes and extracellular vesicles of GRSL cells.

Property[a]	Plasma membranes	Extracellular vesicles
MLr specificity[b]	17	42
5'-nucleotidase (μmoles Pi/ mg protein/h at 37°C)	1.7	3.5
Cholesterol/PL (M/M)	0.32	1.10
Sphingomyelin/total PL (%)	0.80	9.2
'Rigidity' (P at 25°C)	0.261	0.325

[a] Pi, anorganic phophate; PL, phospholipid.
[b] On a protein basis relative to twice-washed cells.

favor vesicle formation, or, alternatively, is the low fluidity of the plasma membranes of the cells due to the formation of the rigid vesicles? How does the concentration phenomenon leading to the rigid vesicles occur?

No difinite answers can be provided as yet, but the following possibilities deserve consideration (for references and additional arguments, the reader is referred to the Discussion in ref. 97; see also refs. 98–100). It should be noted that the amount of vesicular material encountered at any given moment in the ascites fluid is insufficient to cause the low rigidity and low cholesterol and sphingomyelin contents of the plasma membranes of the cells. However, if the vesicles were naturally cleared from the ascites fluid at a reasonably high rate, vesicle formation could indeed contribute to, or condition, the particular state of the GRSL cell surface.

The exfoliation of vesicles containing viral antigen may form a means to escape from immunological control. No evidence has been obtained that a humoral immune reaction is responsible for vesicle formation. For vesicle formation to occur in vivo, certain conditions other than the free state of cells must be met, since rigid Novikoff hepatoma ascites cells do not form vesicles in vivo.

Microvilli on cells represent rigid domains that may be exfoliated. The envelope of the B-type virus particles originating by external budding of the plasma membrane is much more rigid then the membrane itself. Now, GRSL cells contain some A-type virus particles and, though budding of B-type particles is extremely rare, the MLr complex of antigen is expressed on the cell surface. This suggests that insertion of viral glycoprotein into the plasma membrane may impose a local concentration of certain membrane compounds, and form the signal for budding and exfoliation of that part of the membrane as a satellite vesicle; we have previously suggested the term 'abortive virus formation' for this phenomenon. It should be noted that purified GRSL vesicles are devoid of viral particles; in nonpurified preparations a viral particle has only been found very occasionally. This may be otherwise for virus-producing lymphomas, i.e., the Moloney virus-induced lymphoma, especially if raw vesicle preparations are used as in experiments mentioned in ref. 74; these experiments were performed after the senior author had learned of vesicle formation in our laboratory.

The opposite phenomenon to external vesicle formation ('vesicular exocytosis') is endocytosis. In the latter the infolding membrane is more rigid than the remainder of the membrane, which becomes fluidized in the process [101]; also, a certain rigidity, imposed by cholesterol, appears to be required for endocytosis [102]. On this basis very fluid lymphoma cells in the GRSL population might be deficient in endocytosis and this, combined with a deficiency in the cytoskeleton, could have two consequences. First, the cholesterol-containing low-density serum lipoproteins would not be taken up by these cells, which could help to explain the lack of inhibition of cholesterol biosynthesis by exogenous cholesterol in this system. Secondly, mature circulating lymphocytes do not have insulin receptor on their cell surface, whereas activated lymphocytes (blasts) and human leukemic cells do [103]. If insulin or some other growth factor [104, 105] were instrumental in cell proliferation, the insulin-receptor or growth-factor–receptor complex would be internalized by normal blasts, which would provide for a temporary stimulation ('down' regulation), whereas in the very fluid leukemic cells

54

deficient endocytosis might result in more permanent stimulation of cell proliferation. As to other effects, increased fluidity has been found to be correlated with the lack of induction of differentiation in myeloid leukemia cell clones [106]. Phagocytosis by macrophages increases with enhanced unsaturation of membrane PL-fatty acyls [107].

OTHER ALTERATIONS OF THE TUMOR-CELL SURFACE LEADING TO AN ESCAPE FROM IMMUNE CONTROL

In general [108–112], the immunogenicity of a tumor cell is inversely related to its capacity to grow out into a tumor and its metastatic potential. Higher immunogenicity requires the inoculation of more cells to obtain tumor development, and transplantation will be restricted to syngeneic animals, whereas in the reverse case transplantation into allogeneic animals (xeno-transplantation) may become possible.

To enable survival despite host control, tumor cells could conceivably be selected by various mechanisms that lead to the same net effect, as has been shown for the acquisition of resistance to chemotherapeutic agents.

Besides the mechanisms mentioned in the preceding section (see Fig. 4: 1, 2), antigen may be shed [113–116] from tumor cells in soluble form (some-

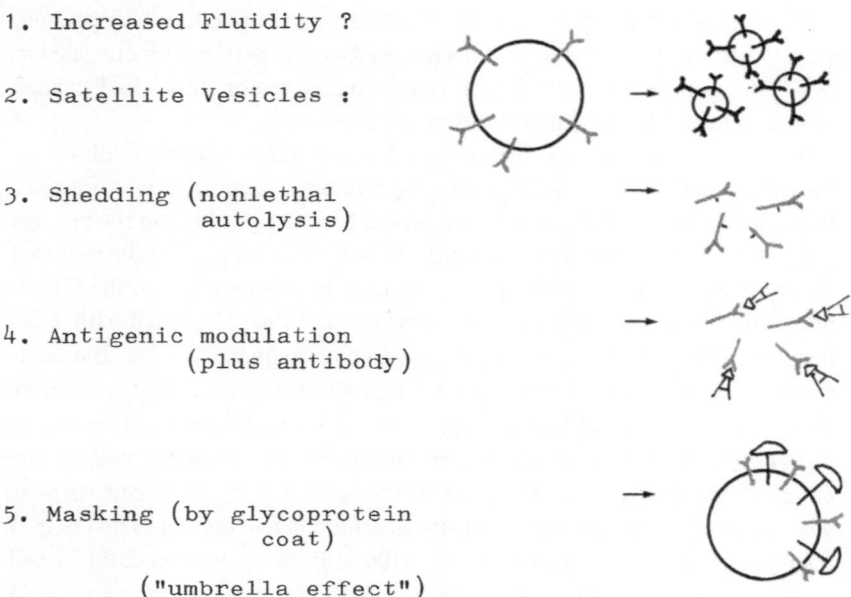

1. Increased Fluidity ?

2. Satellite Vesicles :

3. Shedding (nonlethal
          autolysis)

4. Antigenic modulation
          (plus antibody)

5. Masking (by glycoprotein
          coat)

     ("umbrella effect")

Fig. 4. Schematic representation of escape mechanisms from immunological control.

times together with other proteins or parts thereof — nonlethal autolysis could be a mechanism) or as antigen-antibody complexes; both these forms have been observed for GRSL cells growing in vivo [81]. Antigenic modulation of the viral antigen of GRSL cells by antibody can also proceed in vitro [117]; blebs were formed. Still another mechanism may operate, e.g., in malignant MBVIA mouse lymphoblasts. For tumor-cell systems with analogous or similar behavior, see refs. 110–112, 118, and 119.

MBVIA cells maintained in vivo do not agglutinate with concanavalin A, but when they are grown in vitro the cells become highly agglutinable by the lectin [120]. Unexpectedly, when inoculated into the syngeneic mice, the cells grown in vitro did not form tumors. However, when inoculated into immune-deficient mice, tumors did arise. From these results the conclusion was drawn that blasts grown in vivo carried 'masked' antigen, and 'unmasking' during in vitro growth led to the immunological rejection of the cells inoculated into normal mice. Since mild proteolytic treatment of the cells grown in vivo made these cells highly agglutinable by the lectin, it was concluded that (glyco) protein was in some way involved in the 'masking' phenomenon. Injection of normal mice with the immunogenic cells cultured in vitro yielded a high degree of protection against subsequent challenge with cells grown in vivo [121]. The latter result may indicate that the antigen on the in vivo cells is only slightly immunogenic but that once an immune response is induced (by the in vitro cells) the immune reaction does proceed.

'Masking' may also occur by way of neuraminidase-sensitive sialic acid in glycoprotein [122, 123]. According to an early publication [124], mouse sarcoma cells acquired increased negative electrical surface charge in the selection process of attaining the capacity to grow as ascites cells. Recently, cells of a highly metastatic variant line of polyoma-induced rat renal sarcoma were found to be more highly sialylated than were the cells of a weakly metastatic line [125, 126]. The metastatic cells also showed more clumping [125]; electrostatic interaction by way of Ca^{2+} and sialyl-COO^- could be involved in self-adhesion [126].

A UNIVERSAL MARKER FOR CANCER CELLS?

When tumor cells and homologous normal cells are differentially labeled metabolically with ^{14}C- or ^3H-fucose either in vitro or in vivo and then mildly trypsinized, and the resulting trypsinates combined and exhaustively digested with pronase before gel filtration, a characteristic profile emerges: at least part of the tumor glycopeptides elute ahead of the normal ones (Fig. 5).

To date, this phenomenon has been established for the following animal (A) and human (B) tumor cell systems:

56

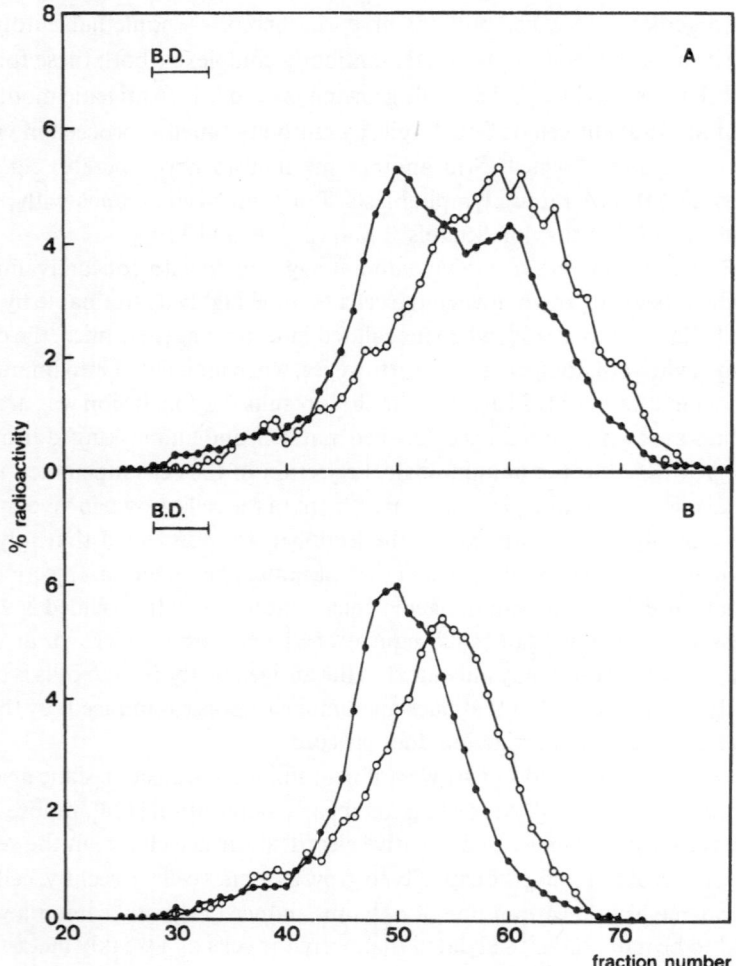

Fig. 5A and B. Gel filtration profile of fucosyl-glycopeptides. The glycopeptides were derived from ³H-fucose-labeled cells from a patient with acute lymphocytic leukemia (●———●) and compared by cochromatography with ¹⁴C-fucose-labeled glycopeptide from normal lympho-cytes (O———O). A = without purification; B = after removal of Con-A-binding glyco-peptides by affinity chromatography. (Courtesy Dr. L.A. Smets, The Netherlands Cancer Institute.)

(A) Virally, spontaneously, and chemically transformed fibroblasts in vitro, which are tumorigenic (three species, oncogenic RNA and DNA viruses, and a total of at least ten cell strains) [128–131]; malignant mouse lymphoblasts MBVIA grown in vivo or in vitro [130, 131]; mouse lymphoma GRSL cells [131]; four rat hepatomas, one of which was studied in two states (solid tissue and ascites cells) [132]; and hormone-independent GR mouse mammary tumors [133].

(B) All types of human leukemia (more than 60 samples from patients; six established cell lines); lymphosarcomas (two samples from patients); Burkitt lymphomas (20 lines); non-Burkitt, non-Hodgkin lymphomas (five lines); gliomas (six lines); osteosarcomas (three lines) [134–137].

The change in glycopeptide profile was not observed in the following cases: rat liver cells proliferating in vitro [130]; regenerating rat liver [131]; late-embryonic rat liver [132]; PHA-stimulated lymphocytes (blasts), nonmalignant human lymphoproliferative disorders, including infectious mononucleosis (19 cases) [134], hormone-dependent primary mammary tumors of the GR/A mouse [133], and SV40-tranformed fibroblasts [138]. The last two cases require comment.

First, if the changed glycopeptide profile reflects change that is invariably associated with tumors (as difined), the hormone-sustained GR/A mammary tumors — which regress after the conditioning hormone is withdrawn — apparently lack this property of tumors. Their mode of growth is that of reversible hyperplasia, being of a diffuse type in pregnancy-induced tumors. The glycopeptide change, on the other hand, is associated with the change to (clonal) autonomous growth, since the autonomous tumors arising in this system show the glycopeptide change, which increases with their autonomy [133].

Secondly, SV40-transformed fibroblasts maintained in vitro apparently contain too few tumorigenic cells for the glycopeptide change to be demonstrable, but after selection of tumorigenic cells by in vivo passage, the glycopeptide change is prominent [138]. The reason for the gradual decrease in the number of tumorigenic cells during in vitro culture has been established: these cells are more sensitive to the mild trypsinization used to detach cells for each subsequent culture than are the transformed, nontumorigenic cells [139]. This effect differs from the above-mentioned instantaneous effect seen when MBVIA cells are cultured.

Thirdly, although cultured MBVIA cells do not yield tumors on transplantation in vivo, the glycopeptide assay demonstrates the tumorigenic character of these cells. This potential of the assay has also been demonstrated for human lymphoblastoid cell lines (= human B-lymphocytes infected with Epstein-Barr virus in vitro) [137], and in cases of uncertain clinical diagnosis where malignant disease was indicated by the assay before it became clinically manifest [127].

The glycopeptide alteration in the tumor-cell surface is expressed in many glycopeptide fractions. This pleiotropic effect is reminiscent of the action of the *sarc*. gene responsible for cell transformation by avian sarcoma virus that codes for a phosphorylating enzyme (protein kinase) acting on a number of cellular and membrane proteins [140, 141]. In an analogous manner the glycoprotein changes could be installed by an altered activity or localization of a carbohydrate-transferring enzyme forming the oligosaccharide side-chains of different glycoproteins.

At least three chemical factors, according to the tumor type studied, appear to be involved in the glycopeptide change [131, 132]. In most tumors the alteration is due to a higher sialic acid density in glycoprotein than normal: treatment with neuraminidase before chromatography results in a coincidence of the profiles of tumor and normal glycopeptides. Besides neuraminidase-sensitive sialic acid, neuraminidase-insensitive sialic acid (released by very mild acid treatment) is also a determinant, but in a smaller number of tumors. As shown previously, the latter type of change may be dictated by the mode of growth of the tumor cells (solid versus ascites) alone, in which case the change (neuraminidase-insensitive) occurs at the expense of the former type (neuraminidase-sensitive). In the few cases encountered so far (H35-hepatoma, Burkitt lymphoma, and chronic myelocytic leukemia in man), a third, as yet undefined, chemical change dominates the tumor glycopeptide profile.

CONCLUSION

The general absence of a consistent pattern of change in tumor cell phenotypes is conspicuous. However, according to present knowledge, the glycopeptide change would qualify as a general marker of the tumorigenicity/malignancy of cells. Whether it is also a causal change remains to be established.

With today's emphasis on the cell surface as a site — or even the main site — at which the genetic changes underlying the tumorigenic character of cells are expressed and mediated, it should be kept in mind that the glycopeptide alteration is coordinately expressed throughout the tumor cell, including the intracellular membranes [128]. The same applies to the lipid and glycolipid compositions and contents of tumor membranes [142].

However, it has been established that events at the cell surface involving (glyco)protein may regulate normal growth, e.g. the effects of hormones [143, 144], proteolytic enzymes [145, 146], and various growth factors [147] which, by sole interaction with cell-surface components, induce DNA synthesis and cell proliferation. That alteration in the cell surface at the level of carbohydrate insertion into glycoprotein may regulate growth is shown by the following recent finding [148]. A cell-surface component (X) isolated from resting 3T3 cells inhibited DNA synthesis when added to growing 3T3 cells, which do not exhibit X activity. Prior incubation of resting cells with uridine diphosphate-N-acetyl glucosamine-GlcNAc (but not with three other sugar dinucleotides) gave a preparation without inhibitory X activity, but treatment of this preparation with N-Ac-glucosamidase restored its inhibitory function. Thus, reversible glycosylation with N-Ac-glucosamine residues on the cell surface might serve as a regulatory factor in DNA synthesis. Blockade of this process at the tumor-cell surface — due to substitution of acceptor sites by sialylation or the more general type of masking discussed in the previous paragraph, or by proteolytic activity — might give rise to uncontrolled growth.

Although the exact mechanisms are still unknown, sufficient evidence has been collected in recent years to support the view that altered surface processes participate in mediation of the tumorigenic state of cells. Yet this may only be part of the story. Therefore, the cell surface should not be looked at in splendid isolation since in between the cell surface and the nucleus other controls may also be operative and be altered, the first candidates for such function being ectoplasmic or subsurface filaments.

REFERENCES

1. Emmelot P: Biochemical properties of normal and neoplastic cell surfaces; a review. Eur J Cancer 9: 319–333, 1973.
2. Nicolson GL: Transmembrane control of the receptors on normal and tumor cells II. Surface changes associated with transformation and malignancy. Biochim Biophys Acta 458: 1–72, 1976.
3. Gahmberg CG: Cell surface proteins: changes during cell growth and malignant transformation. In: Post G, Nicolson GL (eds) Dynamic aspects of cell surface organization. Amsterdam, North-Holland, 1977, pp 371–422.
4. Scherer E, Emmelot P: Kinetics of induction and growth of precancerous liver-cell foci, and liver tumour formation by diethylnitrosamine in the rat. Eur J Cancer 11: 689–696, 1975.
5. Emmelot P, Scherer E: The first relevant cell stage in rat liver carcinogenesis; a quantitative approach. Biochim Biophys Acta 605: 247–304, 1980.
6. Losa G, Morell A: Plasma membrane linked enzymes in lymphoproliferative diseases. Proc Am Assoc Cancer Res 30: 29 (117), 1979.
7. Check W: Cancer, chromosome changes intertwinted. JAMA 240: 335–337, 1978.
8. Steel CM, Woodward HA, Davidson C, Philips J, Arthur E: Non-random chromosome gains in human lymphoblastoid cell lines. Nature 270: 349–351, 1977.
9. Anderson NG, Coggin Jr JH, Cole E, Holleman JW (eds): Embryonic and fetal antigens in cancer, vol 2. Oak Ridge, Oak Ridge Natl Lab, 1972.
10. Fishman WH, Busch H (eds): Methods in cancer research, vol 18: Oncodevelopmental antigens. New York, Academic Press, 1979.
11. Ibsen KH, Fishman WH: Developmental gene expression in cancer. Biochim Biophys Acta 560: 243–280, 1979.
12. Baldwin RW: Immunological aspects of chemical carcinogenesis. Adv Cancer Res 18: 1–75, 1973.
13. Baldwin RW, Embleton MJ, Pimm MV: Neoantigens in chemical carcinogenesis. In: Griffin AC, Shaw CR (eds) Carcinogens: identification and mechanisms. New York, Raven Press, 1979, pp 365–379.
14. Scherer E, Emmelot P: Multihit kinetics of tumor cell formation and risk assessment of low doses of carcinogen. In: Griffin AC, Shaw CR (eds) Carcinogens: identification and mechanims. New York, Raven Press, 1979, pp 337–363.

60

15. Chan EPH, Ball JK, Sergovich FR: Trisomy no. 15 in murine thymomas induced by chemical carcinogens, X-irradiation and endogenous leukemia virus. J Natl Cancer Inst 62: 605–610, 1979.
16. Emmelot P, Visser A, Benedetti EL: Studies on plasma membranes VII. A Leucyl-β-naphthylamidase-containing repeating unit on the surface of isolated liver and hepatoma plasma membranes. Biochim Biophys Acta 150: 364–375, 1968.
17. Emmelot P, Bos CJ: Studies on plasma membranes X. A survey of enzyme activities displayed by plasma membranes isolated from mouse liver and three mouse hepatoma strains. Int J Cancer 4: 723–734, 1969.
18. Emmelot P, Bos CJ: Differences in the association of two glycolytic enzymes with plasma membranes isolated from rat liver and hepatoma. Biochim Biophys Acta 121: 434–436, 1966.
19. Davidova SY, Shapot VS, Solowjeva AA: Hexokinase activity and glycolytic capacity of plasma membranes of hepatomas. Biochim Biophys Acta 158: 303–305, 1968.
20. Bhatty RS, Hickie RA: Absence of hexokinase activity in plasma membranes of Morris hepatoma 5123 t.c. Biochem Biophys Res Commun 44: 1443–1448, 1971.
21. Inoue S, Skoryna SC: Intercellular junctions in human breast cancer. Proc Am Assoc Cancer Res 20: 29 (114), 1979.
22. Emmelot P, Benedetti EL: On the possible involvement of the plasma membrane in the carcinogenic process. In: Carcinogenesis: a broad critique. Baltimore, Williams and Wilkins, 1967, pp 471–533.
23. Weinstein RS, Merk FB, Alroy J: The structure and function of intercellular junctions in cancer. Adv Cancer Res 23: 23–89, 1976.
24. Pauli BH, Knettner KE, Weinstein RS: Intercellular junctions in FANFT-induced carcinomas of rat urinary bladder in tissue culture: in situ thin-section, freeze-fracture, and scanning electron microscopy studies. J Microscopy 115: 271–283, 1979.
25. Pauli BH, Weinstein RS, Alroy J, Arai M: Ultrastructure of cell junctions in FANFT-induced urothelial tumors in urinary bladder of Fischer rats. Lab Invest 37: 609–621, 1977.
26. Loewenstein R: Intercellular communication in normal and neoplastic tissues. In: Cellular membranes and tumor cell behavior. Baltimore, Williams and Wilkins, 1975, pp 239–248.
27. Dexter DL, Konalski HM, Blazar BA, Fligiel Z, Vogel R, Heppner GH: Heterogeneity of tumor cells from a single mouse mammary tumor. Cancer Res 38: 3174–3181, 1978; cf. Proc Am Assoc Cancer Res 20: 61(246), 1979.
28. Dexter DL, Fligiel Z, Vogel R, Calabresi P: Heterogeneity of neoplastic cells from a single human colon carcinoma. Proc Am Assoc Cancer Res 20: 199(804), 1979.
29. Olsson L, Ebbesen P: Natural polyclonality of spontaneous AKR lymphoma and its consequences for so-called specific immunotherapy. J Natl Cancer Inst 62: 623–627, 1979.
30. Gerber MA, Thung SN, Sarno E: Emergence of heterogenous cell populations in hepatocellular carcinoma. Lab Invest 40: 256, 1979.
31. Neri A, Ruoslahti E, Nicolson GL: Relationship of fibronectin to the metastatic behavior of rat mammary adenocarcinoma cell lines and clones. J Supramol Struct [Suppl] 3: 181(444), 1979.
32. Fidler IJ, Kripke ML: Metastasis results from pre-existing variant cells within a malignant tumor. Science 197: 893–895, 1977.
33. Weiss L, Harlos JP: Differences in the peripheries of Walker cancer cells growing in different sites of the rat. Cancer Res 39: 2481–2485, 1979.
34. Fidler IJ: Selection of successive tumor lines for metastasis. Nature [New Biol] 242: 148–149, 1973.
35. Tao T-w, Burger MM: Non-metastasing variants selected from metastasing melanoma cells. Nature 270: 437–438, 1977.
36. Brunson KW, Beattie G, Nicolson GL: Selection and altered tumor cell properties in brain-colonizing metastatic melanoma. Nature 272: 543–545, 1978.
37. Tao T-w, Matter A, Vogel K, Burger MM: Liver-colonizing melanoma cells selected from B-16 melanoma. Int J Cancer 23: 854–857, 1979.
38. Reading V, Nicolson GL: In vitro selection of lymphosarcoma variant with altered

malignancy in vivo. J Supramol Struct [Suppl] 3: 183(450), 1979.

39. Nicolson GL, Winkelhake JL: Organ specificity of blood-borne tumor metastases determined by cell adhesion? Nature 255: 230–232, 1975.

40. Nicolson GL, Brunson KN, Fidler IJ: Specificity of arrest, survival and growth of selected metastatic variant cell lines. Cancer Res 38: 4105–4111, 1978.

41. Ambrus JL, Ambrus CM, Gastpar H: Tumor metastasis and platelet aggregation. Proc Am Asso Cancer Res 19: 83(329), 1978.

42. Bubenik J, Perlmann P, Fenyo EM, Janlova T, Suhajova E, Malkovsky M: Inverse relation between cell-surface adhesiveness and malignancy in mouse fibroblastoid cell lines. Int J Cancer 23: 392–396, 1979.

43. Brunson KW, Nicolson GL: Cell surface components of malignant melanoma variants selected for organ specificity: J Supramol Struct [Suppl] 3: 181(443), 1979.

44. Fogel M, Gorelik E, Segal S, Feldman M: Differences in cell surface antigens of tumor metastases and those of the local tumor. J Natl Cancer Inst 62: 585–588, 1979.

45. Gorelik E, Fogel M, Segal S, Feldman M: Tumor-associated antigenic differences between the primary and the descendant metastatic tumor cell population. J Supramol Struct [Suppl] 3: 184(452), 1979.

46. Shin S, Freedman VH, Risser R, Pollack R: Tumorigenicity of virus transformed cells in nude mice is correlated specifically with anchorage-independent growth. Proc Natl Acad Sci USA 72: 4435–4439, 1975.

47. Stanbridge EJ, Wilkinson J: Analysis of malignancy in human cells: malignant and transformed phenotypes are under separate genetic control. Proc Natl Acad Sci USA 75: 1466–1469, 1978.

48. Smets LA, Van Beek WP Van Rooy H, Homburg Ch: The relationship between membrane glucoprotein alterations and anchorage-independent growth in neoplastic transformation. Cancer Biochem Biophys 2: 203–208, 1978.

49. Lang WE: Anchorage-independent growth and plasminogen activator production by bovine endothelial cells. Proc Am Assoc Cancer Res 20: 96(385), 1979.

50. Freedman VH, Shin S: Isolation of human diploid variants with enhanced colony forming efficiency in semisolid medium after a single-step chemical mutagenesis. J Natl Cancer Inst 58: 1873–1875, 1977.

51. Tökes ZA: Proteolysis available at the surface of viable normal and transformed fibroblasts. Proc Am Assoc Cancer Res 19: 145(580), 1978.

52. Harris ED, Faulkner CS, Wood S: Collegenase in carcinoma cells. Biochem Biophys Res Commun 48: 1247–1253, 1972.

53. DeVore DP, Houchens DP, Ovejera AA, Hutson TB: Noninvasiveness of human tumors in the athymic (nude) mouse. Proc Am Assoc Cancer Res 20: 5(18), 1979.

54. Wang BS, McLoughlin GA, Richie JP: Correlation of plasminogen production with tumor metastasis. Proc Am Assoc Cancer Res 20: 161(648), 1979.

55. Kramer RH, Nicolson GL: Metastatic tumor cells induce the in vitro degradation of endothelial extracellular matrix. J Supramol Struct [Suppl] 3: 181(445), 1979.

56. Nathanson, SD, Morton DL, Sarna GP: Inhibition of antibody-induced lysis of human melanoma cells by fibrinolysin (plasmin). Proc Am Assoc Cancer Res 20: 217(880), 1979.

57. Cohen IK, Moncure CW, Witorsch RJ, Diegelmann RF: Collagen synthesis in capsule surrounding dimethylbenzanthracene-induced rat breast tumors and the effect of pretreatment with β-aminopropionitrile. Cancer Res 39: 2923–2927, 1979.

58. Dvorak HF, Dvorak AM, Manseau EF, Wiberg L, Churchill WH: Fibrin gel investment associated with line 1 and line 10 solid tumor growth, angiogenesis and fibroplasia in guinea pigs. Role of cellular immunity, myofibroblasts, microvascular damage, and infarction in line 1 tumor regression. J Natl Cancer Inst 62: 1459–1472, 1979.

59. Critchley DR, Vicker MG: Glycolipids as membrane receptors important in growth regulation and cell-cell interaction. In: Poste G, Nicolson GL (eds) Dynamic aspects of cell surface organization. Amsterdam, North-Holland, 1977, pp 307–370.

60. Oncology overview. Selected abstracts on glycosphingolipids, US Department of Health, Education and Welfare, National Institutes of Health, National Cancer Institute, 1979.

62

61. Koppel TM, Morré DJ, Cherry JM, Jacobson LB: Surface characteristics of metastatic and nonmetastatic cell from single hepatocellular carcinomas. J Supramol Struct [Suppl] 3: 182 (451), 1979.
62. Taki T, Hirabayashi Y, Ishiwata Y, Matsumoto M, Kojima K: Biosynthesis of different gangliosides in two types of rat ascites hepatoma cell with different degrees of cell adhesiveness. Biochim Biophys Acta 572: 113–120, 1979.
63. Ishimaru Y, Kudo K, Koga Y, Hayashi H: A possible mechanism for island formation by rat ascites hepatoma cells with special reference to the function of aggregation factor at the cell surface. J Cancer Res Clin Oncol 93: 123–136, 1979.
64. Lingwood CA, Ng A, Hakomori S: Monovalent antibodies directed to transformation-sensitive membrane components inhibit the process of viral transformation. Proc Natl Acad Sci USA 75: 6049–6053, 1978.
65. Sela BB, Raz A, Geiger B: Antibodies to ganglioside GM_1 induce mitogenic stimulation and cap production. In: Program and Abstracts 12th International Leukocyte Culture Conference, Beersheba, Israel, 1978, p 66.
66. O'Keefe E, Cuatrecasas P: Persistence of exogenous, inserted ganglioside GM_1 on the cell surface of cultured cells. Life Sci 21: 1649–1653, 1977.
67. Siperstein MD, Fagan V: Deletion of the cholesterol-negative feedback system in liver tumors. Cancer Res 24: 1108–1115, 1964.
68. Chen HW, Kandutsch AA, Heiniger HJ: The role of cholesterol in malignancy. Prog Exp Tumor Res 22: 275–316, 1978.
69. Van Hoeven RP, Emmelot P: Studies on plasma membranes XVIII. Lipid class composition of plasma membranes isolated from rat and mouse liver and hepatomas. J Membr Biol 9: 105–126, 1972.
70. Barclay M, Terebus-Kekish O, Dnistrian AM, Archibald FM, Stock CC: Lipoproteins isolated from plasma membranes of Morris hepatoma 5123. Cancer Res 38: 1774–1781, 1978.
71. Dnistrian AM, Barclay M, Archibald FM, Terebus-Kekish O, Morris HP: Cholesterol and fatty acid profiles in plasma membranes from Morris hepatomas of varying degrees of malignancy. Proc Am Assoc Cancer Res 17: 3(10), 1976.
72. Dnistrian AM, Barclay M, Terebus-Kekish O, Archibald FM, Morris HP: Serum lipoproteins of rats bearing Morris hepatomas of different degrees of differentiation. Cancer Biochem Biophys 3: 81–84, 1979.
73. Van Blitterswijk WJ, Emmelot P, Hilkmann HAM, Oomen-Meulemans EPM, Inbar M: Differences in lipid fluidity among isolated plasma membranes of normal and leukemic lymphocytes and membranes exfoliated from their cell surface. Biochim Biophys Acta 467: 309–320, 1977.
74. Rosenfeld C, Jasmin C, Mathé G, Inbar M: Dynamic and composition of cellular membranes and serum lipids in malignant disorders. Recent Results Cancer Res 67: 67–77, 1979.
75. Van Hoeven RP, Van Blitterswijk WJ, Emmelot P: Fluorescence polarization measurements on normal and tumour cells and their corresponding plasma membranes. Biochim Biophys Acta 551: 44–54, 1979.
76. Diatlovitskaia EV, Einisman EB, Goloshchapov AN, Buvlakova EB: Microviscosity of intracellular membranes of rat liver and rat hepatoma. Biofizika 23: 1104–1106, 1978.
77. Van Hoeven RP, Emmelot P, Krol JH, Oomen-Meulemans EPM: Studies on plasma membranes XXII. Fatty acid profile of lipid classes in plasma membranes of rat and mouse livers and hepatomas. Biochim Biophys Acta 380: 1–11, 1975.
78. Burns CP, Luttenegger DG, Dudley DT, Buettner GR, Spector AA: Effect of modification of plasma membrane fatty acid composition on fluidity and methotrexate transport in L1210 murine leukemia cells. Cancer Res 39: 1726–1732, 1979.
79. Hilgers J, Van Der Sluis PJ, Van Blitterswijk WJ, Emmelot P: Membrane fluidity, capping of cell-surface antigens and immune response in mouse leukaemia cells. Br J Cancer 37: 329–336, 1978.
80. Van Blitterswijk WJ, Hilkmann H, De Veer G, Hilgers J, Feltkamp CA, Emmelot P:

Shedding of rigig vesicles involved in the increase of plasma membrane fluidity by transplantation of leukemia cells. Protides Biol Fluids Proc Colloq 27: 201–204, 1980.

81. Van Blitterswijk WJ, Emmelot P, Hilgers J, Kamlag D, Nusse R, Feltkamp CA: Quantitation of virus-induced (*MLr*) and normal (*Thy 1.2*) cell surface antigens in plasma membranes and the extracellular fluid of mouse leukemia cells. Cancer Res 35: 2743–2751, 1975.

82. Borochov H, Abott, RE, Schachter D, Shinitzky, M: Modulation of erythrocyte membrane proteins by membrane cholesterol lipid fluidity. Biochemistry 18: 251–255, 1979.

83. Shinitzky M, Rivnay B: Degree of exposure of membrane proteins determined by fluorescence quenching. Biochemistry 16: 982–986, 1977.

84. Borochov H, Shinitzky M: Vertical displacement of membrane protein mediated by changes in microviscosity. Proc Natl Acad Sci USA 73: 4526–4530, 1976.

85. Humphries GMK, McConnell HM: Antigen mobility in membranes and complement-mediated immune attack. Proc Natl Acad Sci USA 72: 2483–2487, 1975.

86. Brûlet Ph, McConnell HM: Lateral hapten mobility and immunochemistry of model membranes. Proc Natl Acad Sci USA 73: 2977–2981, 1976.

87. Parce JW, Henny N, McConnell HM: Specific antibody-dependent binding of complement component C1q to hapten-sensitized lipid vesicles. Proc Natl Acad Sci USA 75: 1515–1518, 1978.

88. Brûlet Ph, McConnell HM: Structural and dynamical aspect of membrane immunochemistry using model membranes. Biochemistry 16: 1209–1217, 1977.

89. Hafeman DG, Parce JW, McConnell HM: Specific antibody-dependent activation of neutrophils by liposomes containing spin-label lipid haptens. Biochem Biophys Res Commun 86: 522–528, 1979.

90. Lewis JT, McConnell HM: Model lipid bilayer membranes as targets for antibody-dependent, cellular-, and complement-mediated immune attack. Ann NY Acad Sci 308: 124–136, 1978.

91. Yasuda T, Daucey GF, Kinsky SC: Immunogenicity of liposomal model membranes in mice: dependence on PL composition. Proc Natl Acad Sci USA 74: 1234–1236, 1977.

92. Gillette RW, Boone CW: Augmented immunogenicity of tumor cell membranes produced by surface budding viruses: parameters of optimal immunization. Int J Cancer 18: 216–222, 1976.

93. Dahl JS, Dahl ChE, Levine RP: Role of lipid fatty acyl composition and membrane fluidity in the resistance of Acholeplasma laidlawii to complement-mediated killing. J Immunol 123: 104–108, 1979.

94. Shin ML, Paznekas WA, Mayer MM: Effect of membrane fluidity on efficiency of sheep erythrocyte lysis by terminal complement proteins. Fed Proc 38: 1468(6549), 1979.

95. Clark WR, Gill R, Shimizu S, McVey E: Effect of membrane lipid composition on immune cell function. Fed Proc 38: 1166(4958), 1979.

96. Van Blitterswijk WJ, Van Der Sluis PJ, Hilgers J, Hilkmann HAM, Feltkamp CA. Emmelot P: High lipid fluidity of leukemic cell membranes through host immune response and shedding of tumor antigen-enriched plasma membrane regions. In: Bentvelzen P, Hilgers J, Yohn DS (eds) Advances in comparative leukemia research. Amsterdam, Elsevier/ North-Holland Biomed, 1978, pp 341–344.

97. Van Blitterswijk WJ, Emmelot P, Hilkmann HAM, Hilgers J, Feltkamp CA: Rigid plasma-membrane derived vesicles enriched in tumor-associated surface antigens (*MLr*) occurring in the ascites fluid of a mouse leukemia (GRSL). Int J Cancer 23: 62–70, 1979.

98. Stewart GJ, Gasic GJ, Gasic T, Catalfalmo JL: Membrane activity of mouse mammary tumor 15091A cells in vivo: blebbing and shedding of membrane vesicles. J Supramol Struct [Suppl] 3: 187(462), 1979.

99. Lange Y, Steck TL: Cholesterol, spectrin and the vesiculation of human erythrocyte membranes. Fed Proc 38: 794(2981), 1979.

100. Lutz HU, Barber R, McGuire RF: Glycoprotein-enriched vesicles from sheep erythrocyte ghosts obtained by spontaneous vesiculation. J Biol Chem 251: 3500–3510, 1976.

101. Berlin RD, Fera JP: Changes in membrane microviscosity associated with phagocytosis:

effects of colchicine. Proc Natl Acad Sci USA 74: 1072–1076, 1977.

102. Heiniger H-J, Kandutsch AA, Chen HW: Deletion of L-cell sterol depresses endocytosis. Nature 263: 515–517, 1976.

103. Krug U, Krug F, Cuatrecasas P: Emergence of insulin receptor on human lymphocytes during in vitro transformation. Proc Natl Acad Sci USA 69: 2601–2608, 1972.

104. Das M, Fox CE: Molecular mechanism of mitogen action: processing of receptor induced by epidermal growth factor. Proc Natl Acad Sci USA 75: 2644–2648, 1978.

105. Fox CR, Wrann M, Vale R: Mitogenic hormone-induced comodulation of EGF receptor. J Supramol Struct [Suppl] 3: 176(434), 1979.

106. Simon I: Differences in membrane unsaturated fatty acids and electron spin resonance in different types of myeloid leukemia cells. Biochim Biophys Acta 556: 408–422, 1979.

107. Schroit AJ, Gallily R: Macrophage fatty acid composition and phagocytosis: effect of unsaturation on cellular phagocytic activity. Immunology 177: 989–991, 1979.

108. Klein G, Klein E: Rejectability of virus-induced tumors and non-rejectability of spontaneous tumors: a lesson in contrasts. Transplant Proc 9: 1095–1104, 1977.

109. Kennel SJ: Characterization of a tumor cell surface protein with heterologous antisera to a spontaneous BALB/c lung carcinoma. Cancer Res 39: 2934–2939, 1979.

110. Cooper AG, Codington JF, Miller DK, Brown MC: Loss of strain specificity of the TA3-St subline; evidence for the role of epiglycanin in mouse allogeneic tumor growth. J Natl Cancer Inst 63: 163–169, 1979.

111. Codington JF, Cooper AG, Miller DK, Slayter HS, Brown MC, Silber C, Jeanloz RW: Isolation and partial characterization of an epiglycanin-like glycoprotein from a new non-strain-specific subline of TA3 murine mammary adenocarcinoma. J Natl Cancer Inst 63: 153–161, 1979.

112. Carraway KL, Huggins JW, Sherblom AP, Chesnut RW, Buck RL, Howard SP, Ownby CL, Carraway CA: Membrane glycoproteins of rat mammary gland and its metastasizing and nonmetastasizing tumors. ACS Symp Ser 80: 432–445, 1978.

113. Kim U, Baumles A, Carruthers C, Bielat K: Immunological escape mechanism in spontaneously metastasizing mammary tumors. Proc Natl Acad Sci USA 72: 1012–1016, 1975.

114. Chatterjee SK, Kim U, Bielat K: Plasma membrane associated enzymes of mammary tumors as the biochemical indicators of metastasizing capacity. Analysis of enriched plasma membrane preparations. Br J Cancer 33: 15–26, 1976.

115. Chatterjee SK, Kim U: Galactosyltransferase activity in metastasizing and nonmetastasizing rat mammary carinomas and its possible relationship with tumor cell surface antigen shedding. J Natl Cancer Inst 58: 273–280, 1977.

116. Beddison WE, Palmer JC: Development of tumor cell resistance to syngeneic cell-mediated cytotoxicity during growoth of ascitic mastocytoma P815y. Proc Natl Acad Sci USA 74: 329–333, 1977.

117. Feltkamp CA, Wilschut IJC, Van Blitterswijk WJ, Hilgers J, Sonnenberg A: Modulation of virus-induced tumor antigens (MLr) on murine leukemia cells. In: Bentvelzen P, Hilgers J, Yohn DS (eds) Advances in comparative leukemia research. Amsterdam, Elsevier/North-Holland Biomed, 1978, pp 345–348.

118. Miller DK, Cooper AG: Kinetics of release of glucosamine-labeled glycoprotein from the TA3H murin adenocarcinoma cell. J Biol Chem 253: 8798–8803, 1978.

119. Jamasbi RJ, Nettesheim P: Increase in immunogenicity with concomitant loss of tumorigenicity of respiratory tract carcinomas during in vitro culture. Cancer Res 39: 2466–2470, 1979.

120. Smets LA, Broekhuyzen-Davies J: Shielding of antigens and concanavalin A agglutination sites by a surface coat of transplantable mouse lymphosarcoma cells. Eur J Cancer 8: 541–548, 1972.

121. Smets LA, Homburg Ch: Immunogenicity and concanavalin A agglutination in transplantable mouse lymphosarcoma and human leukemia. Eur J Cancer 12: 605–610, 1976.

122. Currie GA, Bagshawe KD: The role of sialic acid in antigenic expression: further studies of the Landschütz ascites tumor. Br J Cancer 22: 843–853, 1968.

123. Bekesi JG, Arneault St, Holland JF: Increase of leukemia L-1210 cell immunogenicity

after neuraminidase treatment. Am Soc Hematol, 13th Annu Mtg Program, no. 115: 78, 1970.

124. Purdom L, Ambrose EJ, Klein G: A correlation between electrical surface charge and some biological characteristics during the stepwise progression of a mouse sarcoma. Nature 181: 1586–1587, 1958.

125. Salk PL, Lanza RP: In vitro growth charateristics, motility and adhesive properties of metastatic variant PW20 cell lines. J Supramol Struct [Suppl] 3: 182(446), 1979.

126. Yogeeswaran G, Sebastian H, Stein BS: Cell surface sialylation of glycoproteins and glycosphingolipids in cultured metastatic variant RNA-virus transformed non-producer BALB/c 3T3 cell lines. Int J Cancer 24: 193–202, 1979.

127. Benedetti EL, Emmelot P: Studies on plasma membranes IV. The ultrastructural localization and content of sialic acid in plasma membranes isolated from rat liver and hepatoma. J Cell Sci 2: 499–512, 1967.

128. Warren L, Buck CA, Tuszynski GP: Glycopeptide changes and malignant transformation. A possible role for carbohydrate in malignant behavior. Biochim Biophys Acta 516: 97–127, 1978.

129. Van Nest GA, Grimes WJ: A comparison of membrane components of normal and transformed BALB/c cells. Biochemistry 16: 2902–2908, 1977.

130. Van Beek WP, Smets LA, Emmelot P: Increased sialic acid density in surface glycoprotein of transformed and malignant cells — a general phenomenon? Cancer Res 33: 2913–2933, 1973.

131. Emmelot P, Van Beek WP, Smets LA: Cell surface carbohydrates and cell transformation: a general change signifying tumorigenicity. In: Popper H, Bianchi L, Reutter W (eds) Membrane alterations as basis of liver injury. Lancaster, England, MTP, 1977, pp 179–196.

132. Van Beek WP, Emmelot P, Homburg C: Comparison of cell-surface glycoproteins of rat hepatomas and embryonic rat liver. Br J Cancer 36: 157–165, 1977.

133. Smets LA, Van Beek WP, Van Nie R: Membrane glycoprotein changes in primary mammary tumors associated with autonomous growth. Cancer Lett 3: 133–138, 1977.

134. Van Beek WP, Smets LA, Emmelot P: Changed surface glycoprotein as a marker of malignancy in human leukaemic cells. Nature 253: 457–460, 1975.

135. Van Beek WP, Smets LA, Emmelot P, Roozendaal KJ, Behrendt H: Early recognition of human leukemia by cell surface glycoprotein changes. Leuk Res 2: 163171, 1978.

136. Van Beek WP, Glimelius B, Nilsson K, Emmelot P: Changed cell surface glycoproteins in human glioma and osteosarcoma cells. Cancer Lett 5: 311–317, 1978.

137. Van Beek WP, Nilsson K, Klein G, Emmelot P: Cell surface glycoprotein changes in Epstein-Barr virus-positive and -negative human hematopoietic cell lines. Int J Cancer 23: 464–473, 1979.

138. Smets LA, Van Beek WP, Van Rooy H: Surface glycoproteins and concanavalin-A-mediated agglutinability of clonal variant and tumour cells derived from SV40-virus transformed mouse 3T3 cells. Int J Cancer 18: 462–468, 1976.

139. Smets LA, Homburg Ch, Van Rooy H: Selective effects of trypsinization on established and tumour-derived mouse 3T3 cells. Cell Biol Int Rep 3: 107–111, 1979.

140. Collett MS, Erikson RL: Protein kinase associated with the avian sarcoma virus Src gene product. Proc Natl Acad Sci USA 75: 2021–2024, 1978.

141. Erikson RL, Brugge JS, Collett MS, Erikson E, Purchio AF: The transforming gene product of avian sarcoma viruses. J Supramol Struct [Suppl] 3: 179(439), 1979.

142. Dnistrian AM, Skipski VP, Barclay M, Stock CC: Glycosphingolipid of subcellular fractions from rat liver and Morris hepatoma 5123 tc. J Natl Cancer Inst 62: 367–370, 1979.

143. Selinger RC, Civen M: ACTH diazotized to agarose: effects on isolated adrenal cells. Biochem Biophys Res Commun 43: 793–799, 1971.

144. Cuatrecasas P: Interaction of insulin with the cell membranes: the primary action of insulin. Proc Natl Acad Sci USA 63: 450–457, 1969.

145. Carney DH, Cunningham DD: Initiation of chick cell division by trypsin action at the cell

surface. Nature 268: 602–606, 1977.

146. Carney DH, Cunningham DD: Role of specific cell surface receptors in thrombin-stimulated cell division. Cell 15: 1341–1349, 1978.

147. Levine S, Pictet R, Rutter WJ: Control of cell proliferation and cytodifferentiation by a factor reacting with the cell surface. Nature [New Biol] 246: 49–52, 1973.

148. Natraj CV, Datta P: Control of DNA synthesis in growing BALB/c 3T3 mouse cells by a fibroblast growth regulatory factor. Proc Natl Acad Sci USA 75: 6115–6119, 1978.

6. MORPHOLOGY AND CYTOCHEMISTRY
OF THE CELL COAT

J.H.M. TEMMINK

THE CELL SURFACE

The cell surface is the outermost part of the cell that forms a semipermeable barrier. It maintains the cell's integrity as a biologically functioning unit and at the same time facilitates several regulating contacts with neighbouring cells and/or the microenvironment. It consists of the plasma membrane, the extracellular membrane-associated components, and the intracellular membrane-associated components. At present, the most generally accepted membrane model is that of Singer and Nicolson [1]. According to this fluid-mosaic model, cell membranes consist of a viscous lipid bilayer with integral proteins intercalated between the lipid molecules of both leaflets and penetrating more or less deeply into the hydrophobic centers of the bilayer. Both the lipid and the protein molecules are mobile in the plane of the membrane. Many of the lipid and integral protein molecules of the outer leaflet of the plasma membrane carry oligosaccharide chains differing in length and composition (glycolipids and glycoproteins). This moiety at the outer cell surface forms the most specific part of the extracellular membrane-associated components, and is further composed of more or less firmly adhering glycosaminoglycans or mucopolysaccharides (mixture of oligosaccharides and hexosamines) and small peripheral proteins. Some of these components are produced by the cell itself, others are more or less permanently adsorbed from the fluids surrounding the cell. Without trying to distinguish through nomenclature the origin or degree of adhesion of the extracellular, membrane-associated substances, we call the total of these substances the cell coat or glycocalyx. The intracellular membrane-associated components, finally, consist of the peripheral proteins (e.g., enzymes), which are permanently linked to the inner cell membrane leaflet, and of transiently linked filamentous proteins of the cytocortical network.

The thickness of the cell coat can differ considerably. Whereas the cell coat of most cells is too thin to be detected by conventional electron-microscopic

---

Abbreviations: 3T3, established line of nontransformed mouse cells; Con A, Concanavalin A; WGA. wheat-germ agglutinin; Fer, ferritin; HC. hemocyanin; HRP, horseradish peroxidase; MP, microperoxidase; aIg, anti-immunoglobulin.

techniques, the cell coat of the brush border of intestinal epithelium can be made visible without using special cytochemical techniques. Furthermore, the cell coat of many transformed cell lines appears to be thicker than that of their nontransformed counterparts. Even local differences in the thickness of the glycocalyx on the same cell seem to occur, probably depending on phase of the cell cycle, adhesion to a substrate, and other parameters.

A vast amount of biological data has implicated the cell surface as primary site for the control of cell growth, division, development, communication, differentiation, and death [2, 3]. In addition, cancer research has recognized the important role of the cell surface in loss of growth control, escape from host immunological surveillance, and metastasis [4–6]. Knowledge of the specific cell-surface molecules such as receptors and antigens is therefore of interest in many fields and cytochemistry of the cell coat is one of the tools for obtaining that knowledge.

CYTOCHEMICAL TECHNIQUES

Over the years a number of cytochemical techniques have been developed for the detection of the carbohydrate moiety of the cell coat [7, 8]. For light-microscopic detection, these include the periodic acid–Schiff (PAS) technique for glycoproteins and the use of cationic dyes such as Alcian blue, colloidal iron, or ruthenium red for acidic carbohydrates of glycoproteins and mucopolysaccharides. For use in electron microscopy, these techniques have been adapted and some similar methods have been added. For instance, the periodic acid–silver methenamine, the periodic acid–chromic acid–silver methenamine, and the periodic acid–thiocarbohydrazide–osmic acid techniques are adapted PAS techniques. Colloidal iron and thorium and ruthenium red are also used in electron microscopy, as are phosphotungstic acid at low pH and lanthanum. Figure 1 shows the results obtained with ruthenium red for the detection of acid carbohydrates of the cell coat of normal mouse fibroblasts. Local differences in thickness of the cell coat (Fig. 1a), partial detachment of less firmly adhering components (Fig. 1b), and the presence of the coat between contacting cells and endocytotic uptake (Fig. 1c) are illustrated. More recently, cationized ferritin has been used to label negatively charged cell-surface components, primarily their terminal sialic acid.

In addition to these strictly cytochemical techniques, a number of immunocytochemical techniques have been developed. In these techniques, which provide a much higher degree of specificity, an antibody against a cell-surface antigen or a lectin with affinity for certain cell-surface monosaccharide residues is used as label. The membrane molecules to be labeled are called receptor molecules; the specifically binding label is called ligand. To make the

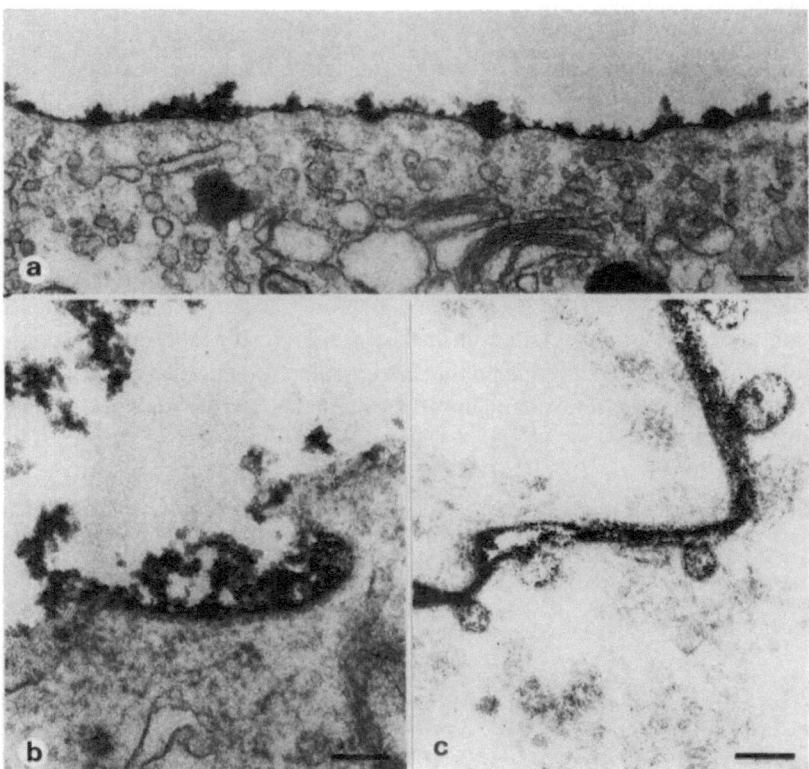

Fig. 1. (a) Cell surface of 3T3 cell treated with ruthenium red for detection of acid mucopoly-saccharides. Notice the uneven distribution of the flocculent reaction product. Bar: 0.2 μm. (b) Higher magnification of cell surface stained with ruthenium red. Part of the loosely adhering material has become detached. Bar: 0.1 μm. (c) Intercellular localization of cell surface material by ruthenium red. Stain is also present in vesicles that seem to be involved in endocytosis. Bar: 0.1. μm.

label visible, marker molecules are attached to the ligand. This attachment can take place in different ways. If, after specific attachment to the cell surface, the ligand has specific binding sites left for receptors on the marker molecule, coupling occurs spontaneously, e.g., coupling of hemocyanin (HC) or horseradish peroxidase (HRP) to Concanavalin A (Con A) via mannose or glucose residues. When the marker molecule does not have the ligand-specific receptors, they can sometimes be applied, e.g., glycosylation of ferritin (Fer) with mannose residues for Con A. Alternatively, the marker is covalently coupled to a label by a cross-linking agent, for instance glutaraldehyde. In that case, detection can be realized by a direct method, the marker being attached to the primary label, or by an indirect method, the marker being covalently bound to a secondary label with specificity for the primary label. In the latter, called the sandwich method, the secondary label generally is an antibody specific for the primary label. Some marker molecules can be recognized individually by their shape or electron density; others are detected by the presence of an electron-dense reaction product. Table 1 shows some frequently used label and marker molecules. Several recent review articles describe the methodology in greater detail [9–12].

The methods mentioned above are not exclusively used in conventional transmission electron microscopy. Enzyme markers (peroxidases; phosphatase) can be used in light microscopy; fluorescent markers are employed in fluorescence microscopy; radioactive labels are visualized in light- and electron autoradiography. At the ultrastructural level, the label-marker conjugates can be detected not only in the scanning electron microscope, but also in freeze-etched preparations and in surface replicas in the transmission electron microscope.

Table 1. Some of the label and marker molecules used in the immunocytochemistry of cell-surface components.

LABEL MOLECULES	*Antibodies:*	Anti-immunoglobulins (aIg)
		Antihistocompatibility antigens
		Anti-theta antigen
		Antilectins
	Lectins:	Concanavalin A (Con A)
		Wheat-germ agglutinin (WGA)
		Lens culinaris lectin (LcL)
		Ricinus communis agglutinin (RcA)
MARKER MOLECULES	*Particulate:*	Ferritin (Fer)
		Hemocyanin (HC)
		Iron-dextran
		Colloidal gold
		Plant viruses
	Enzymes:	Horseradish peroxidase (HRP)
		Microperoxidase (MP)

Some applications are illustrated in Figs. 2–7, all taken from previous work by the present author and several coworkers. For instance, the lectin Con A has been used to detect glucose and mannose residues on the surface of normal and transformed cells of an established murine cell line in vitro (3T3). These residues were made visible by the combination of Con A with various marker molecules, such as HRP (Fig. 2a), Hc (Fig. 2b), Fer (Fig. 2c), and microperoxidase (MP) (Fig. 2d). To show that serum-derived components were also detected, substrate without growing cells was labeled with Con A-HC (Fig. 3a) and Con A-Fer (Fig. 3b). This complicates the interpretation of

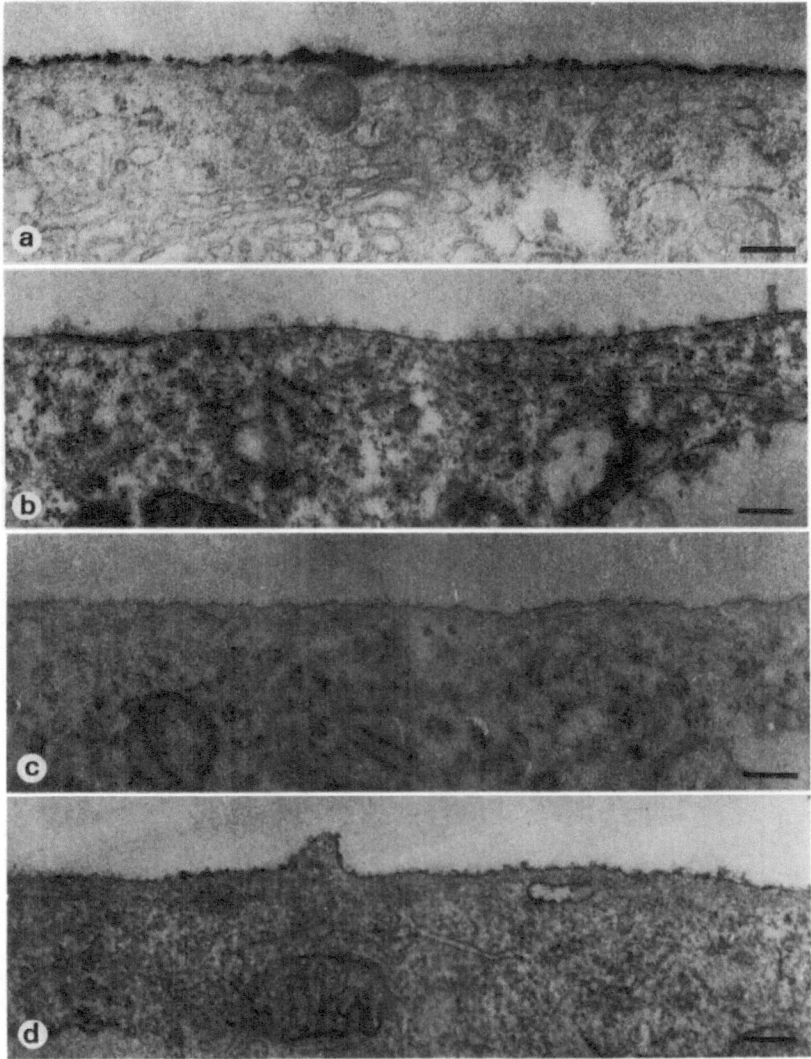

Fig. 2. (a) Cell surface of 3T3 cell labeled with Con A-HRP. In spite of nonparticulate reaction product, some irregularity in cell-surface layer is observable. Bar: 0.2. μm. (b) Cell surface of 3T3 cell labeled with Con A-HC. Irregular distribution of Con-A receptors is apparent. Bar: 0.2. μm. (c) Cell surface of 3T3 cell labeled with Con A-Fer, showing same irregular distribution of Con-A receptors. Bar: 0.2 μm. (d) Cell surface of 3T3 cell labeled with Con A-MP, resulting in relatively small patches of reaction product at Con-A binding sites. Bar: 0.2 μm.

72

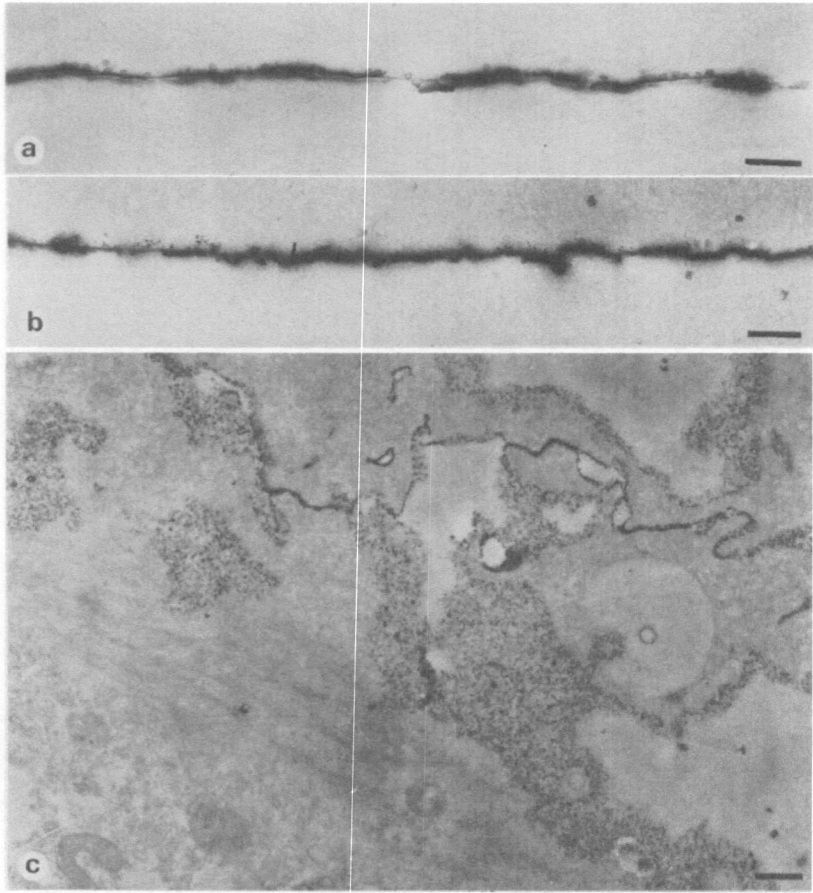

Fig. 3. (a) Detection of Con A- specific serum components by labeling substrate with Con A-HC prior to seeding of 3T3 cells. Bar: 0.2 μm. (b) Detection of same serum components with Con A-Fer. Bar 0.2 μm. (c) Distribution of Can A-HRP on substrate under growing 3T3 cells and between 3T3 cells. Relative contribution of cell-derived products and serum components is unclear. Bar: 0.5 μm.

labeling data on 3T3 cells attached to the substrate (Fig. 3c). The next figure shows that detection of sugar residues via a nonparticulate enzyme reaction product (Fig. 4a) does not allow quantification, whereas detection via a particulate marker (Fig. 4b) does, at least in principle. If the marker molecule is sufficiently large, the general surface distribution can be detected in surface replicas of Con-A-labeled cells (Fig. 5a), and at higher magnification the individual marker molecules can be recognized (Fig. 5b). In Fig. 6 the surface distribution of marker molecules has been influenced by endocytotic uptake

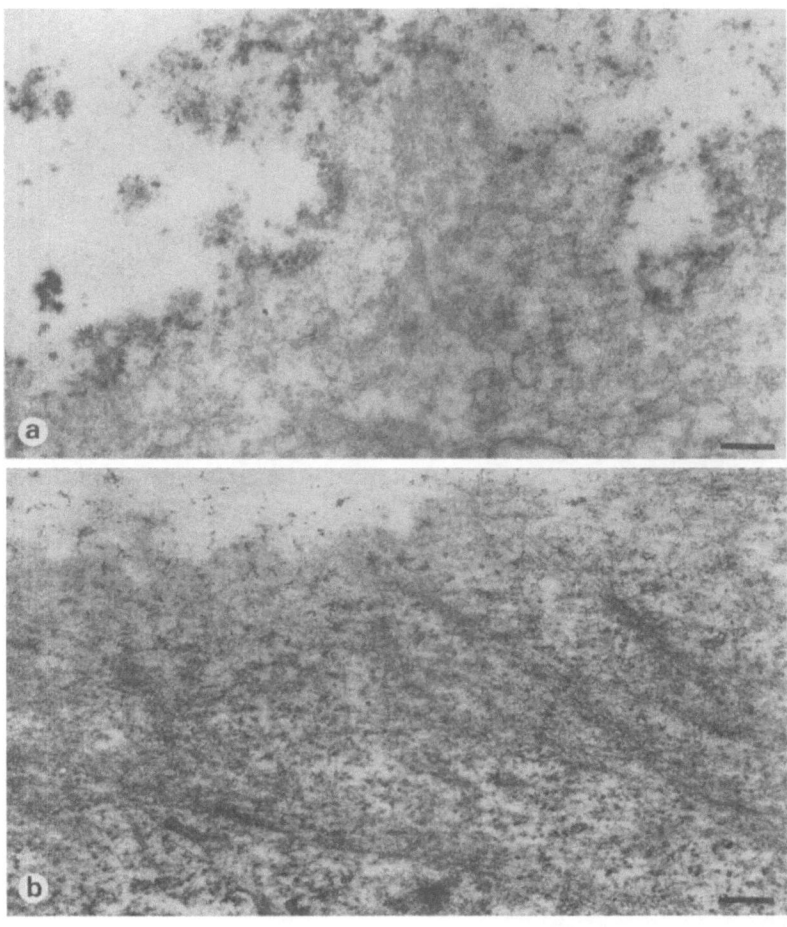

Fig. 4. (a) Con A- HRP distribution on substrate-attached surface of 3T3 cell. Number of Con A-labeled receptors cannot be established. Bar: 0.2 μm. (b) Con A-Fer distribution on substrate-

of the ligand-receptor complex. Intracellular vesicles with HRP-reaction product (Fig. 6a), with Con A-HC complex (Fig. 6b), or with Con A-Fer (Fig. 6c) can be seen. Finally, the distribution of receptors can also be influenced by active or passive movement induced by the binding of ligand to receptor. This is shown in Fig. 7, where receptors on human lymphocytes of a patient with hairy-cell leukemia have capped upon labeling with complexes of anti-immunoglobulin (aIg) and Fer.

74

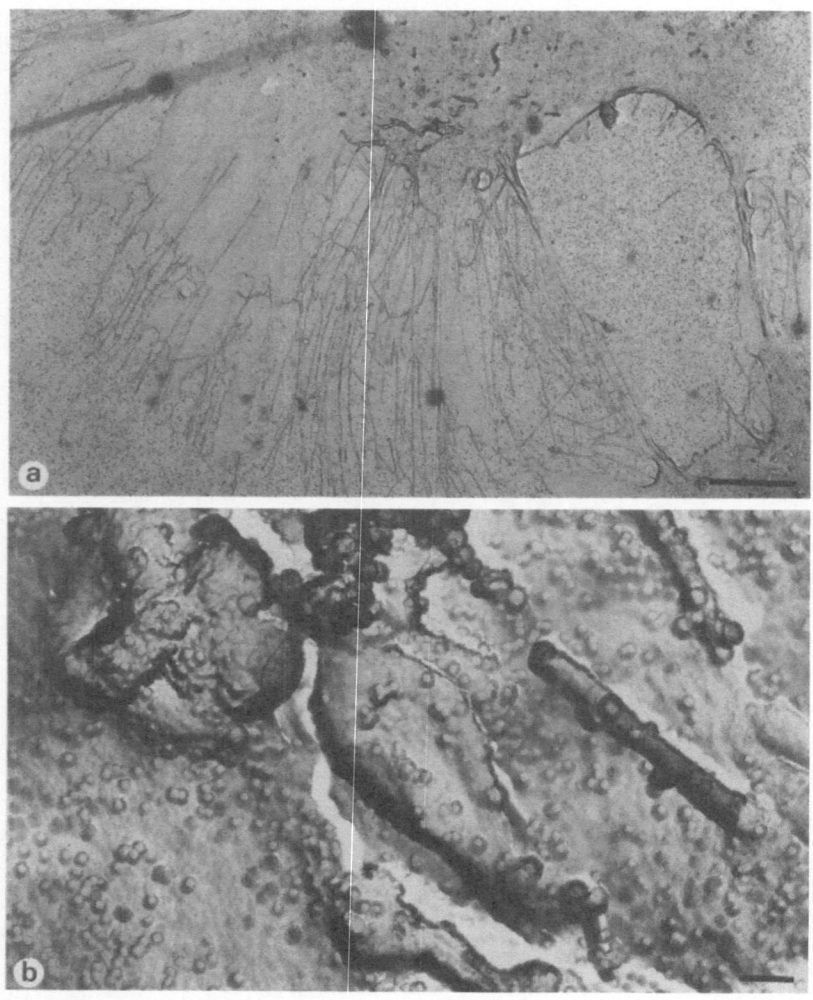

Fig. 5 (a) Distribution of Con A-HC complexes on cell-surface replica of 3T3 cell. In spite of heavy nonspecific background labeling, differences between cell body and lamellipodia are observable. Bar: 2.0 μm. (b) Higher magnification of Con A-HC labeled cell-surface replica. Individual HC molecules can be recognized by their shape. Bar: 0.2 μm.

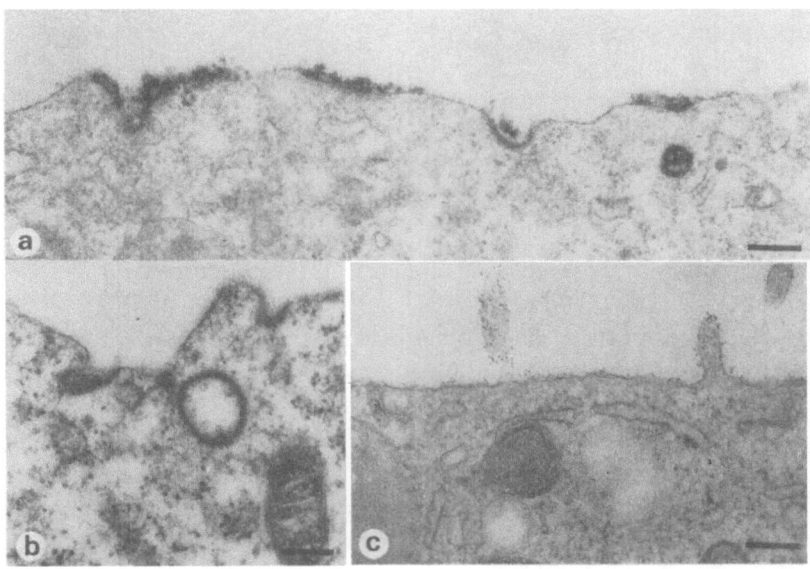

Fig. 6. (a) Endocytotic vesicles with Con A-HRP complexes in 3T3 cell. Bar: 0.2 μm. (b) Endocytosis of Con A-HC complexes from surface of 3T3 cell. Bar: 0.2 μm. (c) Endocytotic uptake of Con A-Fer complexes in 3T3 cell. Microvilli are also labeled. Bar: 0.2 μm.

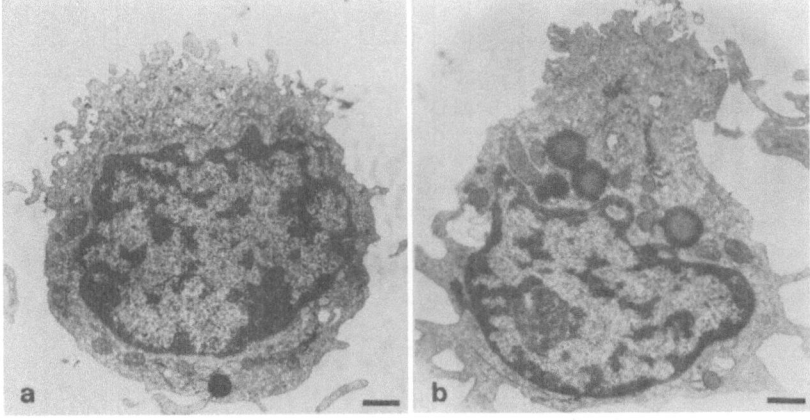

Fig. 7a and b. Cells of patient with hairy cell leukemia showing capped (a) and endocytosed (b) aIg-Fer complexes. Bar: 0.5 μm.

LIMITS OF APPLICABILITY

Cytochemical and immunocytochemical techniques are, in principle, capable of providing the answers to three important questions:

a) What molecule is present in or on the cell? (Identification)
b) Where in or on the cell is that molecule present? (Localization)
c) How many of these molecules are present? (Quantitation)

However, each of the techniques has its limitations with respect to applicability as well as the type of information supplied [13, 14]. Many of these limitations are listed in Table 2. Figure 8 is an on-scale schematic representation of two glycoprotein molecules with different Con-A-marker combinations labeling some terminal sugar residues. This figure is based on Marchesi's [15] model of glycophorin; although in reality glycophorin does not have exposed Con-A receptors, it is included to help visualizing the limiting mechanisms as briefly discussed below. The effect of some of the factors involved has already been mentioned in connection with the description of the electron micrographs.

The problem of identification is essentially a matter of labeling specificity. As mentioned above, many of the cytochemical techniques detect classes of substances rather than specific molecules. With the advent of immunocyto-

Table 2. Some of the factors limiting the usefulness of cytochemistry for the study of cell-surface receptors.

Identification:	Specificity of labeling
Localization:	Specificity of labeling
	Exposure of receptor sites
	Nonparticulate marker
	Active receptor movement
	Passive receptor movement
	Endocytosis and shedding
Quantitation:	Specificity of labeling
	Exposure of receptor sites
	Nonparticulate marker
	Active receptor movement
	Passive receptor movement
	Endocytosis and shedding
	Label-to-marker ratio
	Size of label and marker molecules
	Valency of label molecule
	Affinity and avidity of binding
	Type of bond between label and marker
	Number of sugar residues on marker
	Pliability of oligosaccharide chains

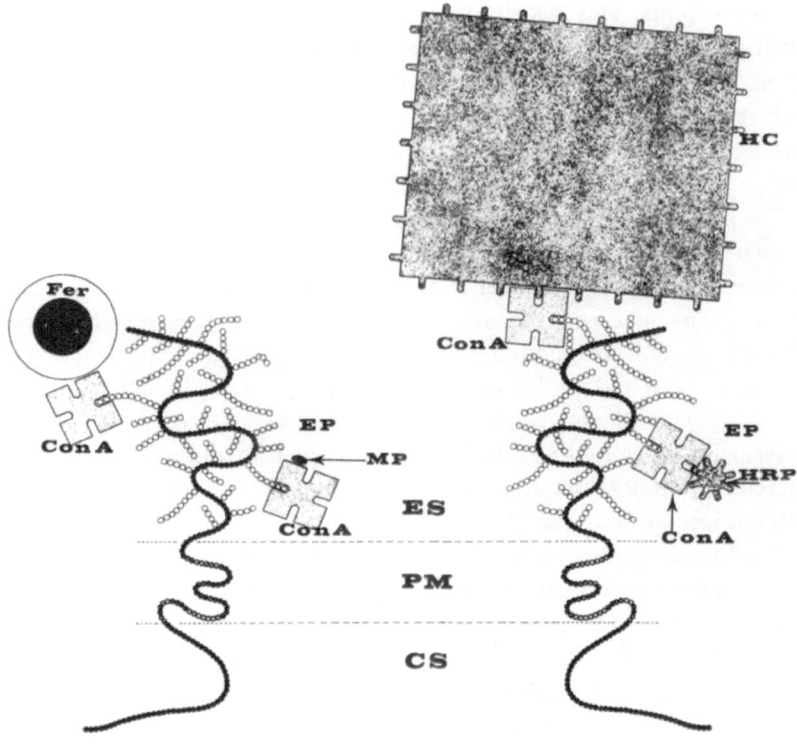

Fig. 8. Schematic representation of integral glycoprotein molecules in plasma membrane labeled with various Con A-marker complexes. Con A, Concanavalin A; CS, cytoplasmic space; ES, extra-cellular space; EP, enzyme reaction product; Fer, ferritin; HC, hemocyanin; HRP, horse-radish perodixase; MP, microperoxidase; PM, plasma membrane.

chemistry the labeling specificity has been increased considerably, provided the proper controls for a specific binding are included in the experiments. Immunocytochemistry at the electron-microscopical level enables much higher resolution in the localization of substances on the cell surface. Nonetheless, it is limited by the degree of exposure of the macromolecules: local differences in thickness of the glycocalyx and accessibility of specific sites for the labeling molecules may lead to absence of label in certain areas. Two other factors adversely influence the results. The use of enzymes as markers limits high-resolution localization, because the diffuse electron-dense enzyme product spreads over a more or less extended area around the labeled macromolecules. In addition, the binding of multivalent label and marker molecules very often induces lateral movement of the receptors through the lipid matrix of the membrane, thus causing misinterpretations about the original location of the receptors. This receptor movement can be caused by cross-linking of different glycoprotein molecules (passive) or by inducing attachment of the receptor to the cytocortical network and contraction of this network (active). This may even lead to local loss of the receptor molecules from the surface due to shedding into the extracellular space or endocytotic uptake in the cytoplasm.

The limitations with respect to the localization of receptor sites also apply to their quantitation (Table 2). Loss of receptor sites and inaccessibility cause underestimation of the number. Nonparticulate markers obviate counting of the receptors underneath the reaction product. Induced receptor movement also affects results of quantitative experiments. This is due to the fact that the size of the label and marker molecules prohibits labeling of all specific sites, especially when these have been brought close together by induced lateral movement. When many of the same specific sites are present on one glycoprotein, this underestimation due to the size of label and marker occurs even without receptor movement.

Finally, there are a number of factors related to the valency of the label and marker molecules and the techniques employed to couple them. With increasing valency of the label molecules and in combination with the size of the label molecule or the distance between the binding sites, one ligand may bind several receptors, especially when the pliability of the receptor-bearing oligosaccharide chains is sufficient to enable movement toward the binding sites of the ligand. If the label molecule has multispecific binding sites the relative avidities for the different receptors will determine whether all are detected and to what extent. In situations where the marker molecule is bound to the label by similar specific ligand-receptor interactions, the avidity for these bonds also influences the detection of specific binding sites on the cell surface. In addition, more than one sugar residue on the marker molecule may result in the attachment of one marker to several specifically bound label molecules. Likewise, the formation of covalent label-marker bonds by cross-linking may result in ligands with more than one marker molecule or marker molecules bound to several label molecules, depending on the ratio between label and marker in the cross-linking mixture. Special procedures and chromatographic purification of the reaction product are employed to reduce this effect to acceptable levels. Because many of the other factors mentioned play a role that is also difficult to quantitate, continuous efforts are being made to decrease their effect. It is in this light that the development of monovalent lectins, monospecific antibodies, univalent antibody fragments, and smaller electron-dense markers should be considered.

The attention paid to the factors limiting the applicability of cytochemical techniques might suggest that the use of these methods has very little value, but many publications are there to prove that this is not the case. Cytochemistry has contributed considerably to our knowledge of the cell surface and its receptors, and it will undoubtedly continue to do so in the future as well. The results of cytochemical experiments are important biological data, provided they have undergone careful and critical interpretation.

Acknowledgments. The author is grateful to the editors of the Journal of Cell Biology, Journal of Cell Science, Biologie Cellulaire and Experimental Cell Research for the right to use micrographs previously published in their journals.

REFERENCES

1. Singer SJ, Nicolson GL: The fluid mosaic model of the structure of cell membranes. Science 175: 720–731, 1972.
2. Cuatrecasas P: Membrane receptors. Annu Rev Biochem 43: 169–214, 1974.
3. Singer SJ: Molecular biology of cellular membranes with applications to immunology. Adv Immunol 19: 1–66, 1974.
4. Nicolson GL: Transmembrane control of the receptors on normal and tumor cells. I. Cytoplasmic influence over cell surface components. Biochim Biophys Acta 457: 57–108, 1976.
5. Nicolson GL: Transmembrane control of the receptors on normal and tumor cells. II. Surface changes associated with transformation and malignancy. Biochim Biophys Acta 458: 1–71, 1976.
6. Rapin AMC, Burger MM: Tumor cell surfaces: general alterations detected by agglutinins. Adv Cancer Res 20: 1–91, 1974.
7. Martinez-Palomo A: The surface coats of animal cells. Int Rev Cytol 29: 29–75, 1970.
8. Rambourg A: Morphological and histochemical aspects of glycoproteins at the surface of animal cells. Int Rev Cytol 31: 57–114, 1971.
9. Brown JC, Hunt RC: Lectins. Int Rev Cytol 52: 277–349, 1978.
10. Nakane PK: Ultrastructural localization of tissue antigens with the peroxidase-labelled antibody method. In: Wisse E, Daems WTh, Molenaar I, Duijn P van (eds) Electron microscopy and cytochemistry. Amsterdam, North-Holland, 1974, pp 129–143.
11. Roth J: The lectins. Molecular probes in cell biology and membrane research. Jena, Gustav Fischer, 1978.
12. Williams MA: Autoradiography and immunocytochemistry. In: Glauert AM (ed) Practical methods in electron microscopy, vol 6. Amsterdam, North-Holland, 1977, pp 5–72.
13. Temmink JHM: Application of cytochemical methods in electron microscope investigations on cell surface receptors. Biol Cell (in press) 1979.
14. Temmink JHM, Collard JG, Spits H, Roos E: A comparative study of four cytochemical detection methods on Concanavalin A binding sites on the cell membrane. Exp Cell Res 92: 307–322, 1975.
15. Marchesi VT: The structure and orientation of a membrane protein In: Weismann G, Claiborne R (eds) Cell membranes. Biochemistry, cell biology and pathology. New York, HP, 1975, pp 45–53.

7. RECEPTORS IN DISEASED STATES

H.M.J. KRANS AND Tj. WIERINGA

INTRODUCTION

Protoplasm-membrane receptors are recognition elements on the outer surface of the cell membrane. They form an integral part of the structure of the
membrane. They are identified by the binding of specific molecules present in
the extracellular fluid, i.e., substances normally present in the blood such as
(peptide) hormones, lipoproteins, or immunoglobulins, or substances only
present in specific situations such as toxins or drugs. The term 'ligand' is often
used to designate substances that bind specifically.

The structure of the ligand is often well known. The receptor is less well
defined. The only receptor to have been isolated in pure form is the acetylcholine receptor. Other receptors have been partially defined by various
properties. Without exact knowledge of the receptor and the interaction of
the receptor with the ligand in physiological states, it is impossible to establish
pathological changes exactly.

Changes in receptors are seen in many diseases and the concept that
receptors play a role in disease is quite popular at present. In this chapter,
attention will be given mainly to changes in the hormone receptor on the
plasma membrane as part of the endocrine system.

Peptide hormones can exert intracellular effects without entering the cell.
The first step in their action is binding to specific sites [1]. A general idea of
the transformation of signals from peptide hormones is given in Fig. 1.
A hormone floating in the extracellular fluid is recognized by a specific
receptor site. The reaction generates a signal which is transferred through the
membrane of an effector system. A single hormone may generate different
responses in two or more effector systems. The process of coupling of the
receptor with the effector may be direct or mediated by changes in the
physical or chemical state of the membrane. Three steps can be distinguished
[2, 3] in the transfer of the message of the hormone through the membrane: (1)
hormone (H) receptor (R) interaction, (2) formation of hormone-receptor
complex (HR) which elicits (3) a physiological response (E). These three steps
do not occur in all receptor systems. For the binding of immunoglobulins, the
third step is often missing.

W.Th. Daems et al. (eds.), Cell Biological Aspects of Disease, 81–95. All rights reserved.
Copyright © 1981 by Martinus Nijhoff Publishers bv, The Hague/Boston/London.

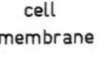

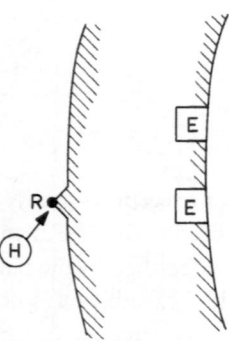

H = Hormone

R = Receptor

E = Effector

Fig. 1. Scheme indicating the relation between hormone (H), receptor (R), and effector (E). Note that the relation between receptor and effector(s) is interrupted, indicating a variety of potential coupling mechanisms.

THE LIGAND

The principal ligands are drugs, immunoglobulins, and hormones. Pharmacologists were pioneers in the thinking on binding [4]. Agonists, antagonists, and partial agonists in binding are examples of the specific role of drugs in the expression of catecholamines [3, 5]. The surprising finding of a specific opiate receptor in the brain led to the discovery of the enkephalins and endorphins [6] as neurohormones.

Circulating immunoglobulins or antigens are often 'caught' by immunoreactive cells, such as lymphocytes, and are bound to specific receptor sites. The steric effect of a bound large immunoglobulin molecule differs from the effect of smaller ligands. A specific property of the interaction of immunoglobulins with receptors is the induction of a type of network formation that leads to an accumulation of all binding material on one side of the cell (capping).

The binding of hormones will be discussed in some detail. Two factors characterize binding: (a) affinity, which can be determined by varying the concentration of hormone in the system under study, and (b) the maximum number of binding sites. The latter factor must be estimated, which can be done by incubation with such high concentrations of the hormone that all available sites are occupied. The affinity and the maximum number of binding sites do not necessarily change in parallel. A change in binding during disease may be only a change in affinity without a change in the maximum number of binding sites (see Fig. 6). This makes it imperative to measure binding at various ligand concentrations and for various intervals when differences between normal and diseased states are investigated.

The structure of small peptide hormones and glucagon does not differ between most mammalian species, whereas peptide hormones of high molecular weight such as insulin or growth hormone differ in animo acid composition in different species of animals. Structural differences affect both action and binding. Hormones with a naturally chemically modified structure show a decreased binding affinity compared with the native hormone. Beef insulin shows the greatest affinity for bovine tissues. A remarkable exception concerns such animals as the cavia, the coypu, the chinchilla, and the casiragua. Casiragua insulin differs from beef insulin in 20 of the 51 amino acids. In fat cells of the rat, casiragua insulin is less effective and shows decreased binding. But even in the casiragua, bovine insulin is more effective and binds better than the casiragua insulin [7].

It has long been postulated that the formation of abnormal hormones may cause endocrine diseases. Very recently, this was demonstrated for the first time when an exceptional form of altered glucose tolerance was found in a patient who produced an abnormal form of insulin [8]. Excessive aberrant hormone may occupy normal receptor sites and block hormonal action. The abnormal hormone has lost its potency to elicit secondary actions. Experimental examples are more abundant. Glucagon which is depleted of the N-terminal amino acid histidine can bind to liver membranes; it inhibits the binding of glucagon but does not activate adenylate cyclase [9].

Injected hormones can induce the formation of antibodies. Hormone-antibody complexes do not bind. But receptors can generate specific antibodies as well. These antibodies bind at hormone binding sites and thus prevent the binding of hormone. Binding of receptor antibodies can have two effects: they can block or can stimulate the action of the ligand. Blocking antibodies against acetylcholine receptors are seen in myasthenia gravis [10]. Antibodies against insulin receptors are found in some rare forms of diabetes displaying a very high degree of insulin resistance [11]. After removal of the antibodies the binding sites show normal hormone binding and the sensitivity for insulins is restored [12]. This indicates that the receptor itself is normal and that the antibody causes the insulin resistance. Other types of antibody can induce hormonelike activity (e.g., nonsuppressible insulinlike activity, NSILA) [13]. This type of antibody occupies the receptor and acts as a hormone, but destroys the regulatory mechanism when hormone is secreted. The antibody changes the structure of the binding site such that the binding site acts as

84

though it was stimulated by the hormone. A stimulatory effect of antibodies on target cells is also seen in the thyroid, where thyroid stimulatory immunoglobulins (TSI) occupy TSH receptors in the thyroid gland and stimulate hormone secretion. The autonomous hormone secretion leads to the hyperthyroidism seen in Graves' disease [14]. The factor responsible for initiating the immune responsiveness on receptors remains unclear.

THE RECEPTOR

The receptor must be defined by its binding characteristics and specific effects. Binding is specific, which means that there is no competition for the binding site by substances unrelated to the hormone. This is in contrast to receptors for immunoglobulins, where immunoglobulins with different antibody specifity can bind to the same binding sites. Binding sites form an integral part of the membrane, but they are not preexistent fixed structures. The membrane is constantly changing (see Zwaal, chapter 2). Binding sites are located on the outer surface of the membrane but they may be covered by material adhering to this surface. Furthermore, the sites can be expelled or retracted into the membrane. They are constantly formed and degraded. The covering and uncovering of receptors is partially regulated by the ligands. A hormone can induce the specific structure of its receptor. Factors such as the number of occupied adjacent binding sites, structure of the ligand, temperature, ionic environment (pH), metabolic state of the subject, and the rapidity of the turnover of receptors and hormone determine the actual binding of the hormone.

Binding sites are expected to be situated on the outer surface of the cell, but many substances can bind indiscriminately to other biological materials. Therefore, the critical reader of any report on a binding study must consider a number of points. How pure was the (labeled) preparation and did it have the same biological activity as the native substance? Was the binding studied in tisssues, cells, cell membranes, tissue pieces, or subcellular fragments? How pure were these substances? Does the ligand have a physiological action on the target studied, and which physiological response can be measured? Isolated cells have to be treated carefully; otherwise, they may be a source of misinterpretation. Cells may rupture during preparation or incubation unless they are handled very carefully. Intracellular temperature-dependent proteases may be released from broken cells or isolated membranes and lower the apparent hormone concentrations in the medium. An example is given in Fig. 2.

Factors affecting hormone binding can be divided into two categories: (a) effects related to receptor turnover, and (b) immediate effects.

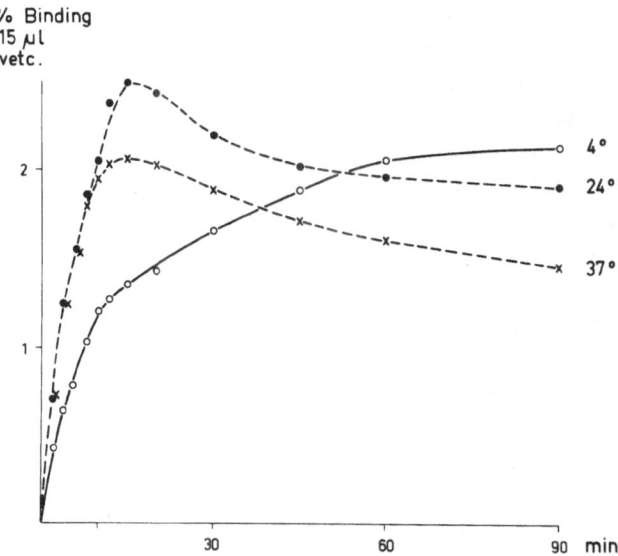

Fig. 2. A typical example of the course in time of binding of insulin to badly prepared fat cells. The decrease in binding after an optimum has been reached is caused by the decrease in actual hormone concentration induced by liberated endoproteases from ruptured fat cells.

a) The turnover of membrane constituents is influenced by protein synthesis in the nucleus. Cyclohexamide and inhibitors of DNA and RNA change receptor turnover. Steroid hormones, e.g., cortisol, do not affect the binding during short in vitro incubation. However, glucocorticoids are known to interfere with hormonal effects of peptide hormones in patients. Cortisol excess, as seen in Cushing disease, induces an insulin-resistant form of diabetes mellitus. In animals, cortisol excess leads after a few days to a reduction of the amount of insulin bound and a decrease of the stimulation of glucose transport [15]. Estrogens may have a strong effect on the binding and activity of LH, FSH, and prolactin. Quantitation of this action is difficult [16]. Increased sensitivity on the receptor level is seen in thyrotoxic states. Excess of thyroid hormone increases the binding [17] and the effect on the heart rate of catacholamines.

Excess of hormone can also induce a reduction of the available binding sites (desensitization). This has also been shown in vitro for insulin binding to cultured lymphocytes [18]. In the adrenergic system, tonic stimulation by adrenal hormones or adrenergic drugs leads to desensitization [5] and similar stimulation by antagonists to sensitization. Effects of food intake [19] and diurnal variations [20] have been reported for insulin binding sites.

b) Immediate effects of binding may be seen in both in vivo and in vitro systems. A classic approach to investigation of the interaction of certain substances involving hormone binding concerns the effect of guanosinetriphosphate (GTP) on the binding of glucagon and the release of bound glucagon. Addition of GTP in very small doses induces a decrease in binding (Fig. 3), and bound glucagon is released much more easily when GTP is added [21]. The involvement of GTP in the binding of many hormones seems to be a general phenomenon [22]. Factors such as ions, GTP, etc., do not regulate the synthesis or destruction of receptors but affect the state of the receptor. The adapt the binding sites in such a way that they can bind hormone and accept the message of the hormone. The shape of the binding site is determined by the structural configuration of membrane proteins (hydrophobic or hydrophylic areas) and of the phospholipids as well.

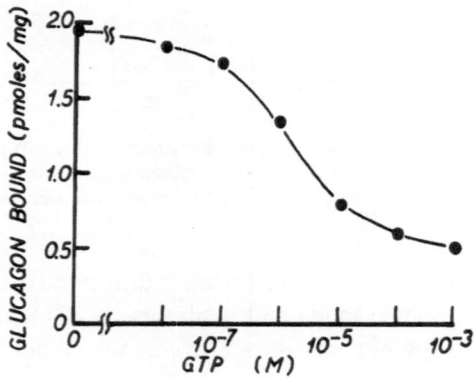

Fig. 3. The effect of GTP on binding of glucagon to purified liver membranes (see ref. 21).

Most binding studies have been performed in vitro. When the relation between the amount of hormone in the incubation medium and the amount bound is plotted graphically, the result is a concave curve (Fig. 4). These curves are often transformed mathematically according to Scatchard [23]. The ratio of bound to free hormone is plotted against the amount of bound hormone per unit of tissue. This makes it easier to determine whether one or more classes of binding sites are present. The class with the highest affinity often has a low capacity, but incubation with hormone concentrations found in the blood in physiological and pathological situations usually only shows occupation of the high-affinity sites.

The question of two classes of binding sites is still under dispute. De Meyts et al. [24] have postulated that the curvilinear Scatchard plot is caused by negative cooperativity. This means that if a binding site is occupied by a hormone, it is more difficult for other hormone molecules to reach the neighboring binding sites. It is not clear whether the hormone-receptor com-

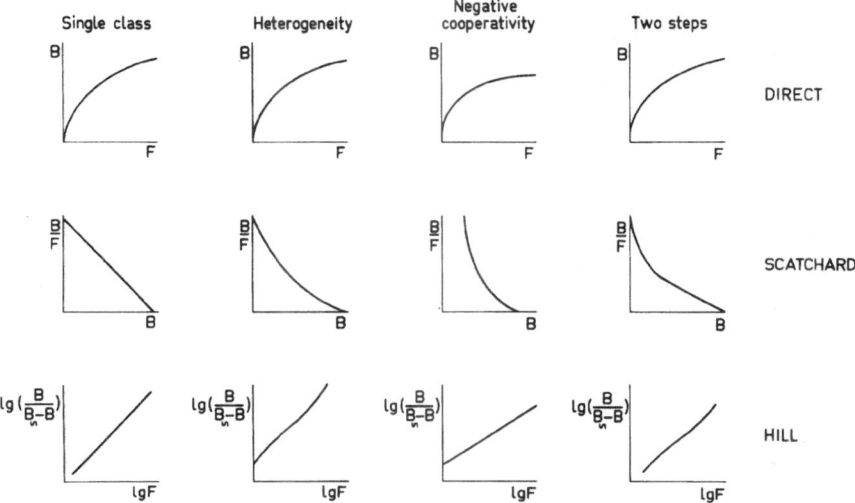

Fig. 4. Computer-simulated graphical analysis of binding of hormone to membrane receptors. The top horizontal row represents the relationship between the amount of free and bound hormone plotted for the given possibilities of receptor behavior. The second and third horizontal rows represent data subjected to mathematical transitions according to Scatchard and Hill (adapted from ref. 25). A broken Scatchard plot can be caused by a two-step reaction in which the product of the first step of the reaction is the substrate for the second step. The effect of a change in affinity without an increase in the total number of binding sites is shown in Figs. 5 and 6.

plex can attract adjoining binding sites in a way comparable to the capping phenomenon known in immunology, but some support has been obtained in electron-microscopic studies on membranes on which hormones coupled to ferritin were bound. A discussion of this problem does not lie within the present scope, but Boeynaems and Dumont [25] have given a comprehensive review on the interpretation of the various mathematical transformations of binding data (see Fig. 4). Our studies on the effect of phospholipase treatment of fat cells on binding of insulin suggest the existence of more than one class of binding sites [35].

The number of binding sites can be regulated by the hormone in question. When an excessive amount of hormone circulates, the number of apparent binding sites decreases (down regulation). The apparent number of insulin receptors is decreased in cases of obesity, a state often accompanied by high insulin levels in the blood. Up regulation is the reverse phenomenon: a rise in the number of apparent binding sites, when hormone levels are low. An example of this is our finding [26] that in rats made diabetic by destruction of the B cells, binding of insulin increased after 48 h (Figs. 5 and 6). This increase is only due to a change in affinity without any change in the maximal number of binding sites. An increase in the total number of binding sites is seen after a

88

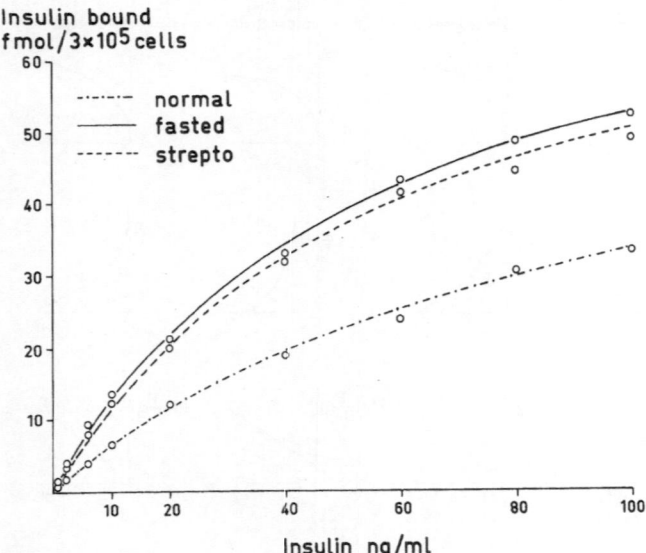

Fig. 5. Binding of hormone to adipocytes isolated from normal rats, from fasted rats and from rats which had been diabetic for two days. The curve concerns only insulin concentrations in man. At high insulin concentrations the three lines will coincide (for experimental details, see ref. 26).

Scatchard plot

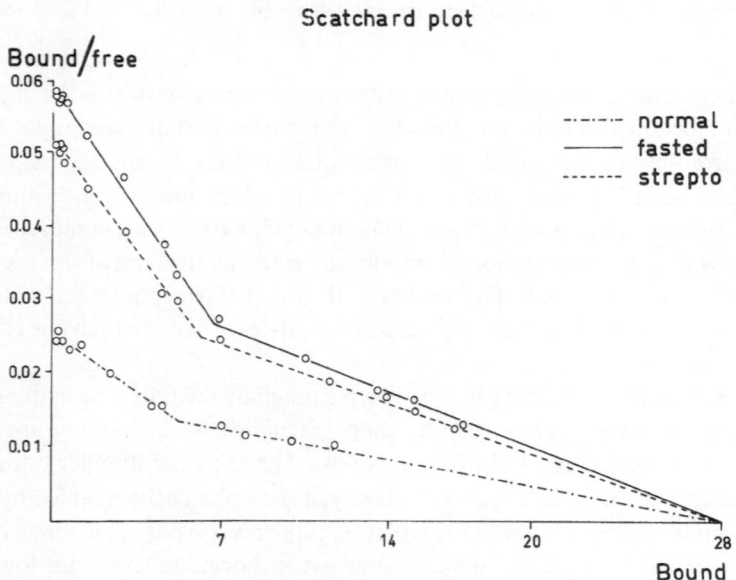

Fig. 6. Scatchard tranformation of the binding data given in Fig. 5, indicating heterogeneity of the binding sites. The lines cross the x-axis at the same point, an indication that the total number of potential binding sites has not changed. The amount of bound insulin is plotted on the abscissa in ng $\times 10^{-8}$/cell.

week [27]. This indicates that the feedback of changes in hormone level on the binding sites involves structural changes in the membrane, which may be a consequence of changes in cellular metabolism. Up regulation and down regulation are complex situations. Binding sites are constantly synthesized and degraded. The degradation of binding sites might be related to the occupation or internalization of the hormone-receptor complex.

COUPLING BETWEEN BINDING AND INTRACELLULAR RESPONSES

The binding of hormone must be followed by other steps before the metabolic actions are expressed. In the stimulation of the production of CO_2 from glucose by insulin, a cascade of activated enzymatic reactions is involved. The first metabolic step in such a cascade will be the one most directly related to binding. Sutherland, who was the first to show that intracellular cAMP levels are influenced by many different hormones, called cAMP the second messenger of hormone action. Later studies have revealed that the relation between hormone and cAMP levels can also depend on other regulatory systems besides the activation of adenylate cyclase. Direct hormonal effects on phosphodiesterase and protein kinases have been demonstrated to influence cAMP levels [28]. Thus, cAMP has lost its unique position as single second messenger. The formation of cyclic-GMP, a shift in calcium ion concentration, stimulation of glucose transport, amino acid transport, activation of K/Na ATPase, or changes in ionic fluxes can all serve as secondary messenger systems as well.

The receptor must be connected with a functional site before it can act as a unit, but the quantitative effects of factors affecting the coupling are difficult to establish. The relation between receptor occupancy and action is not a simple one. In the first place, glucagon binding on liver membranes is saturated at molar concentration of 10^{-6} [29]. For instance, the maximal effect of glucagon on adenylate cyclase stimulation is seen at molar concentrations of 10^{-8} M. In the second place, the equilibrium for binding is not reached before 15 min, but the secondary effect of adenylate cyclase stimulation is maximally expressed or turned off within 15 s (Fig. 7) [2, 30]. A similar relation can be demonstrated for insulin binding and the stimulation of glucose transport, which is directly related to an action of insulin expressed on the membrane level [31]. Glucose transport in isolated fat cells is maximally stimulated within 3 min by insulin concentrations of 100 μU (or 5 ng) /ml. But at these concentrations less than 10% of the potential binding sites are occupied after 15 min. Occupation of only some of the binding sites is sufficient to express the full activity of the hormone. The remaining binding sites seem to be superfluous. Much confusion could be avoided in the literature if the terms binding sites

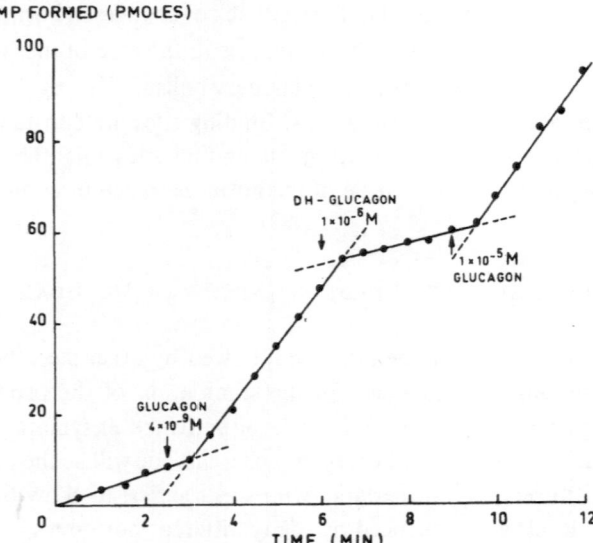

Fig. 7. Relationship between adenylate cyclase activity and glucagon. Stimulation occurs between 15 and 45 s after addition of glucagon. Blocking of the binding sites by the non-stimulating glucagon derivate DH-glucagon switches the stimulation off within 30 s (for details, see ref. 2 or 30).

and receptors were not used as synonyms. The term receptor should be reserved for the binding sites that are related to biological actions. The other sites could be designated as spare receptors or binding sites. The function of 'spare' binding sites is not clear. The 'spare' binding site may be an expression of the biological redundancy often seen in cascades of metabolic processes: it might be just a site for storage or it could be related to other biological functions elicited by the hormone [2].

RECEPTOR CHANGES IN PATHOLOGICAL CONDITIONS

Changes in binding and in intracellular actions have been reported in pathological states, but these changes are not parallel. In vivo we see that the mean insulin levels in obesity are elevated but the number of binding sites for insulin is reduced. Studies in genetically obese animals have revealed that reversal of the hyperinsulinemic state reverses the binding abnormalities [32] and that the decrease in binding sites develops concomitantly with hyperinsulinism [33]. Cultured human lymphocytes incubated with high levels of insulin show a decrease in the number of binding sites [18]. Thus chronic, but not acute, elevation of the insulin levels induces a reduction of the binding sites (down regulation).

In obese patients, weight reduction induces an increase of the estimated number of binding sites. The apparent decrease in the number of binding sites has been used to explain the decreased effect of insulin in obesity. But the reduction of binding sites in obesity amounts to only 20%–50%. Insulin effects can, however, be demonstrated when about 2% or less of the binding sites are occupied and less then 10% occupation accounts for maximal effect. Therefore, in obesity the decrease in receptors must be accompanied by alterations behind the receptor [34, 35] or in the coupling between the insulin-receptor complex and secondary reactions. In states with reduced insulin levels, for instance during prolonged fasting or in diabetes induced by destruction of the B cells in the islets of Langerhans by streptozotocin, the binding of insulin is increased [26] (up regulation). Insulin deprivation appears to make the cells less sensitive to insulin. In spite of the increase in binding, the action is decreased. But this only holds for maximal stimulation. The maximal stimulatory effect of insulin in cells of diabetic animals is reached at lower insulin concentrations than in normal cells (Fig. 8). Concentration/activity curves show that the cells of diabetic animals are relatively more sensitive to insulin at submaximal insulin concentrations. The higher number of binding sites in up regulation is paralleled by a relatively increased sensitivity for insulin in general, but the overall insulin effect is a combination of effects on and behind the receptor level and postreceptor level [26]. No direct parallelism between numbers of binding sites or receptors and metabolic responses is seen. It is therefore incorrect to use changes in binding as the measure of altered responsiveness to the hormone. Changes in hormone levels may induce changes in the membrane and in the postmembrane metabolic pathways as well.

Perturbation of membranes with enzymes changes the binding pattern.

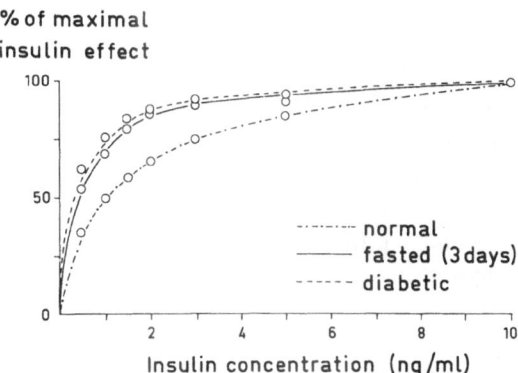

Fig. 8. In adipocytes isolated from animals after a prolonged period of low insulin levels (fasting or diabetes), insulin stimulates 2-deoxyglucose transport relatively more at low insulin levels (for experimental details, see ref. 26).

Proteolytic enzymes decrease the binding and may decrease the hormonal stimulation of metabolic processes. Membrane phospholipids are involved as well. If fat cells are exposed to very pure phospholipase A_2 [36], an enzyme which appears to attack phosphatidyl choline in particular, changes in insulin binding and glucose transport are seen. With respect to glucose transport it has been found that phospholipase treatment stimulates the basal uptake of glucose, which can pass the membrane more easily. But as in insulin-deprived diabetes, the maximal stimulatory effect of insulin has been decreased. At submaximal insulin concentrations the relative sensitivity increases. The changes in binding differ from the situation in diabetes. After treatment with phospholipase, more binding sites appear to be uncovered. Both the affinity and the number of accessible binding sites are increased, but the changes in affinity and total number are not in parallel. Treatment with 3.6 IU/ml phospholipase increases the total number of binding sites only; but the affinity does not change. Phospholipase in a dose of 1.2 IU/ml also changes the affinity. Phospholipase treatment mimics the effect of diabetes on insulin sensitivity for glucose uptake, but the effect of phospholipase on binding differs from that in diabetes. Phospholipids are involved in the changes in diabetes but the change cannot be mimicked by hydrolysis of a specific phospholipid.

Up and down regulation are not seen in proliferating and differentiating cells, e.g., fibroblasts. Incubation of cultured fibroblasts in the presence of prolactin or insulin induces the formation of additional specific binding sites for these hormones. However, the potentials of growing fibroblasts differ from those of outgrown cells. This case may serve to remind us of the need for caution in drawing conclusions about physiological changes from findings in cells in culture.

Up and down regulation and inhibition of responses by an excess of hormone have been reported for many hormones, including glucagon, TSH, TRH, catecholamines. ACTH, LH, FSH, calcitonin, and vasopressin. Prolactin is an exception, since it appears to induce the formation of its own receptor [16]. Steroids and thyroid hormone too may contribute to membrane changes. In Cushing's disease decreased insulin binding is seen. Hyperthyroidism increases the number of the binding sites for and the sensitivity to beta adrenergic agents [37]. Insulin and glucagon binding sites are also increased in hyperthyroidism [38].

INTERNALIZATION OF RECEPTOR-BOUND MATERIAL

In general, the receptor has been considered as a recognition element which accepts the message of the hormone and transfers it to effectors, but the peptide hormone receptor may have other functions as well. The reaction of low-density lipoproteins with their specific receptors initiates a process of uptake of LDL into the cell [39] (see Thompson, chapter 15). A comparable process has been demonstrated for peptide hormones. Radiolabeled insulin can be internalized after initial association with the membrane, but this material is then concentrated in lysosomal structures [40], which are involved in proteolysis. Whether internalized insulin can preserve its biological activity is a matter of dispute. Goldfine et al. [41, 42] showed that insulin can bind to nuclear and mitochondrial membranes in vitro, but it is not clear whether this is a normal pathway in which insulin can interfere with nuclear metabolism. Many peptide hormones can be internalized, but we do not know if this is a physiological process for the transport of active hormone toward intracellular structures or a way to dispose of hormone by extra inactivation. Internalization of hormone is not restricted to insulin but also occurs for HCG, epidermal and nerve growth factor and beta-melanotrophin [39]. The process of internalization of membrane material and the theoretical problems it presents are discussed by others in this book (see chapters 12–14).

SUMMARY

The relation between receptor occupancy and physiological intracellular responses is treated in terms of the concept that the first action of hormone on cellular level is a reaction with its specific receptor. Phenomena such as up and down regulation, membrane modification, and factors involved in binding and physiological action are discussed, and examples of changes in diseased state are given. The necessity for quantitative studies when binding patterns and physiological responses are related is underscored.

Acknowledgments. Part of the investigation was supported by the Foundation for the Medical Research FUNGO, which is subsidized by the Netherlands Organisation for the Advancement of Pure Research (ZWO). The secretarial assistance of Miss C. v.d. Haak is gratefully acknowledged.

REFERENCES

1. Rodbell M, Birnbaumer L, Pohl SL, Krans HMJ: Regulation of glucagon action and its receptor. In: Margoulies M, Greenwood FC (eds) Structure-activity relationships of protein and polypeptide hormones. Amsterdam, Excerpta Medica, 1971, pp 199–211.
2. Krans HMJ: The interaction of glucagon with isolated plasma membranes of rat livers: the relevancy of measuring binding sites. In: Dumont JE, Brown BL, Marshall NJ (eds)

Eukaryotic cell function and growth. Nato Advanced Study Institutes Series. New York and London, Plenum, 1976, pp 67–96.

3. Cat KJ, Harwood JP, Aguilera G, Dufau ML: Hormonal regulation of peptide receptors and target cell responses. Nature 280: 109–116, 1979.

4. Ariëns EJ, Beld AJ: The receptor concept in evolution. Biochem Pharmacol 26: 913–918, 1977.

5. Conolly ME, Greenacre JK: The lymphocyte betha-adrenoceptor in normal subjects and patients with bronchial asthma: the effect of different forms of treatment on receptor function. J Clin Invest 58: 1307–1316, 1976.

6. Simons EJ, Hiller JM: In vitro studies on opiate receptors and their ligands. Fed Proc 37: 141–146, 1978.

7. Horuk R, Goodwin P, O'Connor K, Neville RWJ, Lazarus NR, Stone D: Evolutionary change in the insulin receptors of hystricomorph rodents. Nature 279: 439–440, 1979.

8. Tager H, Given B, Baldwin D, Mako M, Markese J, Rubinstein A, Olefsky J, Kobayashi M, Kolterman O, Poucher R: A structurally abnormal insulin causing human diabetes. Nature 281: 122–125, 1979.

9. Rodbell M, Birnbaumer L, Pohl SL, Sundby F: The reaction of glucagon with its receptor: evidence for discrete regions of activity and binding in the glucagon molecule. Proc Natl Acad Sci USA 68: 909–913, 1971.

10. Lindström JM Seybold ME, Lennon VA, Withingham S, Duane PD: Antibody to acetylcholine receptor in myasthenia gravis. Prevalence, clinical correlates, and diagnostic value. Neurology 26: 1054–1059, 1976.

11. Kahn CR, Flier JS, Bar RS, Archer JA, Gorden P, Martin MM, Roth J: The syndromes of insulin resistance and acanthosis nigricans. Insulin-receptor disorders in man. N Engl J Med 294: 739–745, 1976.

12. Muggeo M, Kahn CR, Bar RS, Rechler M, Flier JS, Roth J: The underlying insulin receptor in patients with antireceptor autoantibodies: demonstration of normal binding and immunological properties. J Clin Endocrinol Metab 49: 110–119, 1979.

13. Schoenle E, Zapf J, Froesch ER: Effects of insulin and NSILA on adipocytes of normal and diabetic rats: receptor binding, glucose transport and glucose metabolism. Diabetologia 13: 243–249, 1977.

14. Volpé R: The role of autoimmunity in hypoendocrine and hyperendocrine function. Ann Intern Med 87: 86–99, 1977.

15. Kahn CR, Goldfine ID, Neville DM, De Meyts P: Alterations in insulin binding induced by changes in vivo in the levels of glucocorticoids and growth hormone. Endocrinology 103: 1054–1066, 1978.

16. Tell GP, Haour F, Saez JM: Hormonal regulation of membrane receptors and cell responsiveness: a review. Metabolism 27: 1566–1592, 1978.

17. Williams LT, Lefkowitz RJ, Watanabe AM, Hathaway DR, Besch HR Jr: Thyroid hormone regulation of betha-adrenergic receptor number. J Biol Chem 252: 2787–2789, 1977.

18. Gavin JR, Roth J, Neville DM, De Meyts P, Buell DN: Insulin-dependent regulation of insulin receptor concentrations: a direct demonstration in cell culture. Proc Natl Acad USA 71: 84–88, 1974.

19. De Pirro R, Bertoli A, Greco AV, Gelli As, Lauro R: The effect of food intake on insulin receptor in man. Acta Endocrinologica 90: 473–480, 1979.

20. Beck-Nielsen H, Pedersen O: Diurnal variation in insulin binding to human monocytes. J Clin Endocrinol Metab 47: 385–390. 1978.

21. Rodbell M, Krans HMJ, Pohl SL, Birnbaumer L: The glucagon-sensitive adenyl cyclase system in plasma membranes of rat liver. IV. Effects of guanyl nucleotides on binding of ^{125}I-glucagon. J Biol Chem 246: 1872–1876, 1971.

22. Rodbell M: The role of hormone receptors and GTP-regulatory proteins in membrane transduction. Nature 284: 17–22, 1980.

23. Scatchard G: The attraction of proteins for small molecules and ions. Ann NY Acad Sci 51: 660–672, 1949.

24. De Meyts P, Bianco AR, Roth J: Site-site interactions among insulin receptors. Characterization of the negative cooperativity. J Biol Chem 251: 1877–1888, 1976.

25. Boeynaems JM, Dumont JE: Quantitative analysis of ligands to their receptors. J Cyclic Nucleotide Res 1: 123–142, 1975.
26. Wieringa Tj, Krans HMJ: Reduced glucose transport and increased binding of insulin in adipocytes from diabetic and fasted rats. Biochim Biophys Acta 538: 563–570, 1978.
27. Van Slooten H, Wieringa Tj, Jansen M, Krans HMJ: Effects of fasting and induced diabetes on binding of insulin and glucose transport in isolated rat fat cells. J Endocrinol 72: 48^P–49^P, 1977.
28. Weinryb I: Cyclic AMP as an intracellular mediator of hormone action: Sutherland's criteria revisited. Perspect Biol Med 22: 415–420, 1979.
29. Birnbaumer L: Hormone-sensitive adenylyl cyclases. Useful models for studying hormone receptor functions in cell-free systems. Biochim Biophys Acta 300: 129–158, 1973.
30. Birnbaumer L, Pohl SL, Rodbell M, Sundby F: The glucagon-sensitive adenylate cyclase system in plasma membranes of rat liver. VII. Hormonal stimulation: reversibility and dependence on concentration of free hormone. J Biol Chem 247: 2038–2043, 1972.
31. Gliemann J, Gammeltoft S, Vinten J: Time course of insulin receptor binding and insulin induced lipogenesis in isolated rat fat cells. J Biol Chem 250: 3368–3374, 1975.
32. Assimacopoulos JF, Jeanrenaud B: The hormonal and metabolic basis of experimental obesity. Clin Endocrinol Metab 5: 337–365, 1976.
33. Le Marchand Brustel Y, Jeanrenaud B: Pre- and postweaning studies on development of obesity in mdb/mdb mice. Am J Physiol 234: E568–E574, 1978.
34. Jeanrenaud B: Insulin and obesity. Diabetologia 17: 133–138, 1979.
35. Baxter D, Stanton K, Lazarus NR, Keen H: The relation between insulin and adipocyte insulin receptors during treatment of human obesity. Eur J Clin Invest 8: 361–372, 1978.
36. Krans HMJ, Wieringa Tj: The effect of diabetes and phospholipase treatment on binding of insulin and glucose transport in isolated adipocytes. In: Hessel LW, Krans HMJ (eds) Lipoprotein metabolism and endocrine regulation. Amsterdam, Elsevier/North-Holland Biomedical, 1979, pp 225–231.
37. Jacobs S, Cuatrecasas P: Cell receptors in disease. N Engl J Med 297: 1383–1386, 1977.
38. Madsen SN, Sonne O: Increase of glucagon receptors in hyperthyroidism. Nature 262: 793–795, 1976.
39. Goldstein JL, Anderson RGW, Brown MS: Coated pits, coated vesicles, and recepter-mediated endocytosis. Nature 279: 679–685, 1979.
40. Carpentier JL, Gorden P, Barazzone P, Freychet P, Le Cam A, Orci L: Intracellular localization of ^{125}I-labeled insulin in hepatocytes from intact rat liver. Proc Natl Acad Sci USA 76: 2803–2807, 1979.
41. Goldfine ID, Jones AL, Hradek GT, Wong KY, Mooney JS: Entry of insulin into human cultured lymphocytes: electron microscope autoradiographic analysis. Science 202: 760–763, 1978.
42. Vigneri R, Pliam NB, Cohen DC, Pezzine V, Wong KY, Goldfine ID: In vivo regulation of cell surface and intracellular insulin binding sites by insulin. J Biol Chem 253: 8192–8197, 1978.

8. THE MECHANISMS OF CELL-MEDIATED CYTOTOXICITY

C.J. SANDERSON

INTRODUCTION

Cell-mediated cytotoxicity is an important part of the effector function of the immune system, and can be divided into two parts: firstly, the activity of immune cytotoxic T cells, which bear specific antigen receptors; and secondly, the antibody-dependent cell-mediated systems. These include macrophages, granulocytes, and lymphoid K cells which have receptors for the Fc piece of antibody (see Fig. 1). It should be noted that there is another class of lymphoid effector cell, known as natural killer cells (NK cells). Evidence is accumulating that K cells and NK cells are closely related and probably identical cell populations. They differ in that K cells are dependent on antibody, whereas NK cells bear receptors for undefined antigens on certain cell types. In this presentation no attempt will be made to provide a comprehensive review of the literature, but rather to outline work on T and K cells, based in my laboratory, and other work relevant to the points I wish to make. Readers requiring a wider introduction to the literature are referred to earlier reviews [1–3].

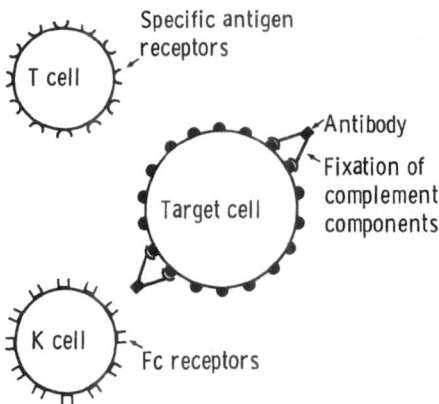

Fig. 1. Diagram showing three mechanisms of target-cell killing. Immune T cells making contact via specific receptors for antigen. Lymphoid K cells making contact via receptors for the Fc piece of antibody, coating the target cell. Complement-mediated lysis via antibody and the fixation of complement components.

W.Th. Daems et al. (eds.), Cell Biological Aspects of Disease, 97–116. All rights reserved.
Copyright © 1981 by Martinus Nijhoff Publishers bv, The Hague/Boston/London.

CYTOTOXIC SYSTEMS

T-cell system

The mouse allograft system was used [4] in which mastocytoma (P815) cells of DBA/2 origin are injected into C57.B6 (H2b) mice. After 10 or 11 days the tumour has been rejected and the spleen and peritoneal cavity contain significant numbers of cytotoxic T cells. The T cells can be easily purified from the peritoneal exudate by using carbonyl iron or nylon wool columns to remove adherent cells. The activity of the T cells can be assayed on the P815 cells or on any other cell type bearing the H2d antigen. Thus macrophages from Balb/c mice have been used as targets in some experiments.

K-cell system

To allow direct comparison with the T-cell system, cells of the same P815 type have been used as targets. A gus strain rat spleen provides the source of K cells, and a rat anti-P815 antiserum the source of antibody. The K cells were enriched by taking the lymphoid cells from the interface of Ficoll-Hypaque density gradient separation, and passing them through nylon wool. The K cells are non-adherent. This preparation would of course also contain rat T cells, but since the animals are not immunised the T cells are not active, so that no cytotoxicity occurs in the absence of antibody [5].

KINETIC EXPERIMENTS, T-CELL CYTOTOXICITY

^{51}Chromium release

The most widely applied technique for the assay of cytotoxicity is the release of ^{51}chromium from prelabelled target cells. The chromate ion diffuses into the cell, where it is reduced to the chromic ion. This ion cannot pass across the membrane and so is retained by viable cells. When the cell dies, about 80% of the chromium is released into the medium. The remaining unreleasable fraction is presumably complexed to cell debris. The 80% of releasable chromium is held in the cell as a small molecule probably chelated by dicarboxylic acid members of the Krebs cycle (e.g. citrate) [6]. This is an important point because it has often been assumed that chromium is complexed to macromolecules, but there is no experimental evidence to support this.

Cell contact

With this assay system it has been shown that close contacts must be established between the T cell and the target cell before killing can occur. On the one hand, killing does not occur in tubes kept on a slow roller (one revolution in 3 min), whereas killing is rapidly initiated if the cells are centrifuged together [7]. On the other hand, 'bystander' cells (that is, cells not bearing the target antigen) are not killed even when centrifuged together with T cells and the relevant target. Therefore, close apposition is not sufficient; there must be specific interaction between the effectors and target cells. This makes it unlikely that any form of lymphotoxin is released into the medium to kill targets at a distance.

The fact that significant number of contacts are not formed in free suspension (slow rolling) but are formed under conditions of vigorous shaking, rocking, or centrifuging, indicates that the time course of chromium release will be markedly affected by the technique used in setting up the assay. The most obvious example is that when cells are allowed to settle under gravity, there will be a lag phase followed by an increasing rate of release until all the cells have settled to the bottom of the tube, when the maximum rat of killing will be achieved until a plateau is reached as chromium release approaches the maximum. The resulting sigmoidal curve cannot be regarded as a fundamental property of the mechanism of killing. This simple technical fact has resulted in much controversy and misunderstanding, because many authors have interpreted contact-limiting factors as fundamental indicators of the mechanism of killing.

Conclusions

When these technical factors are taken into account, an analysis of chromium release [7, 8] shows three basic characteristics:

1) With a constant number of target cells and maintaining a constant number of lymphocytes (by adding normal lymphocytes), chromium release is directly proportional to the number of effector cells.
2) There is no significant lag phase (i.e., it is less than 5 min).
3) Release is approximately linear with time.

These data allowed three statements to be made about the kinetics of killing:

1) Killing requires only one effector cell.
2) Killing can occur within a few minutes of contact, or up to several hours after contact.

3) Target cell death results in the rapid release of chromium, i.e. death is explosive.

Since these statements have been confirmed by a number of different approaches, it is unnecessary to go into the arguments used to derive them [7].

RELEASE OF CELL COMPONENTS

Most other proposals for the mode of target cell death have postulated a leakage of intracellular constituents, starting with small molecules and leading up to the leakage of macromolecules [7, 9, 10]. To test these proposals the release of a number of different cell components was compared by using double-labelling isotope techniques [11]. It was clearly shown that phosporyl choline, sucrose, phosphoryl 3-o-methyl glucose, and chromium (all relatively small molecules) were released at the same rate as macromulecular protein and RNA. The main exceptions were [86]rubidium and DNA. Figure 2 shows these data diagrammatically, and it can be seen that rubidium reaches its maximum within about 15 min, the other cytosol components are released progressively from time zero, and DNA shows a significant lag phase.

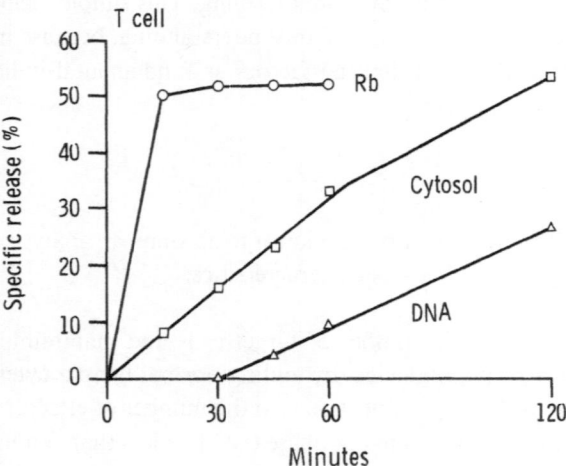

Fig. 2. Diagrammatic representation of the release of different cell components form target cells in T-cell-mediated cytotoxicity. Cytotoxic T cells were mixed with isotope-labeled target cell and centrifuged at time zero to allow contacts to form. Isotope release into the supernatant medium was compared with spontaneous isotope release in the absence of effector cells. Results are expressed as percentage specific release caused by the effector cells. O————O [86]rubidium, □————□ cytoplasmic contents represented by [51]chromium (a range of other cytoplasmic contents showed similar rates of release), △————△ desoxyribonucleic acid. Adapted from [11].

· These results indicate that when lysis occurred all the cytoplasmic contents were released, with no suggestion of a progressive leakage from small to large molecules. The fact that rubidium was released so rapidly after contact suggested that it may be a result of changes in ion fluxes due to contact, and not necessarily the first step in the lytic cycle. The slower release of DNA indicated that nuclear disruption occurred as a post-mortem event after cytoplasmic disruption.

K-CELL CYTOTOXICITY

Relatively little information is available to discuss the K-cell system. Analysis of the kinetics of release of cell components from P815 cells (Fig. 3) shows several similarities with the T-cell system [5]. Firstly, there is an initial rapid release of [86]rubidium; secondly, there is a lag phase before DNA release is detected. The main difference is in the release of [51]chromium and other cytoplasmic contents, which show a rapid release over the first 15–30 min, followed by a slower rate of release. It is important that all the cytoplasmic labels tested showed this type of release. The best interpretation of these data is that killing occurs within 30 min of contact and that the lytic event is explosive, resulting in the loss of all cytoplasmic contents. The slower rate of release after this phase probably represents K cells finding new targets. The slow release of DNA presumably stems from the later breakdown of the nucleus.

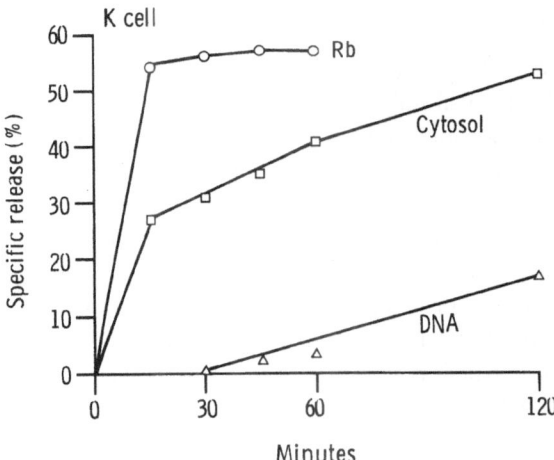

Fig. 3. Kinetics of release of different cell components from target cells in K-cell-mediated cytotoxicity. Methods and symbols as in Fig. 2. Adapted from [5].

THE QUEST FOR COMMUNICATING JUNCTIONS

Many cell types when in contact form specialised junctions which allow the passage of molecules from one cell to the other. It was an attractive proposition that some type of communicating junctions were formed between the T cell and target cell, allowing the passage of a putative toxic material into the target. Results purporting to show the passage of fluorescein from one cell to the other [12] were therefore received with some interest. Unfortunately this claim has not been substantiated, and two separate groups have failed to confirm the observation [13, 14]. To overcome the technical problems associated with working with fluorescein esters, experments were carried out with radioactive tracers and autoradiography [14]. Using a positive control system with cells which were known to form communicating junctions, it was demonstrated that tritiated uridine or choline as well as ^{51}chromium would pass from one cell to the other. However, when these techniques were applied to T-cell/target-cell conjugates, no evidence for transfer was obtained. This was despite the fact that the technique allowed hundreds of conjugates to be examined after various incubation periods.

These experiments show that communicating junctions analogous to those found in other mammalian cells, do not form between T cells and target cells. There is a remote possibility that some specialised junction is formed which allows only the passage of the putative toxin, but, at the present time, there is no experimental or morphological evidence to support this.

UNIDIRECTIONAL NATURE OF KILLING

Important for the functioning of any cell-mediated cytotoxic activity is the question of effector-cell survival. For example, a phagocytic cell is protected against its own lysosomal enzymes, so that target material can be destroyed without self destruction of the effector cell. Cytotoxic T cells are known to survive and recycle to kill further target cells. It was therefore surprising when it was shown that cytotoxic T cells are susceptible to killing by other cytotoxic T cells [15]. These experiments were carried out by mixing two populations of cytotoxic T cells in a primary incubation, and then assaying residual T-cell activity on ^{51}chromium-labelled targets in a second incubation. In this way the survival or destruction of the cytotoxic T cells in the primary incubation is assayed. Thus, when cells with cytotoxic activity (A anti-B) are mixed with cells of strain B, containing cells cytotoxic to a third party (B anti-C), the residual anti-C activity is assayed. It was found that the anti-C activity was decreased, which indicates that these cells had been killed by the anti-B cells.

Another experiment of this type [16] showed that killing proceeded in only the direction receptor to antigen. One population (A anti-B) was mixed with another (B anti-C), and the residual activity of both populations was assayed in a second incubation. It was shown that only the B anti-C cells were killed. Thus, when two cytotoxic cells make contact, only the cell with the antigen is killed. In a third type of experiment [17], two mutually cytotoxic populations were mixed (A anti-B and B anti-A) and the cells forming contacts were isolated by micromanipulation. It was observed that only one of the pair of cells was killed. In this case there is a receptor-antigen interaction in both directions, and yet one cell survives the interaction.

These experiments make it unlikely that there is a toxin generated or delivered at the zone of contact between the two cells.

LETHAL-HIT CONCEPT

Cytochylasin B inhibits ^{51}chromium release if added at time zero, but when added after 1h, there is very little inhibition of the subsequent rate of chromium release [18]. Experiments of this type have been carried out in which the effector has been inactivated by heat [19] or by an alloantibody which lyses the T cells without effect on the target [7, 20]. At first these experiments were interpreted as indicating a slow release of chromium from cells killed soon after contact [19]. However, in view of the kinetic and morphological observations indicating an explosive form of death, it is clear that a lethal-hit concept is a better explanation. This suggests that within 45 to 60 min of contact the target cell is programmed for lysis or has been lethally hit. The effector cell is no longer necessary for the final lytic event.

TIME-LAPSE MICROCINEMATOGRAPHY

With the use of a movie camera attached to an inverted microscope, and exposure of a single frame every 5 s, events taking place over more than 3 h are recorded on a 30-m-long film. This film can then be examined in detail with an analytical projector, which allows each frame to be viewed individually, or the film can be projected forwards or backwards at both slow and fast rates. Events can be timed accurately by means of an automatic frame counter.

Because T-cell killing has so often been compared to the lysis of cells by antibody and complement [21], the first step was to see if the morphological changes in the target cell were the same. In fact they are not [22]. The lysis of P815 cells by antibody and complement shows a progressive darkening of the cytoplasm under phase contrast, indicating changes in the refractive index of the cytoplasmic contents. The cell membrane remains stationary, with no suggestion of swelling. A burst of dark bubbles is seen leaving the cell, and this is followed by swelling of the cell membrane to form a ghost. The time course of these events depends on the amount of complement. With low dilutions of complement, many cells will pass through the lytic cycle within a few minutes, but at dilutions of complement sufficient to lyse about 50% of the targets, some of the cells require more than 30 min for complete lysis.

Morphological changes

In T-cell cytotoxicity there is a period during which the target cell remains morphologically normal, and there is no progressive darkening of the cytoplasm or cell swelling. Suddenly the whole membrane of the target cell starts to form blebs (zeoisis), this lasts for about 5–10 min. Towards the end of this phase of zeiosis, bubbles of material burst out of the cell. The cell then becomes spherical again, and over the next 5–30 min swells and darkens to form a ghost. These morphological changes would suggest a mode of cell death quite different from lysis by antibody and complement, and confirm that death is an explosive phenomenon.

Time analysis

The second problem which could be approached by time-lapse films is the time relationship between contact and killing. Here it is first necessary to define a morphological event consistent with cell death. Probably the best definition of cell death would be the moment when bubbles of cytoplasm leave the cell, but it was easier to record the time of onset of zeiosis, because this is seen more clearly under the low magnification necessary for this type of observation (Fig. 4). This analysis showed that, in some cases, zeiosis occurred within a few minutes of contact by the T cell, whereas in other cases up to 3 h or more elapsed before zeiosis. Similar results were obtained by direct observation of T-cell conjugates with targets that had been isolated by micromanipulation [23]. Thus in confirmation of the suggestions based on kinetic data, there was no fixed relationship between contact and killing. The killing event is unsynchronised. This presents considerable problems for detailed analysis of the intracellular events.

In the phase between contact and lysis the target cell remains morphologically normal, and is able to continue normal membrane movement. Furthermore, cells have been observed to divide while in contact with a T cell.

Target cell cycle phase

Analysis of target-cell size by measuring the area of the cell image on a screen

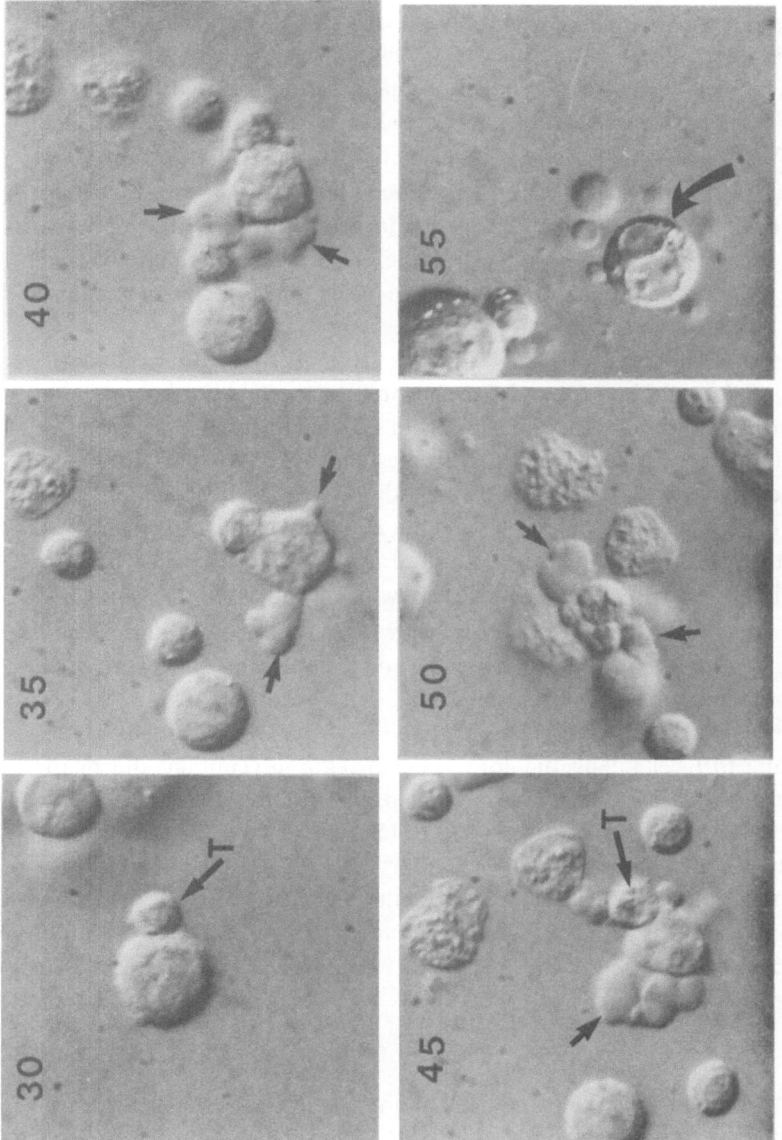

Fig. 4. **Time-lapse sequence of T-cell killing of a P815 cell observed with Nomarski optical system. The numerals represent minutes after** contact was established. At 30 min the P815 cell is normal (T cell indicated by arrow). By 35 min the P815 cell is undergoing zeoisis (blebs indicated by short arrows); this continues through 50 min. The P815 cell explodes to form an empty ghost (curved arrow at 55 min), surrounded by bubbles of cytoplasmic contents.

showed no detectable swelling of the cell during contact. These observations make it unlikely that there is a progressive injury to the target cell culminating in death. However, there was a correlation between target-cell volume and the time between contact and zeiosis [22]. Since cell volume is related to cell-cycle phase, this analysis showed that cells in the G1 phase were killed sooner after contact than were the larger cells in later phases of the cell cycle. This phenomenon was not due simply to changes in antigen density, because antigen density increased until late G1, when it started to decrease. It is known that an unsynchronised population of P815 cells can be totally killed in about 1 h if sufficient effectors are added [24]. This indicates that there is no absolute cell-cycle requirement for target-cell death, only a relative change in susceptibility. A large cell in the G2 phase, which may die only after several hours of contact with a single T cell, must die much sooner if several T cells are in contact with it.

Because a T cell was able to kill cells in the G1 phase sooner than cells in the G2, phase, it could be expected that it would be available to kill a second target sooner; thus a population of cells in G1 should show higher rates of chromium release than cells in G2. To test this directly, P815 cells were separated by velocity sedimentation according to size. This technique gives fractions of cells from the smallest to the largest, which can be shown to correlate with different phases of the cell cycle. There was a decrease in susceptibility as cell volume increased, which confirmed the time-lapse studies. The relative density of H2 antigen was tested at the same time, using limiting dilutions of an anti-H2 antiserum and complement, and it was found to vary independently of susceptibility to T-cell cytotoxicity [25].

On the other hand, a sarcoma cell line (Meth A) which is relatively insusceptible to T-cell killing, did not show changes in susceptibility during the cell cycle. There is no unequivocal explanation for this difference except perhaps that the high susceptibility fo P815 may derive from some special property of cell in the G1 phase. The importance of these experiments lies in the demonstration of changes in susceptibility which are unrelated to membrane antigen density, thus suggesting a contribution from the target cell in the mechanism of killing.

K cells

The time-lapse observations on K-cell killing of P815 cells showed remarkable similarity to the T-cell observations [26]; indeed, it would be impossible for an observer to distinguish the two systems simply by watching a film. K cells are morphologically similar to T cells, and show a similar type of movement. The P815 cells die in a similar way, showing the same spectacular zeiosis. The main difference lies in the fact that most lytic events (defined as the beginning of zeiosis; see *Time analysis*) occur within 15 min of contact. This provides an explanation for the non-linear time course of chromium release (see *K-cell cytotoxicity*). There was no correlation between target-cell size and time between contact and lysis. Thus there was no difference in susceptibility to killing during the cell cycle [25].

When glass-adherent cells (macrophages or human diploid cell line cells [26] were used as targets, the K cell appeared to be over the nucleus immediately before the onset of cell death. The first sign of death was a retraction of the flattened cell membrane towards the nucleus; this was followed by zeiosis. Under high magnification the cell contents could be seen bursting out of the cell during zeiosis.

DETAILED ANALYSIS OF THE T-CELL LYTIC CYCLE

The fact that cell death is an unsynchronised event means that it is not possible to study different phases of the lytic cycle by fixing material at different times. Each time point can be expected to have some cells in zeiosis and some cells pre- and post-zeiosis. However, zeiosis forms such a morphologically distinct phase that it is relatively easy to correlate the time-lapse and electron-microscopic observations. In our initial experiments [27], material was fixed at various times, but obviously the number of target cells undergoing changes was a small proportion of the total. This was overcome to some extent by selecting conditions that would give a very high rate of killing [28]. This was done by using target cells in the G1 phase and selecting cell preparations for the highest rates of killing. Under these conditions the rate of kiling was non-linear: there was a higher rate of chromium release over the first 5 min. Material fixed during this period could be expected to show a greater proportion of cells undergoing lysis.

Contact

The most remarkable features of T-cell contact are firstly the strength of binding, which allows the T cell to move a much larger target cell around with considerable vigour, and secondly its mobility, since the T cell is able to migrate over the surface of an adherent target. There was no suggestion that any particular area of the T cell was involved in making contact. Many cases were observed in which the T cell was in contact with more than one target cell. T cells were observed to break contact with a target without apparently damaging it, and then subsequently contact and kill another cell. The target cell remained morphologically normal throughout the phase of contact, and retained normal movement and the ability to enter mitosis and divide [22].

Electron micrographs showed two distinct forms of contact. One involved only point contacts between the two cells, in the other long areas of close contact occurred. These might be correlated with the formation of weak and tenacious bonds [27] defined by the shearing force necessary to separate the cells. These authors showed that the weak bonds were sufficient for the initiation of killing. It is perhaps the point contacts which allow the T cell to migrate over the surface of the target.

Time-lapse films taken at high magnification clearly show the T cell pushing towards the nucleus of the target cell, so that organelles including the nucleus are distorted. This is a very active process which is impossible to illustrate in still reproduction. As observed in K-cell killing (see *Detailed analysis of the K-cell lytic cycle*), the T cell also appeared to be closely associated with the nucleus of the target cell immediately before the beginning of zeiosis.

Electron micrographs showed that during the phase of contact long projection from the T cell pushed into the target cell [28]. Only the tip of the projection was in close contact with the membrane of the target cell (Fig. 5), and the membrane of the target remained intact. The projections contained microfilaments, but no other organelles. These projections could frequently be seen to distort the outline of a mitochondrion or nucleus in its path. It must be emphasised that to find significant numbers of these projections, it was necessary to set up very high levels of cytotoxicity, as described in this section, and to fix at 37 °C during the first few minutes after contact. If these conditions are not met, projections are very hard to find in sections, even though significant numbers of specific contacts may be observed. It is not possible to observe the projections into target cells under either phase-contrast or Nomarski optical systems. This is not surprising, since there would be little or no difference in refractive index between the projections and the target-cell cytoplasm. Thus it has not been possible to determine directly their speed of movement or their relationship to the beginning of zeiosis. However, surface protrusions from T cells, unrelated to the target cell, can form and disappear within a few seconds. If this also applies to projections into target cells, it would explain why they are relatively difficult to find in fixed sections.

Because the effector cell appeared in close apposition to the target-cell nucleus immediately before death, it appeared possible that the nucleus was in some way directly involved in the lytic process. This has been shown to be unlikely, because isolated cytoplasts are susceptible to killing. However, isolated karyoplasts are more susceptible to killing than intact cells or isolated cytoplasts [29], and so it is possible that some other organelle which is nuclear associated in the intact cell is important in the lytic event.

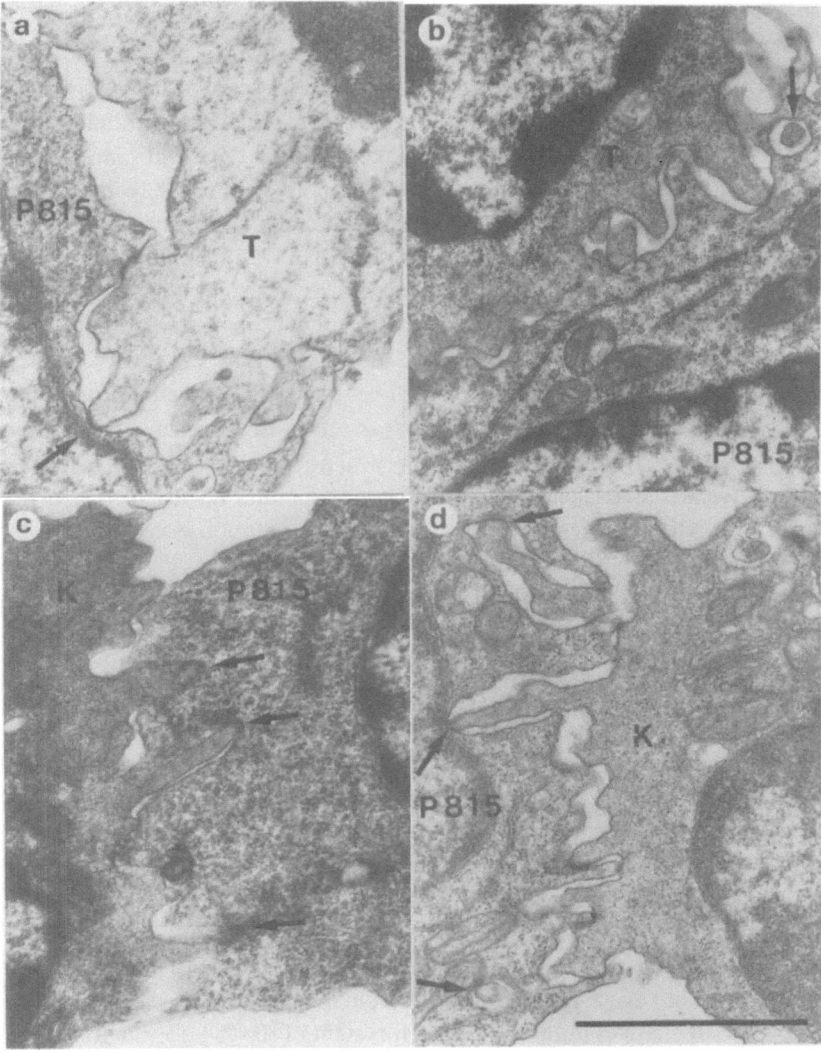

Fig. 5. T-cell contact from [28]. (a) The T-cell projection has pushed towards the nucleus of the target cell. The tip of the projection is in close contact with the plasma membrane of the P815 cell (arrow). Note the microfilaments in the T-cell projection. (b) Several T-cell projections pushing into the P815 cell; one is seen in cross section (arrow) (c, d) K-cell contact with antibody-coated P815 cells from [30]. (c) Three long K-cell projections pushing into a P815 cell (arrows). Note the close contact at the tip of each projection. The projections contain only microfilaments, whereas the interdigitating areas of the P815 cells have a normal distribution of ribosomes. (d) Several K-cell projections (arrows). One has pushed up to the nuclear envelope, and has disorted the outline of the nucleus. Bar represents 0.1 μm.

Zeiosis

Zeiosis is a spectacular and constant feature of the onset of death of P815 cells in T-cell cytotoxicity. The beginning of zeiosis is sudden; in one frame the cell appears normal, and in the next frame, taken 5 s later, the membrane appears ruffled as zeiosis begins. The cell becomes completely misshapen as blebs form and retract (Fig. 4). There is some variation in the appearance and time course of zeiosis. Some cells show little more than ruffling of the membrane, lasting only 2 or 3 min; others show more marked blebbing (as in Fig. 4) lasting up to 20 min. In most cells it lasts from between 5 and 10 min. With good optics the cytoplasmic contents can be seen bursting out of the cell towards the end of the phase. This sometimes appears like a halo diffusing out of the cell; in other cases, the blebs appear to break off the cell and float away.

The fact that significant levels of chromium release can be detected after 5 min indicates that at least in some cases chromium release has occurred during the phase of zeiosis. In all cases that I have observed, the T cell remained in contact through the phase of zeiosis.

Cells in zeiosis can be easily identified under the electron microscope (Fig. 6). The cells are distorted in outline, and frequently the nucleus is misshapen and divided between different blebs of the cell. Cells in zeiosis fall into two clearly defined categories. In the first, in which there are no significant changes in the organelles, the number of ribosomes appears to be normal even in the extremities of the blebs and in some cases stress fibres are visible at the 'focus' of the blebbing movement. In the second category there is vacuolation and loss of organelles (Fig. 7a). This is assumed to be a late phase of zeiosis, after the release of cytoplasmic contents (which can be seen in the time-lapse sequences). This justifies regarding the phase of zeiosis as the time of cell death.

Zeiosis appears to be an important clue to the mechanism of killing. It is not found where cell death results primarily from membrane damage. It seems to be a result of changes in the cytoskeletal system of the cell, for the following reasons:

a) It occurs only in intact cells. Cytoplasts and karyoplasts which have intact membranes but disrupted skeletal systems do not show zeiosis [29].

b) Stress fibres have been observed at the focus of the blebbing of cells dying as a result of T-cell killing [27].

c) It occurs when cells are treated with drugs which disrupt the cytoskeletal system. This effect is reversible, thus indicating that zeiosis itself is not lethal. It is presumably a symptom of some other lethal event in the cell.

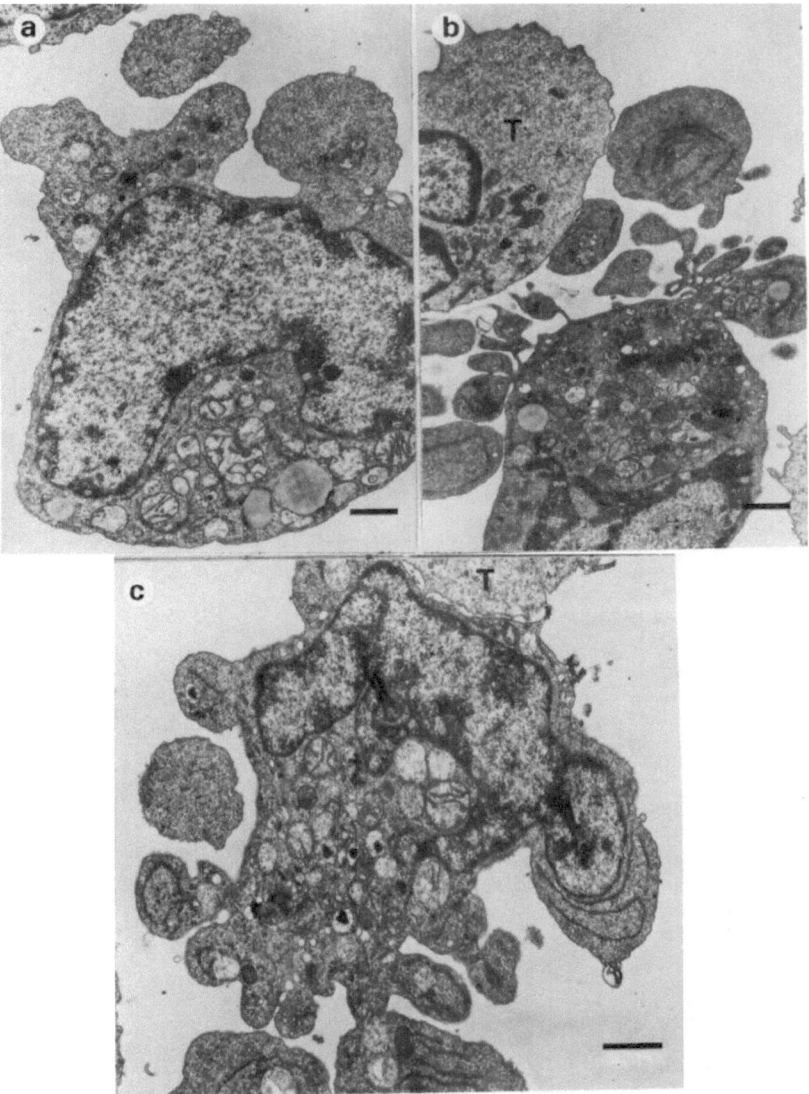

Fig. 6. Electron micrographs from [27] showing P815 cells in the phase of zeiosis. In each case the contents of the cell appear normal, indicating that these were fixed before the loss of cytoplasmic contents. The T cell is indicated (T) in (b) and (c). Bars represent 0.1 μm.

112

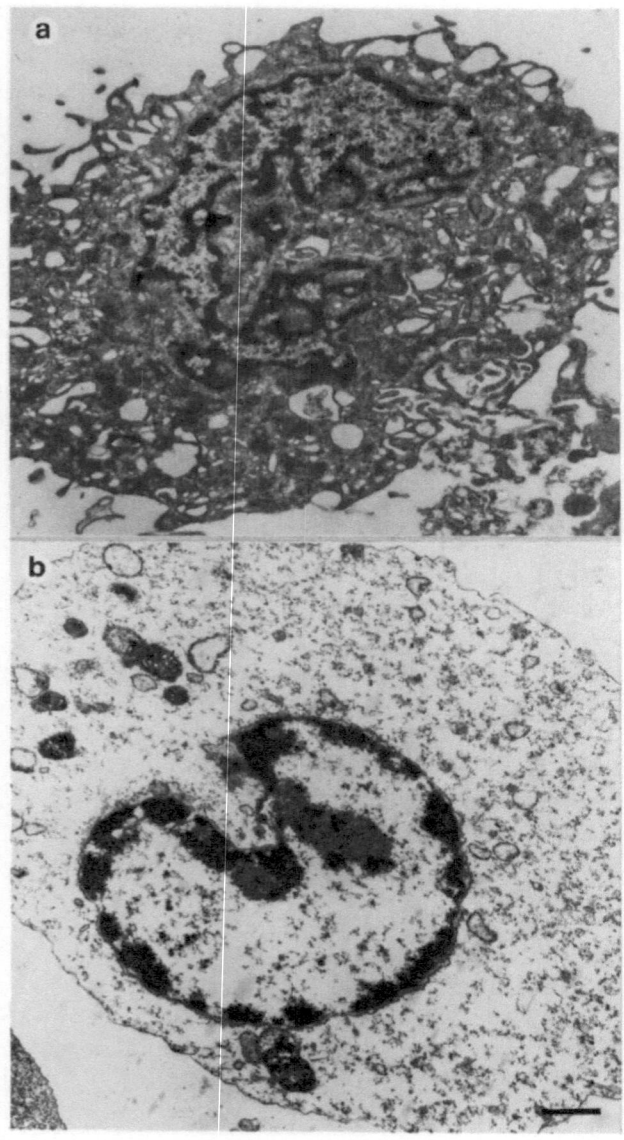

Fig. 7. Final stages of P815 cell death in K-cell killing from [30]. (a) Recognisable as a late stage of zeiosis by the distorted outline of the cell, and the vacuoles suggesting that part of the cytoplasmic contents have burst out of the cell. (b) An empty ghost. Very little of the cytoplasmic contents remains, although some chromatin remains in the nucleus. This is probably equivalent to the phase in Fig. 4 at 55 min. The bar represents 0.1 μm.

Post-zeiosis

This period might well be called the post-mortem phase. Zeiosis ceases abruptly, and no further membrane activity occurs. The cell remains bright under phase contrast, indicating that some refractile material remains in the cell, but darkens as the refractive index of the cytoplasm changes, and finally swells rapidly to form a characteristic ghost. At this time, only the outline of the nucleus and a few refractile inclusions (probably lipid granules) are visible in the cell under phase contrast. Electron micrographs show that the cytoplasm has very few organelles (Fig. 7b), but that some of the nuclear chromatin remains in situ, which explains the slow release of DNA compared to cytoplasmic contents.

DETAILED ANALYSIS OF THE K-CELL LYTIC CYCLE

The fact that K cells kill within 15 min of contact means that material fixed during the first 15 min shows a relatively high proportion of lytic events. Thus, it was in a K-cell system that projections were first observed [30]. This prompted the successful attempts to find projections in the T-cell system (see section on *Contact*). Electron micrographs showed essentially the same phenomena as observed in T-cell cytotoxicity [30]. The K cell is a typical small lymphocyte; it is able to make contact with several target cells at once, and so there seems to be no particular region of the membrane involved in contact. Projections into the target are similar to those produced by T cells (Fig. 5), and appear to be restricted to the zone of contact between the two cells; that is, there is no tendency for the effector cell to produce projections at random, some of which push into the target cell. The tip of the projection is in close contact with the membrane of the target and, in every case observed, the target-cell membrane was intact. Although most areas of contact show only these point contacts, cells are frequently seen where the two membranes are in close apposition over a larger area.

EVIDENCE THAT PROJECTIONS ARE INVOLVED IN KILLING

There are three reasons for supposing that the projections are an active process on the part of the effector cell, and do not result from pulling by the target cell:

a) The visual appearance of effector-cell movement in time-lapse films, which shows an active lymphoid cell moving in relation to a passive target.

b) The projections contain only microfilaments, and no other organelles, whereas target-cell interdigitations between projections contain ribosomes (Fig. 5c).

c) Projections into dead target cells have been observed.

The formation of projections may be analogous to the formation of pseudopodia by phagocytic cells. The interaction of the target with membrane receptors on the phagocytic cell leads to the formation of psueodopodia which envelop the target. T- and K-cell projections appear also to result from contact of the receptors with the target cell. However, unlike the surrounding movements of phagocytosis, the projections push straight into the target cell.

There is no direct evidence that the projections are involved in killing. However, they are of special interest because they do not appear to have been described in any other biological system, apart from lymphoid-mediated killing, and there is circumstantial evidence compatible with their involvement in the killing process:

a) They are found in both T- and K-cell systems, which are mediated by different receptors, but show similar morphological changes in the target cell.

b) Contact by an effector cell does not always result in target-cell death. Effector cells have been observed to break away from one target leaving it intact, and then subsequently kill another cell. Presumably, the projection did not hit the sensitive structures in the first cell.

c) The variation in time between contact and killing, particularly in the T-cell system, indicates that the lytic event is different from initial contact. Furthermore, the fact that susceptibility to killing varies independently of antigen density suggests that an event separate from contact is necessary for killing. The projections are comparable with this.

d) The unidirectional effect of the lytic mechanism is readily explained by an involvement of the projections in killing. Thus, the stimulus for projection formation comes from the effector cell receptors. Even when two cytotoxic T cells make contact, killing is only in the direction receptor to antigen, and if the two cells are mutually cytotoxic then the first cell to deliver the lethal hit survives the interaction.

These arguments do not lead to any clear idea how the target cell is killed. What is the lethal event? It is not clear how the lethal-hit data (see *Lethal-hit concept*) fit into these ideas. How can the effector cell deliver a lethal hit which takes several hours to produce a morphological change in the target cell? This problem is made difficult by the absence of information about what changes in the cell will lead to its death. The cytoplasmic retraction of adherent target cells and zeiosis indicate that one of the first changes in the target cell is in the cytoskeletal system. This could of course be a consequence of some other earlier event, which might involve changes not visible under the electron microscope. Thus one possibility is that projections cause damage to some organelle in the target cell, which releases substances into the cytoplasm causing cell death. More information about other forms of cell death involving zeiosis might assist the understanding of cell-mediated cytotoxicity.

Acknowledgment. I would like to thank Dr. A.M. Glauert of the Strangeways Research Laboratory, Cambridge, for providing the electron micrographs.

REFERENCES

1. Martz E: Mechanism of specific tumor cell lysis by alloimmune T lymphocytes: resolution and characterisation of discrete steps in the cellular interaction. Contemp Top Immunobiol 7: 301–361, 1976.
2. Golstein P, Smith ET: Mechanism of T cell mediated cytolysis: the lethal hit stage. Contemp Top Immunobiol 7: 273–300, 1976.
3. Berke G, Amos DB: Mechanism of lymphocyte mediated cytolysis. Transplant Rev 17: 71–107, 1973.
4. Brunner KT, Mauel J, Cerottini J-C, Chapuis B: Quantitative assay of the lytic action of immune lymphoid cells and ^{51}Cr labelled allogeneic target cells in vitro: inhibition by isoantibody and by drugs. Immunology 14: 181–196, 1968.
5. Sanderson CJ, Thomas JA: The mechanism of K cell (antibody dependent) cell mediated cytotoxicity. I. The release of different cell components. Proc R Soc Lond [Biol] 197: 407–415, 1977.
6. Sanderson CJ: The uptake and retention of chromium by cells. Transplantation 21: 526–529, 1976.
7. Sanderson CJ, Taylor GA: The kinetics of ^{51}Cr release from target cells in cell mediated cytotoxicity and the relationship to the kinetics of killing. Cell Tissue Kinet 8: 23–32, 1975.
8. Berke G, Yagil G, Ginsburg H, Feldman M: Kinetic analysis of a graft reaction induced in cell culture. Immunology 17: 723–740.
9. Henney CS: On the mechanism of T cell mediated cytolysis. Transplant Rev 17: 37–70, 1973.
10. Steinitz M, Weiss DW: Studies on the physiological manifestations of cell mediated cytotoxicity. I. Early metabolic changes in mouse plasmacytoma cells exposed in vitro to sensitised allogeneic splenocytes. Cell Immunol 15: 403–418, 1975.
11. Sanderson CJ: The mechanism of T cell mediated cytotoxicity I. The release of different cell components. Proc R Soc Lond [Biol] 192: 221–239, 1976.
12. Sellin D, Wallach DFH, Fischer H: Intercellular communication in cell mediated cytotoxicity. Fluorescein transfer between H-2d target cells and H-2b lymphocytes in vitro. Eur J Immunol 1: 453–458, 1971.
13. Kalina M, Berke G: Contact regions of cytotoxic T lymphocyte-target cell conjugates. Cell Immunol 25: 41–51, 1976.
14. Sanderson CJ, Hall PJ, Thomas JA: The mechanism of T cell mediated cytotoxicity IV. Studies on communicating junctions between cells in contact. Proc R Soc Lond [Biol] 196: 73–84, 1977.
15. Golstein P: Sensitivity of cytotoxic T cells to T cell mediated cytotoxicity. Nature 252: 81–83, 1974.
16. Kuppers RC, Henney CS: Studies on the mechanism of lymphocyte mediated cytolysis. IX. Relationships between antigen recognition and lytic expression in killer T cells. J Immunol 118: 71–76, 1977.

116

17. Fishelson Z, Berke G: T lymphocyte mediated cytolysis: dissociation of the binding and lytic mechanisms of the effector cell. J Immunol 120: 1121–1126, 1978.
18. Cerotini J-C, Brunner KT: Reversible inhibition of lymphocyte mediated cytotoxicity by cytochylasin B. Nature [New Biol] 237: 272–273, 1972.
19. Wagner H, Rollinghoff M: T cell mediated cytotoxicity: discrimination between antigen recognition, lethal hit and cytolysis phase. Eur J Immunol 4: 745–750, 1974.
20. Martz E, Benacerraf B: T lymphocyte mediated cytolysis: temperature dependence of killer cell dependent and independent phases and lack of recovery from the lethal hit at low temperatures. Cell Immunol 20: 81–91, 1975.
21. Ferluga J, Allison AC: Observations on the mechanism by which T lymphocytes exert cytotoxic effects. Nature 250: 637–675, 1974.
22. Sanderson CJ: The mechanism of T cell mediated cytotoxicity. II. Morphological studies of cell death by time lapse microcinematography. Proc R Soc Lond [Biol] 192: 241–255, 1976.
23. Zagury D, Bernard J, Thierness N, Feldman M, Berke G: Isolation and characterisation of individual functionally reactive cytotoxic T lymphocytes: conjugation, killing and recycling at the single cell level. Eur J Immunol 5: 818–822, 1975.
24. Brunner KT, Mauel J, Rudolf H, Chapuis B: Studies of allograft immunity in mice. I. Induction, development and in vitro assay of cellular immunity. Immunology 18: 501–505, 1970.
25. Sanderson CJ, Thomas JA: The mechanism of T cell mediated cytotoxicity III. Changes in target cell susceptibility during the cell cycle. Proc R Soc Lond [Biol] 194: 417–429, 1976.
26. Sanderson CJ, Thomas JA: The mechanism of K cell (antibody dependent) cell mediated cytotoxicity. II. Characteristics of the effector cell and morphological changes in the target cell. Proc R Soc Lond [Biol] 197: 417–424, 1977.
27. Sanderson CJ, Glauert AM: The mechanism of T cell mediated cytotoxicity. V. Morphological studies by electron microscopy. Proc R Soc Lond [Biol] 198: 315–323, 1977.
28. Sanderson CJ, Glauert AM: The mechanism of T cell mediated cytotoxicity VI. T cell projections and their role in target cell killing. Immunology 36: 119–129, 1979.
29. Sanderson CJ, Thomas JA: The mechanism of T cell mediated cytotoxicity. VII. Lysis of isolated cytoplasts and karyoplasts. Immunology 37: 373–376, 1979.
30. Glauert AM, Sanderson CJ: The mechanism of K cell (antibody dependent) mediated cytotoxicity III. The ultrastructure of K cell projections and their possible role in target cell killing. J Cell Sci 35: 355–366, 1979.

9. CELL BIOLOGY OF SUBPLASMALEMMAL FILAMENTS

J.R. DE MEY

INTRODUCTION

Cells detached from a tissue and brought into tissue culture on a suitable substrate, such as a plastic petri dish or a microscope coverglass, will adhere to this substrate, and in many cases will flatten and spread out to extremely thin cells, not thicker than 1–3 μm. Depending on the cell type and the conditions of cell culture, the cells will be very motile (up to 100 μ/h) or more or less stationary. Such cells therefore provide a very convenient experimental model for investigation of the basic mechanisms underlying cell movement, from creeping over a substrate to internal streaming of cytoplasm and cell organelles, as well as the complex series of events during cell division. A better understanding of these events will eventually give us insight into how cells handle external signals across the cell membrane and control their growth and social behaviour. Only during the last ten years has it been established that all these movements are directed by a limited number of proteins which are the main components of a complex set of different types of filaments. For an excellent recent review, see Lazarides and Revel (1979) [1].

OBSERVATION OF CELL MOVEMENT BY TIME-LAPSE CINEMATOGRAPHY

A detailed discussion of the cell biology of these filaments must be preceded by a description of the sequence of events during cell movement. These events are known from time-lapse cinematography studies on living cells, in which a single cell is followed in the phase-contrast light microscope by taking a picture of it at regular intervals (Figs. 1 and 2). The movie obtained in this way can then be viewed at a speed giving an accelerated version of the events taking place during cell movement.

As cells move in a given direction, they form, towards the direction of movement, delicate, sheet-like extensions of cytoplasm, called lamellipodia, whose leading edge either remains parallel to the substrate or performs upward and backfolding movements producing what are called ruffles. Hence the name of this region: the ruffling membrane. Forward movement of the leading lamella [2] was found to be discontinuous, with phases of standstill, protrusion, and withdrawal. Thus, net advance is the result of a slight and

W.Th. Daems et al. (eds.), Cell Biological Aspects of Disease, 117–131. All rights reserved.
Copyright © 1981 by Martinus Nijhoff Publishers bv, The Hague/Boston/London.

118

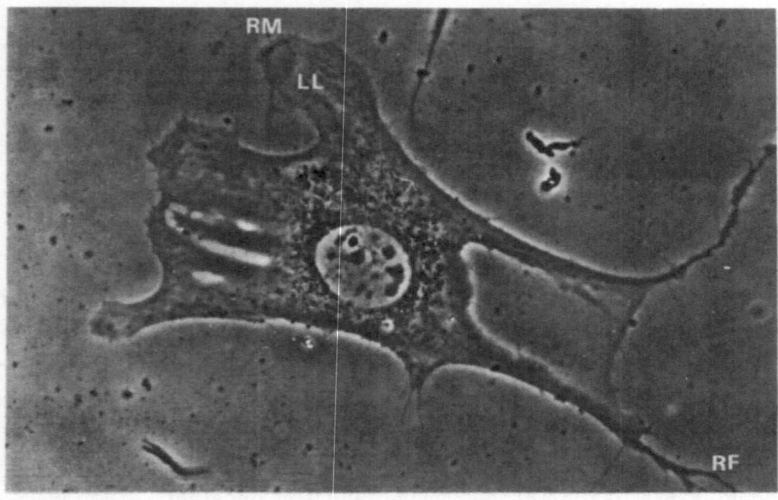

Fig. 1. Single cell growing on a plastic substrate. The cell is moving to the left. The motile pole is characterized by thin leading lamellae (LL) and zones of ruffling membrane (RM). The rear end of the cell shows retractile fibers (RF). × 500. Courtesy of Dr. M. De Brabander, Beerse, Belgium.

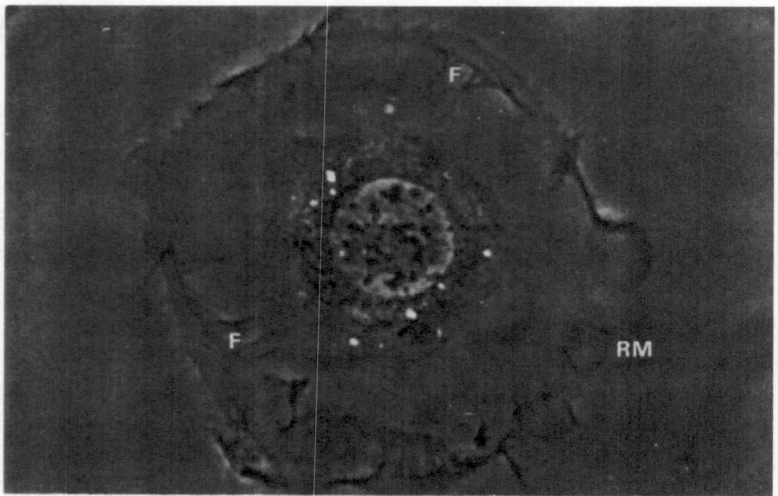

Fig. 2. A single cell 2 h after seeding on a plastic substrate. The cell is spreading actively, is not polarized, and shows ruffling membrane activity all around. Numerous filopodia (F) move freely into the medium and melt back into the cell. A few have formed new attachments and serve as spatial guides between which the membrane follows to form the leading edge (RM). × 630. Courtesy of Dr. M. De Brabander, Beerse, Belgium.

varying excess of protrusion over withdrawal. Interestingly, the formation of ruffles proved to be invariably associated with the phases of withdrawal of the leading lamella. Leading edges are normally limited to one or two regions of the cell, and are the main locomotory organs of the cell. The lamellipodium first extends forward more or less parallel to the substrate. At the level of the ruffling membrane, short finger-like extensions are formed, called filopodia (see Fig. 2). These are highly dynamic structures, capable of changing from a fluid to a rigid state in less than a second. They form spatial guides between which the cell membrane flows to form the leading edge. Newly formed filopodia wave freely in the medium and either attach themselves to the substrate and become rigid or melt back into the cell.

From electron-microscopic studies we know that cells do not simply stick to their substrate but that, instead, there are only a limited number of sites of very close contact, like a hand placed flat on a table with only the finger tips and a few other parts in contact with the table (Figs. 3 and 5). Three types of cell-substratum approach can be discerned: focal contracts, also called adhesion plaques (distance between cell and substratum: 10–15 nm); close contacts (ca. 30 nm), often surrounding focal contacts; and regions of greater separation (100–140 nm). The number of focal contacts varies with the degree of motility of the cell: more motile cells have fewer adhesion plaques [3, 4]. When one looks at moving cells with the interference-reflection microscope, one can actually see the adhesion plaques as dark spots or lines, 0.1–2.0 μm wide and 2–10 μm long (Fig. 3). Combination of this kind of microscopy with time-lapse cinematography has shown that focal contacts are stationary with respect to the substrate, and that new ones appear close to the ruffling membrane, as the cell moves forward, while more posterior focal contacts fade and disappear [5].

MICROFILAMENTS

This brings us to the first filamentous system playing a role in cell movements (Fig. 4). This system can be viewed as the cell's internal musculature and is formed by very thin (5–8 nm) and long fibres, called microfilaments [6] (Fig. 5). These filaments mostly occur just beneath the plasma membrane, and often form long, straight bundles which are visible with phase-contrast light microscopy. These bundles of microfilaments are called stress fibres.

Bundles of microfilaments can form and dissolve very rapidly. Microfilaments also often occur in the form of dense three-dimensional meshworks without any apparent organization. These meshworks are often found in rounded cells and in areas of membrane ruffling (see below), where stress fibres rarely extend (Fig. 6). The two filamentous states are believed to be

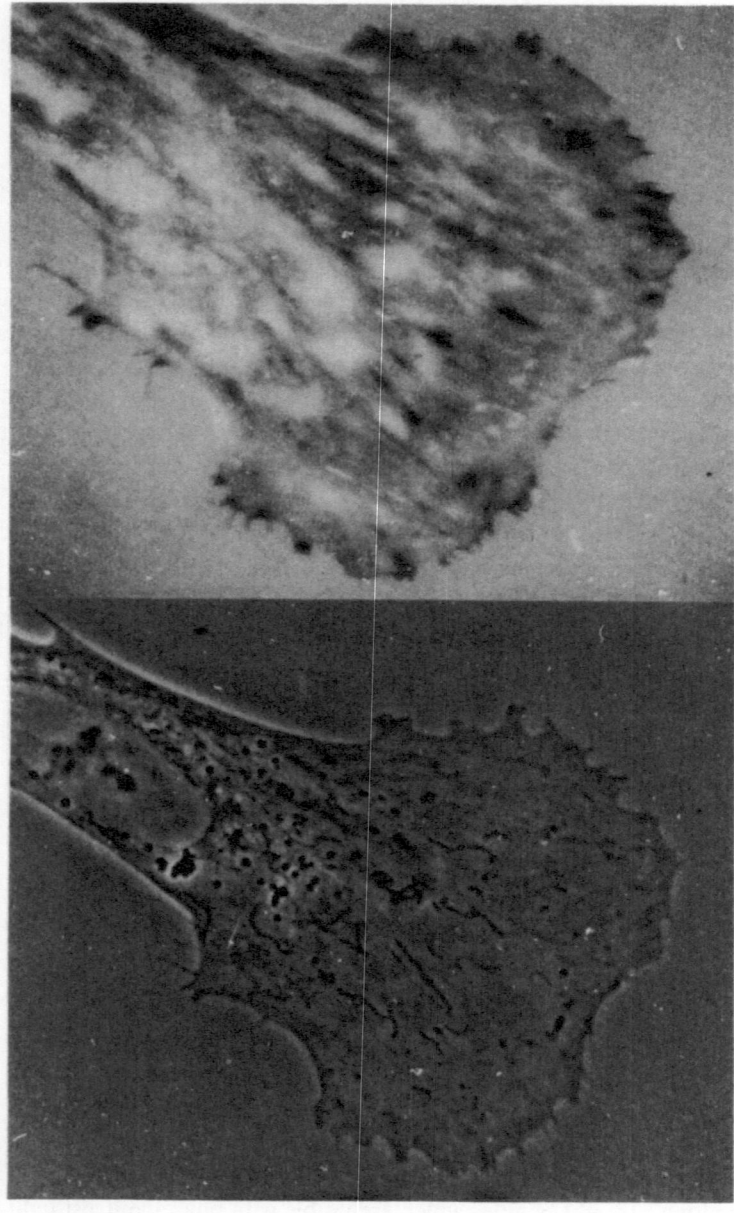

Fig. 3. Primary chick-heart fibroblast as seen in phase-contrast (left) and interference-reflection (IR) microscopy. The darker spots in the IR image represent zones of focal contact (10–15 nm), the grey zones represent regions of close contact ($\pm$ 30 nm), and the white zones indicate regions of wider separation. Courtesy of Dr. J. Heath, Strangeways Laboratories, Cambridge, England.

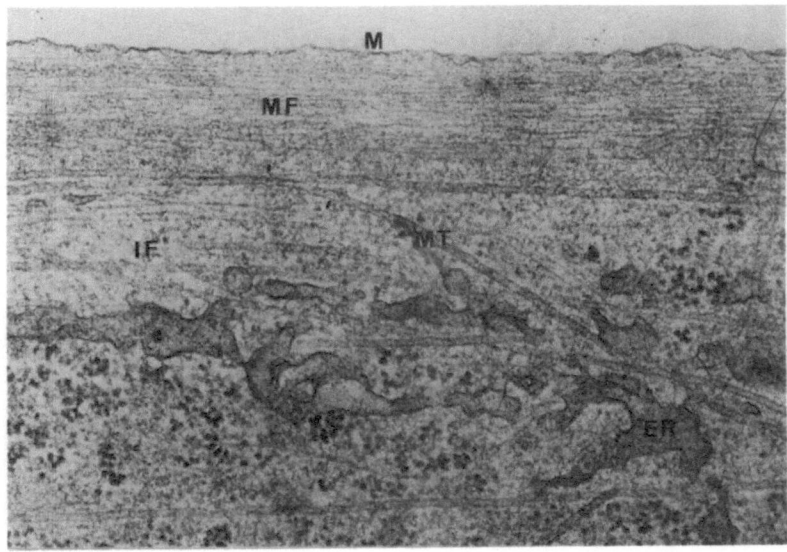

Fig. 4. Vertical section through a cell showing the different types of fibrous elements. Just beneath the plasma membrane (M) there are bundles of microfilaments (MF) lying just above microtubules (MT) and intermediate filaments (IF). Cisternae of endoplasmic reticulum (ER) and polysomes are also visible. × 46, 200. Courtesy of Dr. M. De Brabander, Beerse, Belgium.

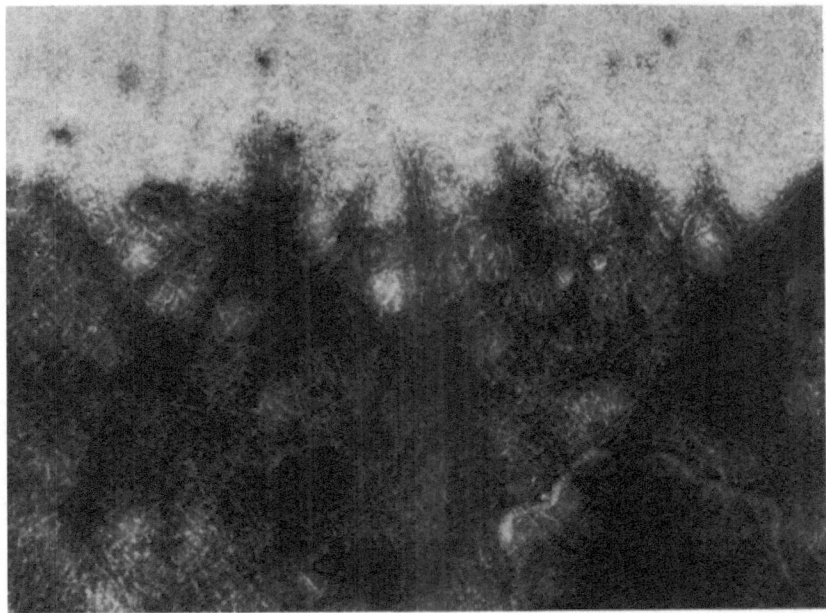

Fig. 5. Negatively stained leading edge of a Triton X-100 extracted hybrid C_1 1D/CHO fibroblast [19]. The delicate meshwork shows diagonally arranged 7–nm actin filaments occurring singly or in bundles. Courtesy of Dr. J.V. Small, Salzburg, Austria.

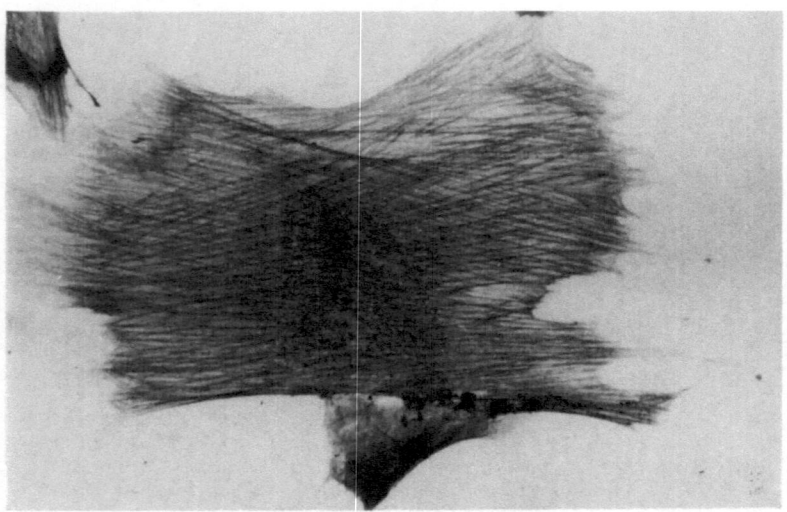

Fig. 6. Cell stained with peroxidase-labelled antibodies to myosin. Myosin is localized mainly on thick stress fibres spanning the whole length of the cell, but shorter bundles are also present.

extremes of a gradient, and the ratio between them is governed by a number of factors including the extent of cell motility, the degree of adhesion to the substrate, the particular region of the cytoplasm in which filaments occur, and the stage of the cell cycle between divisions. With the use of specific fluorescent antibodies to smooth-muscle contractile proteins such as actin, myosin, tropomyosin, and α-actinin, it has been shown that in non-muscle cells, too, microfilaments are made up of actin associated with other proteins, and that stress fibres contain in addition all the other contractile proteins, in an organization that is not yet understood (Fig. 7) [1]. Isenberg et al. [7] have shown that isolated stress fibres are capable of contracting in the presence of ATP, so that is is conceivable that they can develop tension or even be contractile in cells, and that, as in muscle, it is the interaction between myosin and actin that generates the force. It should, however, be kept in mind that no direct evidence of contractile behaviour of stress fibres has been reported yet, and it is also possible that they rather 'stretch' the cell, giving it a certain degree of stiffness.

SYNCHRONOUS FORMATION OF MICROFILAMENT BUNDLES AND ADHESION PLAQUES

In moving chicken embryo fibroblasts, it was clearly shown [3, 5] that adhesion plaques coincide with the distal ends of stress fibres, which terminate in

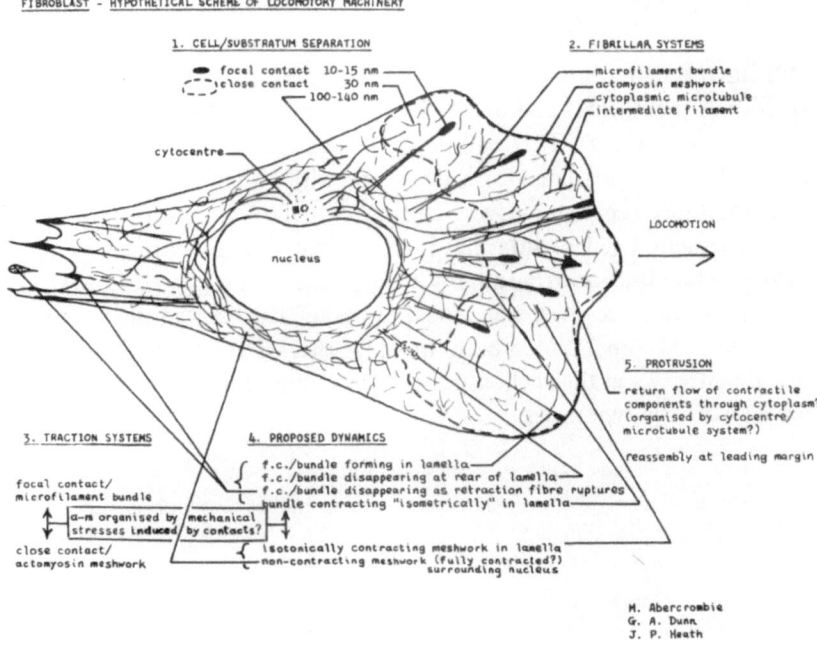

Fig. 7. Hypothetical scheme of the locomotory machinery of a fibroblast. Courtesy of Dr. J. Heath, Strangeways Laboratories, Cambridge, England.

the plasma membrane and pass posteriorly and often obliquely away from the substrate. A recent study in which thick sections were investigated by high-voltage electron microscopy showed [8] that many of these oblique stress fibres, especially those coming from the close contacts near ruffling zones, terminate close to the dorsal surface of the cell, in the perinuclear region. In cells with decreased mobility, however, both ends of a stress fibre were more frequently found to be attached to a focal contact. Furthermore, focal contacts and microfilament bundles were formed synchronously. These findings led to authors to speculate that the formation of a focal contact provides a fixed point with reference to the substrate, and this immediately enables the development of a nearly isometric contraction in the cytoplasm between the adhesion and a relatively stable fibrillar system surrounding the nucleus. Such contraction may then cause a very rapid reorganization of a loose meshwork of cytoplasmic contractile elements into a straight bundle extending from the focal contact to the perinuclear area (Fig. 7). Reorganization of this kind has been demonstrated in the case of isometric contraction in *Physarum*, a primitive slime mold [9].

124

INTERMEDIATE (10–nm) FILAMENTS

One can speculate about the nature of the relative stable fibrillar system which surrounds the nucleus and in which the oblique microfilaments spread out and terminate (Fig. 8). There is indeed a second system of filaments present in cultured cell. This system is formed by fibres with a diameter of 10 nm (Fig. 4). Immunofluorescence studies with antibodies to the major protein component of this system, i.e. vimentin, have shown that it is an extremely resistant system of bundles occurring mainly in the perinuclear region [10] and keeping the nucleus in place, even when most of the cell has been washed away with detergents. No function has been found for this system yet, and the postulation that it serves as the anchorage point for oblique microfilament bundles is only a working hypothesis.

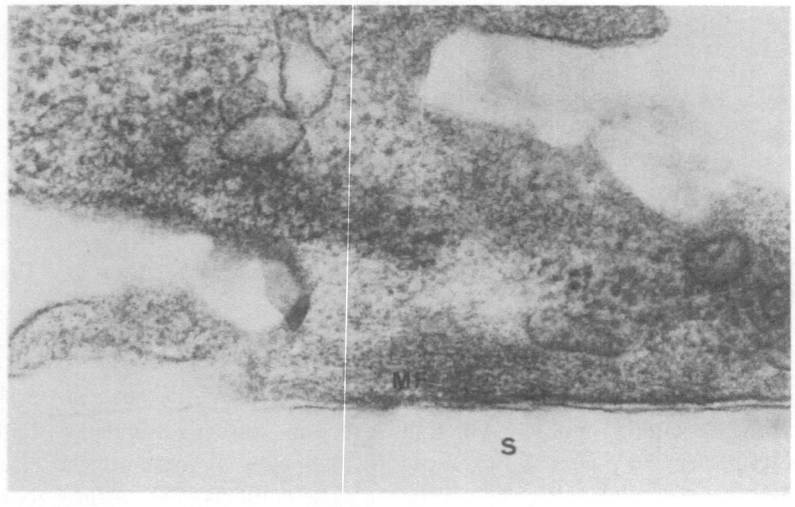

Fig. 8. Vertical section through an adhesion plaque of a cell with its substrate (S). Microfilaments (MF) ending in the plasma membrane, and the space between membrane and substrate is filled with electron-dense material probably containing extracellular fibronectin. × 74, 400. Courtesy of Dr. M. De Brabander, Beerse, Belgium.

ORGANIZATION OF ADHESION PLAQUES: THE FIBRONEXUS

The fact that adhesion plaques coincide with terminations of microfilament bundles into the cell membrane has clearly demonstrated the involvement of the cell's microfilament system in making contact and generating movement (Fig. 10). Recent findings have provided much more information about the organization of adhesion plaques [11]. It was shown with special fluorescent antibody techniques that the distribution of an extracellular fibrillar protein, called fibronectin, and of microfilaments is often coincident, which suggests a transmembrane relationship between microfilament bundles and fibronectin. Fibronectin is a large external protease-sensitive glycoprotein [12] which, when added to transformed malignant cells, causes reappearance of cell adhesiveness and readily visible stress fibres [13]. It has been thought to play a role in keeping cross-linked sulphated proteoglycans at the cell surface. In a subsequent study [14] it was shown at the electron-microscopic level of resolution that fibronectin-containing fibres meet internal microfilament bundle terminations, and this junction was called the fibronexus. Apparently, individual fibronectin-containing fibres were colinear with individual microfilaments, and the fibronexus is thus identical with the cell adhesion discussed above. Therefore, it seems that fibronectin and other proteins in the fibronexus, such as collagen, play an important role in the transmembrane organization of the state of the microfilament system. It has been clearly shown, however, that such communication across the membrane is likely to be two-way, because external fibronectin stimulates internal microfilament bundle formation, whereas breakdown of the bundles by drugs that disrupt microfilament bundles causes release of fibronectin from the cell surface [15]. For a recent review on fibronectin, I refer to reference 16.

OTHER ASPECTS OF MICROFILAMENT FUNCTION

So far I have mainly discussed the microfilament system located at the ventral side of the cell. It should be pointed out that bundles of microfilaments also occur on the dorsal surface. These bundles may play an important role in the control of lateral movement of proteins in the plane of the plasma membrane and in the mechanism by which specific protein or hormones are taken up and delivered to lysosomes [17]. It would lead us beyond the present scope to go into details of this aspect of microfilament function, but it may be as important as its role in cell locomotion and in maintaining cell shape.

MICROFILAMENT ORGANIZATION IN THE ANTERIOR EDGE OF THE LEADING LAMELLA

As we have seen in second section of this article, the most active part of the cell involved in movement is the leading edge or ruffling zone of the leading lamella. Net forward movement is the result of consective protrusion and withdrawal of the leading edge. We still know very little about the exact mechanism underlying this movement, but some advance has been made in defining the structural details of the heading edge. I shall briefly review these studies [18–21], because they can help to at least speculate on the mechanisms of leading edge motility. The leading edge contains a broad band (up to a few microns wide) of thin actin filaments organized in an intricate diagonal meshwork (Figs. 6 and 9). This meshwork often also contains variable numbers of bundles of actin filaments which project from the leading edge. Such bundles form the core of filopodia and microspikes (Fig. 10). Interestingly, transitional stages occur between the diagonal meshwork and the filament bundles. It therefore seems possible that the bundles form by a collection of the ends of individual filaments or of filament groups into foci, at the anterior edge, followed by an inwardly directed lateral aggregation of the filaments into bundles. Since such preparations show extra material at foci as well as at the tips of the filament bundles, it is possible that accessory proteins are involved in this transition (Fig. 11).

It is further speculated that advancement of the leading edge involves a polymerization of actin filaments, probably proceeding inwards from the cell membrane at specific initiation sites. An inward polymerization, bearing

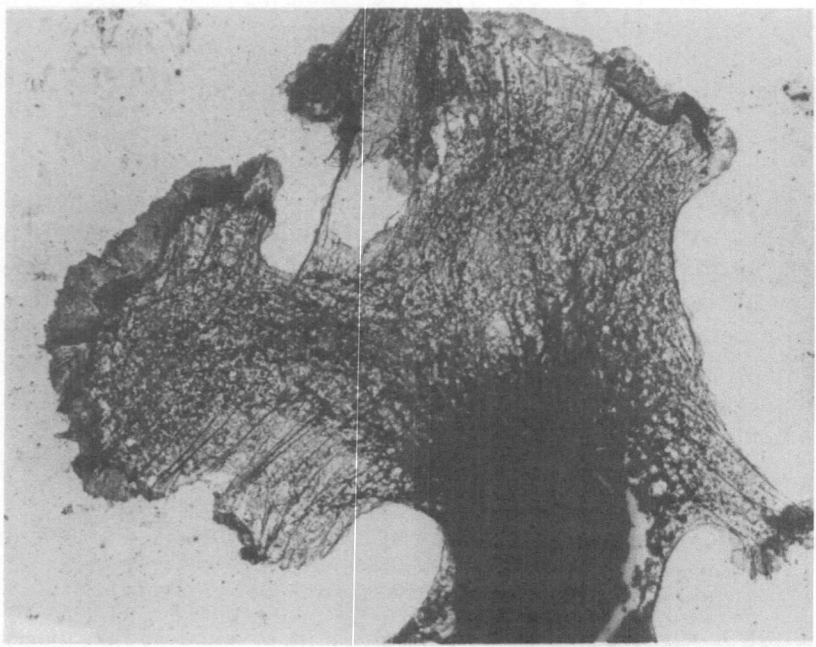

Fig. 9. Negatively stained. Triton X-100 extracted 3T3 cell showing active locomotory activity and prominent leading lamellae with leading edges containing a band of actin filaments organized in a dense meshwork. Courtesy of Dr. J.V. Small, Salzburg, Austria.

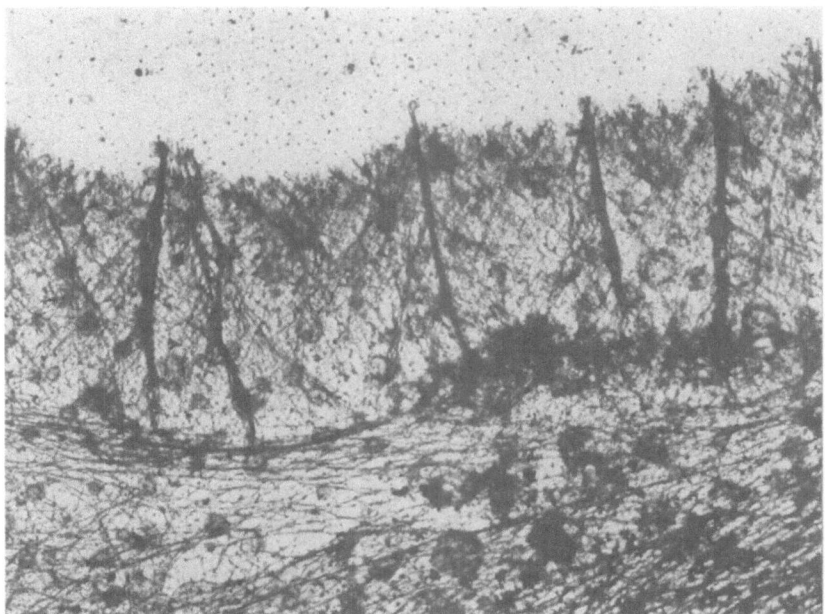

Fig. 10. Leading-edge region of a chick-heart fibroblast showing filament bundles (microspikes) embedded in the diagonal meshwork. Courtesy of Dr. J.V. Small, Salzburg, Austria.

against the inner cytoskeleton, would then produce an outward growth of the leading edge.

In sum, according to these data, the general scheme of events taking place during the various phases of withdrawal and protrusion of the leading edge could involve a controlled polymerization and depolymerization of actin (= actin recycling), coupled with a dynamic rearragement (convergence and divergence) of the filaments comprising the diagonal meshwork (see Table 1).

MICROTUBULES AND THEIR CONTRIBUTION TO DIRECTIONAL LOCOMOTION

To close this chapter on subplasmalemmal filaments, I shall now briefly discuss a very important third kind of fibrillar system: The cytoplasmic microtubular complex (Figs. 4 and 12). Microtubules are hollow tubes with a diameter of 25 nm and built up of 13 protofilaments. Tubulin is the main protein, but several microtubule-associated proteins have been described. Microtubules are very dynamic structures, and are probably continuously formed and broken down. Studies using antibodies to tubulin have shown

128

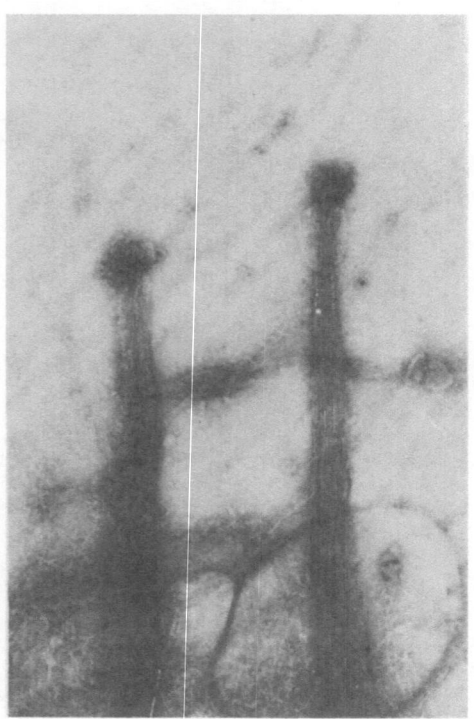

Fig. 11. Detail of the tip of negatively stained microspikes. Extra material is seen to be associated, which suggests that accessory proteins play a role in microspikes formation. Courtesy of Dr. J.V. Small, Salzburg, Austria.

Table 1. Hypothetic microfilament reorganizations in the leading edge, according to Small et al. [20].

Protrusion:	– controlled inward actin polymerization from initiation sites at the cell edge
	– actin source: recycling from actin filaments depolymerizing during withdrawal
	– convergence of actin filaments into microspikes and/or filopodia
	– role of accessary proteins
Withdrawal:	– ruffling = backwards and/or upwards folding of leading edge
	– divergence of bundles and/or depolymerization of actin filaments

that they seem to arise from a region near the nucleus and form an elaborate meshwork of fine bundles of microtubules in the cytoplasm [22, 23]. Antimicrotubule drugs such as colchicine or the vinca alkaloids prevent the polymerization of tubulin into microtubules and have been very useful in studies to determine the function of microtubules. It would take us beyond the scope of this course to try to discuss all of the cellular functions in which

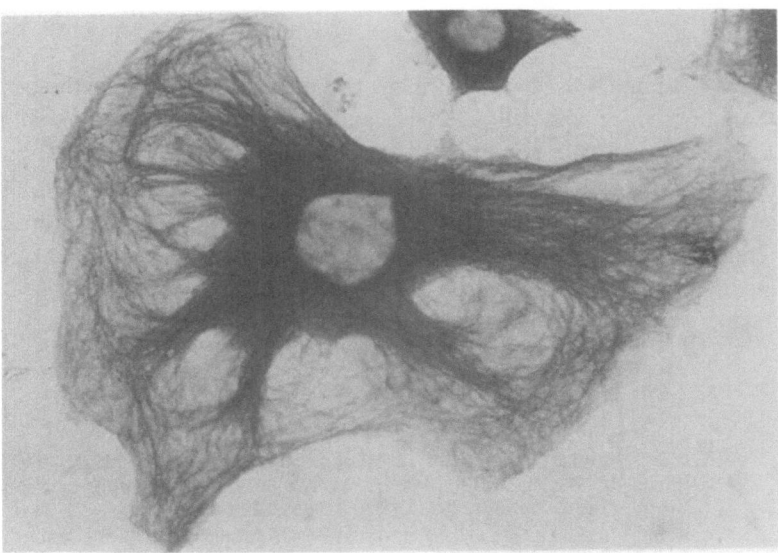

Fig. 12. Cell stained with peroxidase-labelled antibodies to tubulin. Bundles of microtubules radiate out from the nuclear region and form meshworks at the cell edges.

microtubules are involved. I will limit myself here to the role of the micro-tubules in cell locomotion and its probable interaction with the microfilament system. For a very comprehensive review on microtubules, see reference 24.

Treatment of cultured cells with microtubule inhibitors alters the shape that the cells display in the horizontal plane. As we have already seen, in untreated cells the ruffling membrane is mainly confined to one pole of the cell, at the leading edge, while the rear part trails behind. This gives the cell a polarized appearance, which is the result of cell migration in one main direction. Cells treated with microtubule inhibitors remain flat and especially the peripheral parts of the cell remain spread as thin lamellae over the substrate, but the pattern of movement is altered: ruffling membrane activity appears all over the cell periphery. This causes the loss of the polarized shape and of the cell's capacity to migrate in one main direction [25]. It can there-fore be postulated that microtubules play a regulatory role by dividing the contractile microfilament system into parts, some of which are involved in leading-edge formation, and thus give the cell its polarized shape, not merely as a rigid cytoskeleton, but by endowing the cell with the capacity to move in one main direction [26].

130

CONCLUSION

From this limited review, I hope it has become clear that the cell is much more than a bag filled with cell organelles and surrounded with a cell membrane. Each cell has a very complicated set of different types of filaments which seem to play major roles in the coordinated transduction of information, across the membrane, to specific parts of the cytoplasm. However, much remains to be learned about the biochemical and molecular biological mechanisms by which all these activities are made possible.

REFERENCES

1. Lazarides E, Revel JP: The molecular basis of cell movement. Sci Am 240: 88–100, 1979.
2. Abercrombie M, Heaysman JEM, Pegrum SM: The locomotion of fibroblasts in culture. I. Movements of the leading edge. Exp Cell Res 59: 393–398, 1970.
3. Abercrombie M, Dunn GA: Adhesions of fibroblasts to substratum during contact inhibition observed by interference reflexion microscopy. Exp Cell Res 92: 57–62, 1975.
4. Rees DA, Lloyd CW, Thom D: Control of grip and stick in cell adhesion through lateral relationships of membrane glycoproteins. Nature (London) 267: 124–128, 1977.
5. Izzard CS, Lochner L: Cell-to-substrate contacts in living fibroblasts: an interference-reflexion study with an evaluation of the technique. J Cell Sci 21: 129–159, 1976.
6. Buckley IK, Porter KR: Cytoplasmic fibers in living cultured cells. A light and electron microscopic study. Protoplasma 64: 349–380, 1967.
7. Isenberg G, Rothke PC, Hübmann N, Franke NW, Wohlfarth-Bottermann KE: Cytoplasmic actomyosin fibers in tissue culture cells. Direct proof of contractility by visualization of ATP-induced contraction in fibers isolated by laser microbeam dissection. Cell Tissue Res 166: 427–443, 1976.
8. Heath JP, Dunn GA: Cell to substratum contacts of chick fibroblasts and their relation to the microfilament system. A correlated interference-reflexion and high-voltage electron-microscope study. J Cell Sci 29: 197–212, 1978.
9. Fleisher M, Wohlfarth-Bottermann KE: Correlation between tension force generation, fibrillogenesis and ultrastructure of cytoplasmic actomyosin during isometric and isotonic contractions of protoplasmic strands. Cytobiologie 10: 339–365, 1975.
10. Hynes RO, Destree AT: 10 nm filaments in mormal and transformed cells. Cell 13: 151–163, 1978.
11. Hynes RO, Destree AT: Relationships between fibronectin (LETS protein) and actin. Cell 15: 875–886, 1978.
12. Hynes RO: Alteration of cell-surface proteins by viral transformation and by proteolysis. Proc Natl Acad Sci USA 70: 3170–3174, 1973.
13. Ali IV, Mautner V, Lanza R, Hynes RO: Restoration of normal morphology, adhesion and cytoskeleton in transformed cells by addition of a transformation sensitive surface protein. Cell 11: 115–126, 1977.
14. Singer I: The fibronexus: a transmembrane association of fibronectin-containing fibers and bundles of 5 nm microfilaments in hamster and human fibroblasts. Cell 16: 675–685, 1979.
15. Kurkinen M, Wartiovaara J, Vaheri A: Cytochalasin B release a major surface-associated glycoprotein, fibronectin from cultured fibroblasts. Exp Cell Res 111: 127–137, 1978.
16. Lloyd C: Fibronectin: a function at the junction. Nature 279: 473–474, 1979.
17. Anderson R, Vasile E, Mello R, Brown M, Goldstein J: Immunocytochemical visualization of coated pits and vesicles in human fibroblasts: relation to low density lipoprotein receptor distribution. Cell 15: 919–933, 1978.

18. Spooner BS, Yamada KM, Wessells NK: Microfilaments and cell locomotion. J Cell Biol 49: 595–613, 1971.
19. Small JV, Celis JE: Filament arrangements in negatively stained cultured cells: the organization of actin. Cytobiology 16: 308–325, 1978.
20. Small JV, Isenberg G, Celis JE: Polarity of actin at the leading edge of cultured cells. Nature (London) 272: 638–639, 1978.
21. Isenberg G, Small JV, Kreutzberg G: Correlation between actin polymerization and surface receptor segregation in neuroblastoma cells treated with concanavalin A. J Neurocytol 7: 649–661, 1978.
22. Weber K, Pollack R, Biebring T: Antibody against tubulin: the specific visualization of cytoplasmic microtubules in tissue culture cells. Proc Natl Acad Sci USA 72: 459–463, 1975.
23. De Brabander M, De Mey J, Goniau M, Geuens G: Immunocytochemical visualization of microtubules and tubulin at the light and electron-microscopic level. J Cell Sci 28: 283–301, 1977.
24. Dustin P: Microtubules. Berlin, Springer, 1978.
25. De Brabander M, Van de Veire R, Aerts F, Borgers M, Janssen P: The effects of methyl [5-(2-thienyl-carbonyl)-1H-benzimidamidazol-2-yl] carbamate (R 17 934; NCS 238159), a new synthetic antitumoral drug interfering with microtubules on mammalian cells cultured in vitro. Cancer Res 36: 905–916, 1976.
26. De Brabander M, De Mey J, Van de Veire R, Aerts F, Geuens G: Microtubules in mammalian cell shape and surface modulation: an alternative hypothesis. Cell Biol Int Rep 1: 453–461, 1977.

10. REGENERATION DYNAMICS OF THE PLASMALEMMA AND ITS INVAGINATIONS

K.-E. WOHLFARTH-BOTTERMANN

Many cell biological phenomena based on the activity of the cell surface can be favorably studied in free-living cells, e.g., amebae or acellular slime molds. In these as in other cells, the plasma membrane is involved in such important processes as pinocytosis and phagocytosis as well as in cell locomotion. Because cell locomotion is a complex phenomenon that cannot be analyzed without considering the role of the plasmalemma, much of the available information concerns the dynamics of the plasmalemma in proto-

DYNAMICS OF PLASMALEMMA REGENERATION

Restoration of the plasmalemma

Protoplasmic veins are constituents of the plasmodia of acellular slime molds [1], have a diameter of 0.1–2.0 mm, and represent a multinuclear mass of cytoplasm. An ectoplasmic tube envelops a central core in which the low viscous endoplasm is transported (Fig. 1a and b). The ectoplasmic tube is characterized by a complicated system of plasmalemma invaginations [2, 3]. When this tube is punctured with a glass needle, a drop of endoplasm (diameter 0.5–2.0 mm) is pressed out by the vein. When this drop, which contains many nuclei, is isolated from the vein and subcultured under appropriate conditions, it transforms into a new plasmodium. This phenomenon makes it possible to determine how the plasmalemma is regenerated and which morphogenetic events are responsible for the regeneration of the plasmalemma invagination system.

At a drop age of 0 s (Fig. 2), fine-structural investigation [4] reveals that the margin of the cytoplasm is not surrounded by a plasmalemma, but 10 s later this surface is covered by a new membrane. Figure 2 shows the de novo formation of the plasmalemma: numerous vacuoles, which are always present in the flowing endoplasm, move to the drop surface (Fig. 2, age: 1 s), and begin to fuse in a lateral direction (Fig. 2, age: 2 s). As a result, approximately 3 s after drop generation, the surface is bordered by two membranes. The

W.Th. Daems et al. (eds.), Cell Biological Aspects of Disease, 133–143. All rights reserved.
Copyright © 1981 by Martinus Nijhoff Publishers bv, The Hague/Boston/London.

134

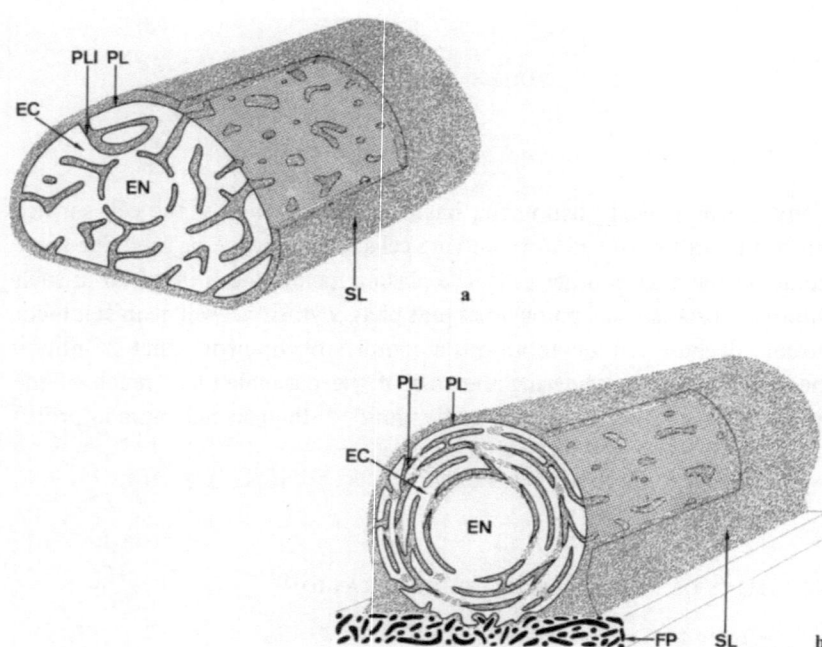

Fig. 1a and b. Plasmalemma invaginations as characteristic constituents of the ectoplasmic tube of protoplasmic veins of *Physarum polycephalum*; (a) in small veins, (b) in large veins [2]. EN, endoplasmic channel; EC, ectoplasmic tube; PLI, plasmalemma invagination; PL, plasmalemma; SL, slime layer; FP, filter paper.

outer membrane (Fig. 2, 3 s, dVM) is discarded together with remnants of dispersed cytoplasm and cell organelles, whereas the inner membrane (Fig. 2, 3 s, pVM) represents the newly formed plasmalemma (Fig. 2, 6 s, p). The velocity of this regeneration, which is accomplished within 6 s, is remarkable. The biological importance of this velocity is obvious, because a naked cytoplasm cannot survive in a nonphysiological environment. This plasmalemma regeneration in a free-living organism shows that biomembranes of a vesicular nature can be transformed into a plasmalemmal structure, and that biomembranes can perform morphological transformations within a time-range of seconds.

Morphogenesis of plasmalemma invaginations

After the regeneration of the plasmalemma as described in the protoplasmic drop performs a series of morphogenetic transformations [5] among which the reconstitution of plasmalemma invaginations is of special interest

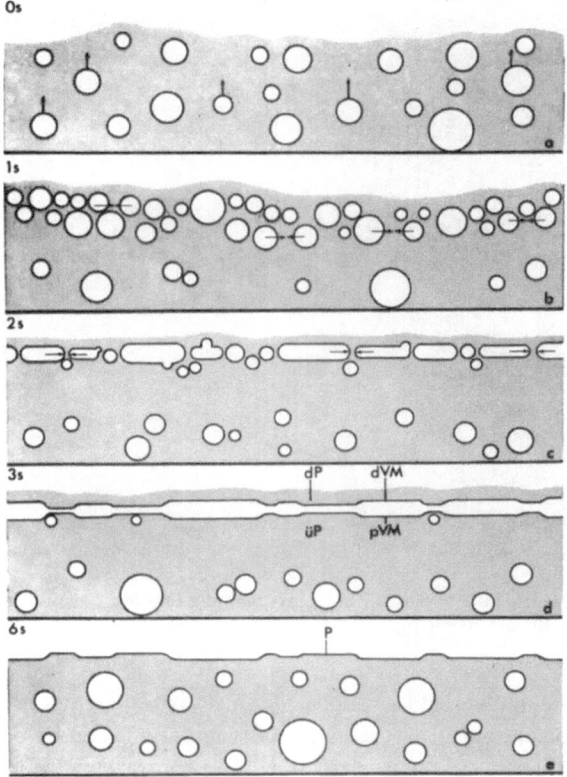

Fig. 2a–e. Regeneration of the plasmalemma in protoplasmic drops of *Physarum* (age: 0–6 s). dP, degenerated and extruded cytoplasm; üP, surviving cytoplasm; dVM, distal, and pVM, proximal membrane of the vesicles fusing in picture c; P, newly formed plasmalemma. Arrows show the direction of movement of the vacuoles in b and c during the fusion process [4].

in this context [6]. Figure 3 shows four stages of this regeneration process (0, 5, 10, and 20 min drop age). In the drop-age period from 0 to 5 min, the small vacuoles, some of which have reconstituted the plasmalemma (compare Fig. 2), fuse to form larger vacuoles (Fig. 3, 5min). At the same time, the reconstituted plasmalemma first shows small indentations. The 10-min-old drops already have deep infoldings of the plasmalemma (Fig. 3). Experimental investigations employing marker substances have shown that the newly formed area of the invaginated plasmalemma is additionally increased by fusion of intracellular vacuoles with true invaginations. This means that the plasmalemma invaginations (Fig. 3, 20 min) are only partially reconstituted by the original plasmalemma membrane; a considerable contribution is made by intracellular vacuoles which extend the invaginations by fusion with

136

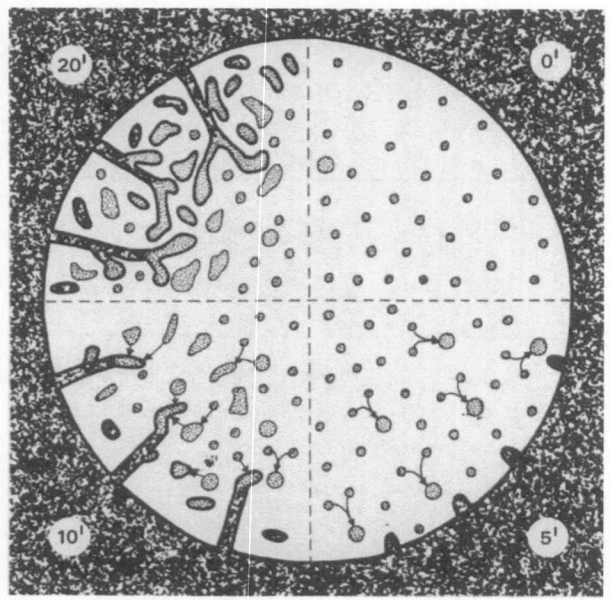

Fig. 3. De novo formation of plasmalemma invaginations in protoplasmic drops of *Physarum*, drop ages: 0, 5, 10, and 20 min [6].

the true plasmalemmal indentations. Quantitative and temporal information about the formation of plasmalemmal invaginations can be obtained from morphometric measurements performed on protoplasmic drops from age 0 min to 60 min (Fig. 4). The results show that 80% of the total amount of interior membranes of light-microscopic size appears within the first 10 min, that the plasmalemmal invaginations lead to a four- to fivefold enlargement of the drop surface, that 5-mM caffeine inhibits the formation of invaginations for 20–30 min, and that this caffeine effect is completely reversible.

The plasmalemmal invaginations in drops (Fig. 3, 20 min) as well as in veins (Fig. 1b) form an extensive extracellular labyrinth with deeply penetrating pockets. The lumen of these invaginations is relatively small. This raises the question of whether they should be regarded, from the standpoint of cell physiology, as an extracellular space within the cell body or whether their interior parts have a closer resemblance functionally to an intracellular compartment, physiologically comparable with the lumen of an endoplasmic reticulum.

Quantitatively, the size of the invagination system in *Physarum* is correlated with the nutritional content of the substrate [3]. The invaginations seem to be concerned with the uptake of nonparticulate food substances. However, the deepest pockets, which immediately surround the streaming

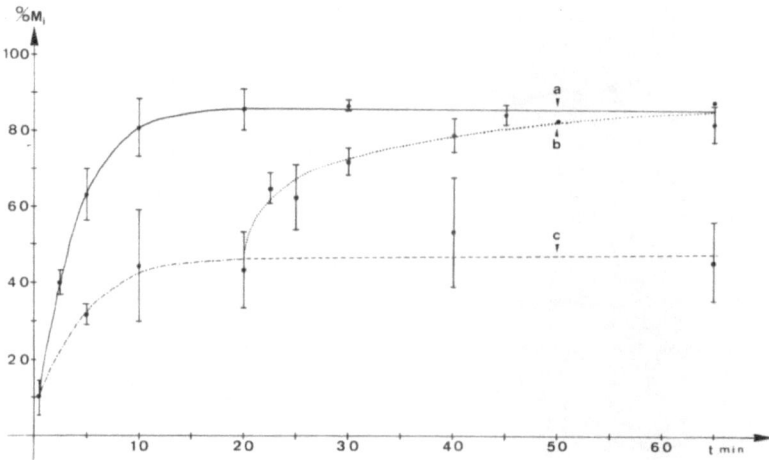

Fig. 4. Morphometric quantitation of time-dependent de novo formation of light-microscopically visible plasmalemma invaginations in normal (curve a) and caffeine-treated drops (curve c) of *Physarum*. Curve b: Effect of drug removal at a drop age of 20 min. Abscissa: drop age in minutes; ordinate: percentage of interior membranes (M_i) in relation to the total amount of membranes (M_i + outer drop profile) [6].

endoplasmic core (Fig. 1), may also have other but still unknown cell physiological functions. Their main function may be related to plasmodial oscillatory contraction activity (for reviews, see refs. 5, 6).

PINOCYTOSIS

Morphology of phenomena

Endocytosis includes pinocytosis and phagocytosis [14]. These phenomena and their function will be discussed thoroughly in other chapters of this book. These processes must be considered in the context of the regeneration dynamics of the plasmalemma, because endocytosis, i.e., intake of peripheral plasmalemma and vesiculation of the endocytotic channel, results in a decrease of the area of the outer plasmalemma and must be compensated for. Otherwise, the plasmalemma surface of the cell would continuously diminish. Figure 5 gives a schematic representation of the phenomenon of induced pinocytosis in *Amoeba proteus* [7, 14]. In these cells the invagination of the plasmalemma, i.e., the formation of pinocytotic channels, is brought about by two simultaneously occurring processes, namely, indentation of the plasmalemma and protrusion of a pseudopod. As shown by differential

138

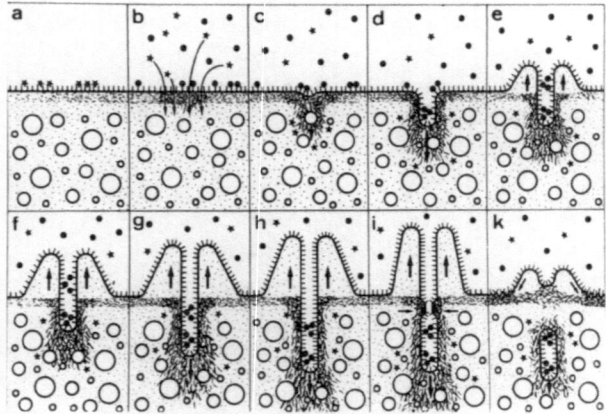

Fig. 5a–k. Successive stages of induced pinocytosis in *Amoeba proteus*; a: situation before activation; b–d: activation of actin filaments and formation of a plasmalemma invagination; e–h: elongation of the pinocytotic channel by extension of hyaline pseudopodia; i–k: vesiculation of the pinocytotic channel and retraction of the pseudopod [7].

interference contrast and phase-contrast microscopy, invagination and pseudopod formation occur in combination (Fig. 5e–i). Only the intra-cellular part of the pinocytotic channel is pinched off (Fig. 5i–k), and this is followed by a retraction of the short-lived pseudopodium (Fig. 5k).

Motive force generation

There is no doubt that cytoplasmic actomyosins deliver the traction force for the invagination process (Fig. 5c–i) as well as for pseudopod formation (Fig. 5e–i) and retraction (Fig. 5k). Presumably these actomyosins are also in-volved in the pinching off of the pinocytotic channel (Fig. 5i–k). Actin filaments insert on the plasmalemma, probably via anchoring molecules such as α-actinin, and this, in combination with the action of oligomeric cyto-plasmic myosin, may be responsible for many movement phenomena of the plasmalemma. At present much research is being done on plasmalemma movements induced by microfilaments [8]. However, the development of a direct tension force between plasmalemma and a cortical layer of cytoplasmic actomyosin (Fig. 5d–f) is only one possible explanation of membrane move-ments. Two other possibilities could explain motility phenomena of the plasmalemma: sliding of the plasmalemma over a stationary cortical acto-myosin network, and the plasmalemma itself moving under its own self-generated motive force, the membrane containing integral proteins resem-bling actin and myosin. Both of these possibilities are under study, and the provisional results indicate that they must be taken into account.

The involvement of cytoplasmic actomyosin in the formation of plasma-lemma invaginations has been established not only in amebae (Fig. 5), but also in *Physarum* (Fig. 1b). In the latter organism, the cytoplasmic acto-myosin fibrils reach light-microscopic dimensions [1], and their insertion on plasmalemma infoldings does not favor another functional interpretation. It would take us beyond the scope of this presentation to discuss motive force generation of plasmalemma motility in detail.

DYNAMICS OF PLASMALEMMA BEHAVIOR IN LOCOMOTING CELLS

Behavior of the plasmalemma

In addition to the main theme of this conference dealing with the importance of endocytotic phenomena in pathology, I should like to point to the im-portance of plasmalemma behavior in locomoting cells in relation to tumor research. The plasmalemma, the cortical cell region, and the locomotive behavior of cells seem to play a decisive role in metastasis [9]. This pathogenic phenomenon justifies all efforts to analyze the basic mechanisms of cell locomotion.

The plasmalemma can be involved in locomotion in very different ways [10, 11] and therefore knowledge gained from one cell type cannot be applied to other cells. Figure 6 shows the divergent behavior of cell membranes in different species of amebae. Three types are distinguished as follows: (1) The plasmalemma glides symmetrically over the ectoplasmic tube, thus steadily accompanying the lengthening of a pseudopod (*Proteus-Chaos* type, Fig. 6a). Because the ectoplasmic tube remains stationary relative to the substrate, there is a shearing movement between plasmalemma and ectoplasm. The velo-city of the forward movement of the plasmalemma is identical with the loco-motion velocity of the cell. (2) A rolling motion is found in the *Vannella-Hyalodiscus* type (Fig. 6b). The plasmalemma and underlying ectoplasm appear to glide over the dorsal cell surface with a velocity twice as high as the velocity of locomotion. (3) The walking motion of amebae (Fig. 6c, *Vam-pyrella* type) is characterized by the extension of pseudopods, their adherence to the substrate, and their subsequent retraction. During pseudopod retrac-tion (contraction), the cell is pulled forward in the desired direction of loco-motion. This type resembles the mode of movement in cultured cells of vertebrates. We have, however, only scanty knowledge concerning the move-ment behavior of the plasmalemma in locomoting cells during tissue culture.

The three examples given above show that plasmalemma behavior during

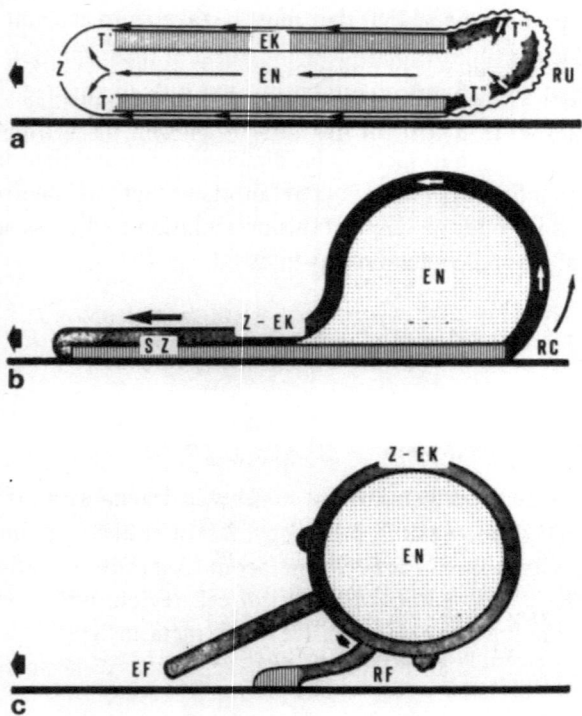

Fig. 6a–c. Plasmalemma behavior in three species of amebae during locomotion [10, 11]. (a) *Proteus-Chaos* type (streaming motion); (b) Vannella-Hyalodiscus type (rolling motion); (c) *Vampyrella* type (walking motion). Hatched areas: stationary ectoplasm (EK); dark gray: nonstationary ectoplasmic components; EN, endoplasm; thick arrows: direction of locomotion.

(a) *Streaming motion*: Maximal motion activity is in the endoplasm (large arrows). Endoplasm begins to stream in the uroid (RU) after transformation from ectoplasm, and stops in the anterior region. Here (T'), it is again transformed into ectoplasm in a second transformation process. The plasmalemma glides symmetrically over the ectoplasmic tube, thus following the elongation of the pseudopod. The contractile ectoplasmic tube constricts, thus generating within the endoplasmic channel a hydraulic pressure gradient between the front and uroid regions. The endoplasm, being less viscous than the ectoplasm, follows this pressure gradient and streams to the open end of the tube, elongating the tube by transforming itself into ectoplasm. EN, quickly streaming endoplasm; EK, ectoplasm; T', zone of EN→EK-transformation; T', zone of EK→EN transformation; RU, retracting uroid; Z, cell surface (plasmalemma).

(b) *Rolling motion*: The maximal motion activity is represented by the gliding of the dorsal cell surface (Z-EK). The gliding rate is double the velocity of locomotion. Motive force is probably generated in the shearing zone between the lower and upper cell surface complexes in the lamellipodium. EN, endoplasm, which performs (1) an unidirectional movement in the direction of locomotion (*Vannella*), or (2) a rolling movement (*Hyalodiscus*). RC, retracting caudal region; SZ, shearing zone in the lamellipodium; Z-EK, cell-surface complex (plasmalemma with underlying ectoplasm).

(c) *Walking motion*: The maximal motion activity is represented by the formation and retraction of filopodia. The cell body shows no distinct motion activity. EN, endoplasm; Z-EK, cell surface complex; EF, expanding filopodium; RF, retracting (contracting) filopodium.

cell locomotion is a highly dynamic phenomenon. One question of interest at present is whether the motive force for plasmalemma movements results from the underlying actomyosin network (possibly related to actin transformations [12]), or whether the plasmalemma itself contains actin- and/or myosin-like proteins. The latter situation would mean that the plasmalemma is able to produce its own motive force. A series of phenomena that cannot be cited here support this hypothesis.

Intracellular plasmalemma membrane turnover

As described in the section on *Morphology of phenomena*, all endocytotic processes lead to a diminution of the area of the outer plasmalemma surface of the cell. This decrease in the surface area must be compensated for by the creation of new plasmalemma, especially in those cases where pinocytosis is a permanent phenomenon bound to locomotion. Permanent pinocytosis in amebae has been shown to be a continuous uptake of cell membrane during locomotion and an inherent phenomenon in the normal migration behavior of these cells [13, 14]. Quantitative investigations [7, 15] revealed that approximately 35% of the total plasmalemma surface of *Amoeba proteus* is internalized in this way within 4–5 h (Fig. 7, lower part). In other words, the

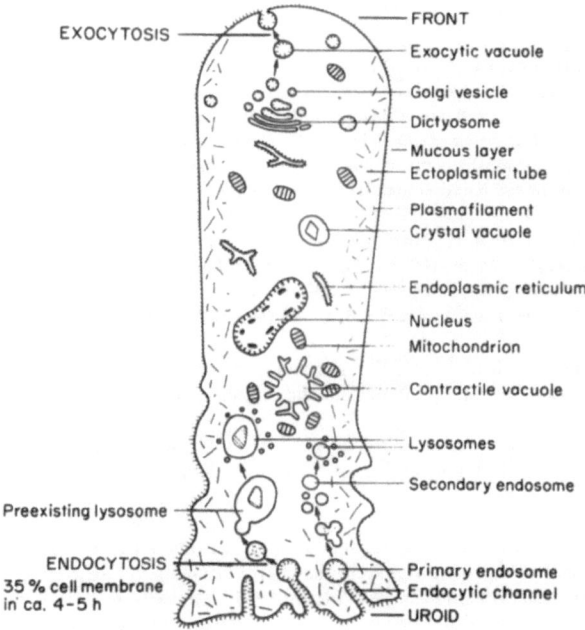

Fig. 7. Membrane turnover during permanent endocytosis in migrating *Amoeba proteus* and the regeneration of outer plasmalemma surface by exocytosis [1, 15].

plasmalemma surface of these cells is completely renewed within half a day. The newly formed membrane is produced by dictyosomes in the form of Golgi vesicles. The Golgi vesicles, whose inner surface is covered by the mucous cell coat, join the outer plasmalemma by exocytosis, and the loss of outer-membrane area by permanent pinocytosis is thereby continuously compensated for (Fig. 7, upper part). During induced pinocytosis, the rate of membrane turnover is much higher (2% of the plasmalemma surface/min), but restricted to a duration of 15–30 min.

In sum, we must take into account a certain degree of permanent membrane turnover of the plasmalemma. This turnover may be of importance for maintenance of the function of the cell coat, which perhaps also requires a certain continuous renewal. This renewal is certainly important especially for free-living cells such as protozoans, which must adapt to varying conditions of their surroundings. Recent research on mammalian cells has, however, revealed that the plasmalemma should also be considered as a highly dynamic and partially ephemeral structure whose behavior is of great importance not only for many phenomena of general cell biology but also for cellular pathology.

REFERENCES

1. Komnick H, Stockem W, Wohlfarth-Bottermann KE: Cell motility: mechanisms in protoplasmic streaming and ameboid movement. Int Rev Cytol 34: 169–249, 1973.
2. Wohlfarth-Bottermann KE: Plasmalemma invaginations as characteristic constituents of plasmodia of *Physarum polycephalum*. J Cell Sci 16: 23–27, 1974.
3. Achenbach F, Naib-Mayani W, Wohlfarth-Bottermann KE: Plasmalemma invaginations of *Physarum* dependent on the nutritional content of the plasmodial environment. J Cell Sci 36: 355–359, 1979.
4. Wohlfarth-Botterman KE, Stockem W: Die Regeneration des Plasmalemmas von *Physarum polycephalum*. Wilhelm Roux Archiv Entwicklungsmech Org 164: 321–340, 1970.
5. Götz von Olenhusen K, Jücker H, Wohlfarth-Bottermann KE: Induction of a plasmodial stage of *Physarum* without plasmalemma invaginations. Cell Tissues Res 197: 463–477, 1979.
6. Achenbach F, Achenbach U, Wohlfarth-Bottermann KE: Plasmalemma invaginations, contraction and locomotion in normal and caffeine-treated protoplasmic drops of *Physarum*. Eur J Cell Biol 20: 12–23, 1979.
7. Klein H-P, Stockem W: Pinocytosis and locomotion of amoebae: XII. Dynamic and motive force generation during induced pinocytosis in *A. proteus*. Cell Tissue Res 197: 263–279, 1979.
8. Bray D: Membranes movements and microfilaments. Nature 273: 265–266, 1978.
9. Sträuli P, Weiss L; Cell locomotion and tumor penetration. Eur J Cancer 13: 1–12, 1977.
10. Haberey M, Hülsmann N: Vergleichende mikrokinematographische Untersuchungen an 4 Amöbenspezies. Protistologica 9: 247–254, 1973.
11. Hülsmann N, Haberey M; Phenomena of amoeboid movement: behavior of the cell surface in *Hyalodiscus simplex* Wohlfarth-Bottermann. Acta Protozool 12: 71–82, 1973.
12. Isenberg G, Wohlfarth-Bottermann KE: Transformation of cytoplasmic actin. Cell Tissue Res 173: 495–528, 1976.

13. Wohlfarth-Bottermann KE: Licht- und elektronenmikroskopische Untersuchungen an der Amöbe *Hyalodiscus simplex* n.sp. Protoplasma 52: 58–107, 1960.
14. Stockem W, Wohlfarth-Bottermann KE: Pinocytosis (endocytosis). In: Lima-De-Faria A (ed) Handbook of molecular cytology. Amsterdam, North-Holland, 1969, pp 1373–1400.
15. Stockem W: Membrane-turnover during locomotion of *Amoeba proteus*. Acta Protozool 11: 83–94, 1972.

11. PATHOLOGY OF CELL MOTILITY

B.A. AFZELIUS

MACHINERIES FOR CELL MOTILITY

Students of cell motility searching for a biochemical machinery responsible for the motility found not one but two. One of these machineries is based on microfilaments, which consist essentially of actin but have associated myosin (and other proteins); and the other system on the microtubules, which are composed essentially of tubulin but also may have associated dynein molecules. One of these systems may be specialized for pulling and the other for pushing movements, and they may be activated by different substances. If this concept is true, the cell can be said to have two types of 'cell muscles', analogous with the body having two types of muscle—flexors and extensors. The microtubules have an ultrastructure which seems suitable for resisting compression, and they may be the likely candidates for any pushing movements, whereas the microfilaments probably exert a pulling force.

Since microfilaments and microtubules are present in virtually all types of cell in the animal or human body, actin and tubulin can be extracted from cells of any type. The richest source of actin is the muscle; that of tubulin is the nervous system. In the neurons there are microtubules (also called neurotubules) along which there is a transport of material, an axonal flow. The axons contain a large number of microtubules with no apparent organization. Large amounts of tubulin are also present in the testis, where each sperm tail contains a well-known 'axoneme' consisting of nine microtubular doublets around two central microtubular singlets (the $9+2$ organelle) (see Fig. 1). Cilia have axonemes of the same $9+2$ structure.

The mechanism underlying ciliary movement (and sperm motility) has been explored in great detail [1, 2]. The bending movements of the cilium and sperm tail (sperm flagellum) are due to a sliding of the nine microtubular doublets relative to one another, and this sliding is effected by work performed by the so-called dynein-arms [3]. Dynein, like myosin, is an ATPase [4]. The mechanism underlying saltatory movements of particles along nerve axons or within the cytoplasm of other cells is a matter of speculation. It has been suggested that the cytoplasmic microtubules may be associated with a dynein-like protein which kicks the particles along the microtubules.

W.Th. Daems et al. (eds.), Cell Biological Aspects of Disease, 145–150. All rights reserved.
Copyright © 1981 by Martinus Nijhoff Publishers bv, The Hague/Boston/London.

PATHOLOGY OF MICROFILAMENTS

It is possible to interfere with the microfilament system of a cell by treating it with drugs such as cytochalasin B or to interfere with the microtubular system with colchicine, vincristine, or other substances, but the action of these drugs is not specific. A better insight into the importance of the microfilamentous or microtubular systems can be obtained by examination of mutants affecting one or another of these two components specifically. Such mutants can be produced in microorganisms such as the unicellular *Chlamydomonas* (see, e.g., ref. 5), but can also be found in man.

A single disorder which seems to be explained by a dysfunctioning of the contractile proteins in the neutrophil leukocytes has been described in man [6]. The patient in question showed an abnormality in the neutrophil behavior and fewer than the normal number of microfilaments and pseudopods in the neutrophils. It is unlikely that all of the cells in the body were equally affected, because, if they had been, the patient would have died at an early embryonic age.

The various forms of inborn muscular atrophy are also likely to be organ-specific rather than generalized, and may not involve the contractile system as such.

PATHOLOGY OF THE CYTOPLASMIC MICROTUBULES

Certain diseases are believed to be caused by a mutation affecting the micro-tubules. This holds for the Chediak-Higashi syndrome, which has been studied more intensively than other microtubular diseases. This syndrome is a disease of man, but animal models of it have been isolated e.g., the beige mouse and the Aleutian mink [7, 8].

Chediak-Higashi syndrome in man (or in animal models) is a congenital disorder characterized clinically by partial albinism, severe recurrent pyogenic infections, and the development of pancytopenia. Diagnosis is based on the findings in blood smears, where the eosinophilic or neutrophilic leukocytes are seen to have giant intracytoplasmic granules [8, 9]. According to Oliver [10], all granule-containing cells show abnormally large granules of this kind, because there is a defect in the regulation of tubulin assembly into micro-tubules. The number of microtubules around the centriole is reduced, and the capacity of the neutrophils to migrate is also diminished in most test systems ([9]; however, see also ref. 10). The Chediak-Higashi syndrome must not be confused with the 'lazy-leukocyte syndrome' [11], where the primary defect of the leukocytes seems to reside in their chemotactic ability rather than in an impaired migratory capacity.

Gallin et al. described another disease which also seemed to be due to abnormal leukocyte functions [12] and which they thought to be caused by increased microtubule assembly. Alzheimer's disease has been related to abnormal bundles of microtubules in the neurons, i.e., the neurofibrillar tangle [13], and this disease, which is a form of presenile dementia, has been attributed to a faulty organization of the microtubules [14]. The disorders mentioned in this section require further investigation.

PATHOLOGY OF CILIA

Inborn disorders affecting the '9 +2 organelle' are relatively easy to diagnose. In men, examination of the spermatozoa may suffice, because the sperm tail belongs to this category of organelles (Fig. 1). The first case to be described was a man with immotile spermatozoa which proved to lack the dynein component associated with the microtubular doublets, i.e., the dynein arms [15]. Other cases were found [16], and it was noticed that whenever the sperm tail had this defect, the cilia had the same defects [17, 18] (Fig. 2). One of the

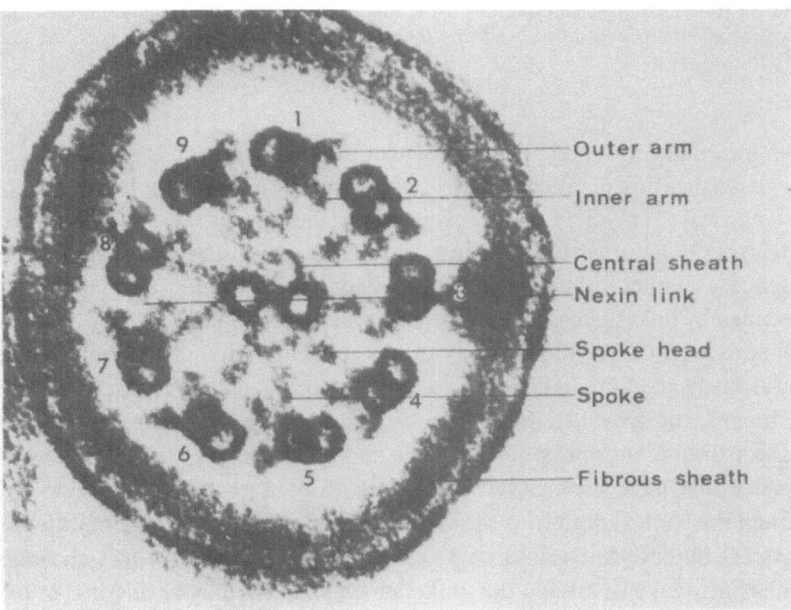

Fig. 1. Electron micrograph of a transversely sectioned human sperm tail. The sperm tail is a motor organelle of great complexity, and the central part has the same structure as that of a cilium. The names of the components are indicated. Reproduced by permission of the *Journal of Ultrastructure Research* (vol. 69, p. 43, 1979).

148

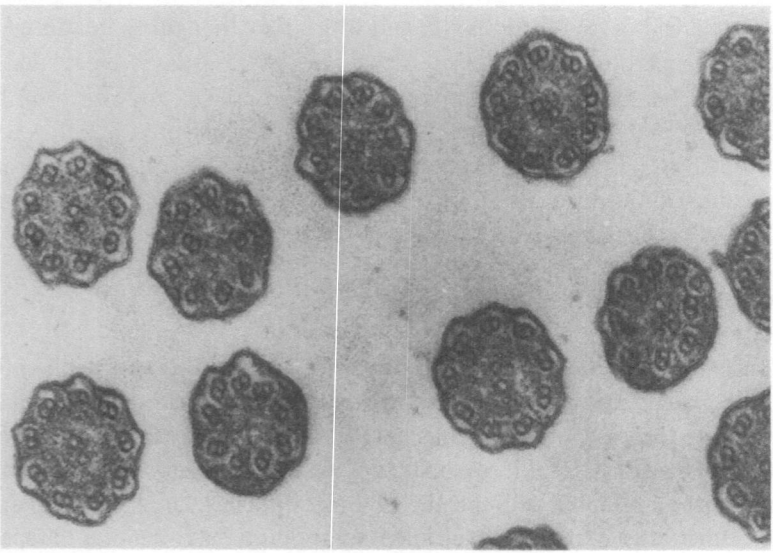

Fig. 2. Electron micrograph of transversely sectioned cilia from the nasal mucosa of a man suffering from immotile-cilia syndrome. Note that in this patient the dynein arms are either absent or greatly reduced in size and that the orientation of the cilia is random rather than ordered.

tests for ciliary functions consists of recording the 'mucociliary clearance,' which is a measure of efficieny of work by the cilia on the mucus blanket in the lower airways. This clearance was found to be absent or almost absent in these patients [19]. Another test is to inspect the ciliary motility — or establish its absence — either by an in situ method or by examining a small biopsy specimen by light microscopy in the living state. This specimen may be taken from any part of the human body that is covered with a ciliated epithelium and is easily accessible: the nasal mucosa, the bronchial mucosa, the middle-ear mucosa, or in women the endometrium of the upper portion of the uterus.

Electron-microscopic studies on cilia and spermatozoa from patients with this disorder have shown that it is a genetically heterogeneous disease. Although the clinical pattern is the same, the cilia may be defective in different ways: the outer dynein arms may be lacking or be abnormally short, the inner dynein arms may be absent, the spokes or spoke heads may be missing, or one or both of the central microtubules may be absent [20]. Many cilia have supernumerary or missing microtubules. In all of these cases the cilia have a random rather than an ordered orientation. The disease has been called the immotile-cilia syndrome [17, 19].

Its clinical manifestations are manifold [21], including chronic sinusitis, chronic bronchitis and often bronchiectasis, a permanently stuffed or permanently running nose, often polyps, often underdeveloped sinuses, and frequent ear infections. Olfaction is poor. Most of the patients have chronic headaches. Men are sterile, but not women. A surprising feature is the frequent association with situs inversus viscerum — probably 50% of the patients with an inborn ciliary immotility also have situs inversus. This curious association may be due to an inability of embryonic cilia to shift the heart to the proper side in fetuses with the immotile-cilia syndrome [17].

Although the number of persons affected by the immotile-cilia syndrome is only just about 1 in 20,000, the number of heterozygotes is as high as about 1 in 30. This is due to the genetic heterogeneity of the syndrome; many genes are needed to code for all proteins required for a functional cilium, and a defect in any one of them will, in a double dose, lead to the immotile-cilia syndrome.

It is not known whether patients with these different subtypes of the immotile-cilia syndrome are equally seriously affected. I disregard here the condition situs inversus, which has no health consequences — unless the inversion of the heart is partial and the heart is malformed. It is conceivable that some types of defective cilia are completely immotile and others have a limited erratic ciliary beat [20]. This would perhaps give clinical symptoms of different severity. It is also conceivable that some cases involve ciliary microtubules only and others both cytoplasmic and ciliary microtubules. To evaluate this possibility we investigated the migratory ability of the neutrophil granulocytes in eight patients suffering from the immotile-cilia syndrome and in the same number of controls. The neutrophils of three of the patients showed a decreased migratory capacity and the number of microtubules in the centriolar area of these cells was also somewhat decreased [22].

CONCLUSIONS

Little is known about the functioning of the biochemical machineries for cell motility. One approach to a better understanding is to isolate and characterize mutants in genetically well-characterized microorganisms (e.g., Chlamydomonas), i.e., mutants with cell-motility defects affecting the cilia or cytoplasmic streaming. A similar approach is to examine analogous inborn diseases in man, i.e., cases of mutants where the primary defect seems to reside in the biochemical machineries for cell motility. The immotile-cilia syndrome seems to be a rather clear-cut example of such a disorder. Other suspected disorders of this type — but involving the cytoplasmic microtubules — are the Chediak-Higashi syndrome, Alzheimer's disease, and possibly other diseases with recurrent severe infections and abnormal leukocyte functions.

150

REFERENCES

1. Satir P: Studies on cilia. II. Examination of the distal region of the ciliary shaft and the role of the filaments in motility. J Cell Biol 26:805–834, 1965.
2. Gibbons IR: Mechanisms of flagellar motility. In: Afzelius BA (ed) The functional anatomy of the spermatozoon. Oxford, Pergamon, 1975, pp 127–140.
3. Afzelius B: Electron microscopy of the sperm tail. Results obtained with a new fixative. J Biophys Biochem Cytol 5: 269–278, 1959.
4. Gibbons IR: Chemical dissection of cilia. Arch Biol (Liege) 76: 317–352, 1965.
5. Luck D, Piperno G, Ramanis Z, Huang B: Flagellar mutants in *Chlamydomonas:* Studies of radial spoke-defective strains by dikaryon and revertant analysis. Proc Natl Acad Sci USA 74: 3456–3460, 1977.
6. Boxer LA, Hedley-Whyle ET, Stossel TP: Neutrophil actin dysfunction and abnormal neutrophil behavior. N Engl J Med 291: 1093–1099, 1974.
7. Prieur DJ, Collier LL: Animal model of human disease. Chediak-Higashi syndrome. Am J Pathol 90: 533–536, 1978.
8. Douglas SD: Disorders of phagocytic function: ultrastructural aspects. In: Greenwalt TJ, Jamieson GA (eds) The granulocyte: function and clinical utilization. New York, Alan R Liss, 1977, pp 141–155.
9. Clawson CC, White JG, Repine JE: The Chediak-Higashi syndrome. Evidence that defective leukotaxis is primarily due to an impediment by giant granules. Am J Pathol 92: 745–754, 1978.
10. Oliver JM: Impaired microtubule function correctable by cyclic GMP and cholinergic agonists in the Chediak-Higashi syndrome. Am J Pathol 85: 395–417, 1976.
11. Miller ME, Oski FA, Harris MB: Lazy-leukocyte syndrome. Lancet 1: 665–669, 1971.
12. Gallin JI, Malech HL, Wright DG, Whisnant J, Kirkpatrick CH: Recurrent severe infections in a child with abnormal leukocyte function: possible relationship to increased microtubular assembly. Blood 51: 919–933, 1978.
13. Wisniewski H, Terry RD, Hirano A: Neurofibrillar pathology. J Neuropathol Exp Neurol 29: 163–176, 1970.
14. Heston LL: Alzheimer's disease, trisomy 21, and myeloproliferative disorders: associations suggesting a genetic diathesis. Science 196: 322–323, 1977.
15. Pedersen H, Rebbe H: Absence of arms in the axoneme of immobile human spermatozoa. Biol Reprod 12: 541–544, 1975.
16. Afzelius BA, Eliasson R, Johnsen Ø, Lindholmer C: Lack of dynein arms in immotile human spermatozoa. J Cell Biol 66: 225–232, 1975.
17. Afzelius BA: A human syndrome caused by immotile cilia. Science 193: 317–319, 1976.
18. Camner P, Afzelius BA, Eliasson R, Mossberg B: Relation between abnormalities of human sperm flagella and respiratory tract disease. Int J Androl 2: 211–224, 1979.
19. Eliasson R, Mossberg B, Camner P, Afzelius BA: The immotile-cilia syndrome. A congenital ciliary abnormality as an etiologic factor in chronic airway infections and male sterility. N Engl J Med 297: 1–6, 1977.
20. Afzelius BA, Eliasson R: Flagellar mutants in man; on the heterogeneity of the immotile-cilia syndrome. J Ultrastruct Res 69: 43–52, 1979.
21. Afzelius BA: The immotile-cilia syndrome and other ciliary diseases. Int Rev Exp Pathol 19: 1–43, 1979.
22. Afzelius BA, Ewetz L, Palmblad J, Udén AM, Venizelos N: Structure and function of neutrophil leukocytes from patients with the immotile-cilia syndrome. Acta Med Scand 208: 145–154, 1980.

12. ENDOCYTOSIS AND THE LYSOSOMAL APPARATUS: RECENT DEVELOPMENTS

P.J. JACQUES

Important advances have been made in recent years in knowledge concerning the structural and functional organization of two frequently cooperating cellular entities: the plasma membrane and the lysosomal apparatus, their respective involvement in physiologic and pathologic processes, and in their exploitation for medical or other aspects of applied biology.

If it is not surprising that a substantial part of that progress can be attributed to its traditional sources, e.g., cellular and molecular biology in both the normal and the diseased states, one is nevertheless impressed by the growing contribution of other disciplines or approaches such as immunology, parasitology, and cytopharmacology, which are almost newcomers in this field. Even more, the science of inflammation and, more generally, of host-defence mechanisms is causing a shattering *reconquista* of the field. It indeed recalls the inspiring concern which, more than a century ago, prompted Metchnikoff to give the first decisive impetus to this whole branch of biology by concentrating his attention on the important, though inconstant, functional axis now known as *endocytosis and lysosomes.*

This encouraging *retour aux sources* being duly recognized, one wonders whether the circumstances have not at last become propitious for envisaging endocytosis, which is but one of the many cytotic phenomena involving the plasma membrane, apart from the lysosomal apparatus. It seems to us rewarding and urgent to adopt this seemingly revolutionary and certainly debatable perspective for as long as necessary to counteract the increasing damage caused by the longlasting overemphasis put on the association of endocytosis with lysosomes. That damage is expressed in the relative lack of interest in other cytotic processes, namely those taking place at the cell periphery and usually involved in bulk discharge or uptake. It assumes dramatic proportions, we feel, in the field of medically applied lysosomology, an exciting an potentially useful domain of research which will soon sink into full discredit if the approaches used most frequently at present are not rapidly reconsidered in the light of modern cell biology.

This preoccupation merges the organizational highlights of this Boerhaave postgraduate course, in imposing the particular structure of the present short and thus highly eclectic essay. Also, when compiling the bibliography, the primary concern was to help the reader to acquire a general view of a few topics, rather than to do justice to the many workers who have made this field what it is: fascinating.

ENDOCYTOSIS

The concept of endocytosis covers the familiar notions of phagocytosis and pinocytosis, except that there is an increasing tendency to restrict it to the uptake act per se, whatever the postengulfment series of events may be. Endocytosis differs distinctly from other processes for the bulk uptake of extracellular material, in that the latter is sequestered within a discrete vacuole (*endosome, heterophagosome*) during the very process of its uptake (Fig. 1). In contrast, material taken up after membrane perforation or through reverse cellular budding finds itself free in the extravacuolar cytoplasm immediately after uptake. Not infrequently can it be found later within a cytoplasmic vacuole, but the mechanism of that secondary sequestration has nothing to do with endocytosis.

Endocytosis has been reviewed from various points of view in a host of recent articles [1–10], and is the subject of two papers in this book (Glaumann and Marzella, chapter 13; Kaplan, chapter 14). Considerable progress has been made toward the understanding of the intimate mechanism of endocytosis, which involves microfilaments [1, 11] and electro-ionic activity [12, 13]. These findings should permit selective modulation of endocytotic activity by means of pharmacologic agents [14].

Very much like recent work on the lysosomal apparatus, that on endocytosis has been profoundly influenced by immunology, its methods and its problems (Kaplan, chapter 14). A striking example is that of selective ve-

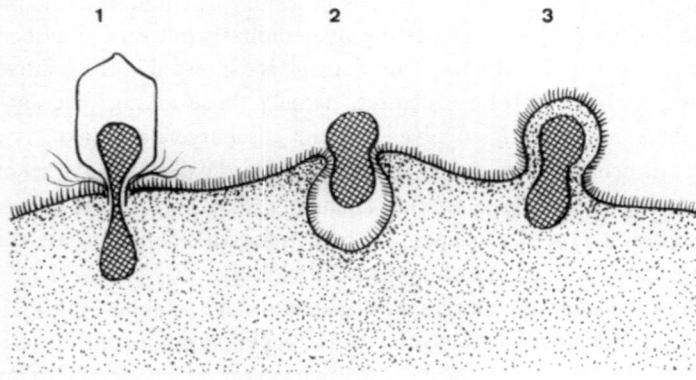

Fig. 1. Varieties of bulk uptake: 1, membrane perforation; 2, endocytosis; 3, reverse cellular budding. (Simplified from Jacques, ref. 2; courtesy of the Academic Press.)

sicular transcellular transport of immunoglobulins from mother to young. The first theory was put forward by Brambell [15] and involved complexing of the immunoglobulins with Fc-receptors located on the plasma membrane, endocytosis followed by discharge of the complex into the lysosomes, and there: selective proteolysis of the immunoglobulins depending on the respective stability, in the lysosomal microenvironment, of their complex with the receptors. The theory is, however, silent on the crucial point of subsequent transport, from the lysosomes to the extracellular space on the side of the young, of the globulins that have resisted intralysosomal peptidase action; besides, other properties of endocytosis, cytotic redistribution of phagosome contents, and determinism of phagosome-lysosome fusion offer several alternative potential mechanisms of selective uptake-digestion-transfer, other than those considered by the theory and exposed to experimental assessment [3, 16, 17]. A more comprehensive model was proposed on experimental grounds by Wild [18]. This model involved two structurally different types of phagosome, also differing in the functional sense by their ability or incapacity to discharge their contents into the lysosomes or to exocytose them outside the cell. More precisely, all the immunoglobulins would be sequestered within usual phagosomes and then transferred to and degraded within the digestive vacuoles (Fig. 2, route 12). In contrast, only those immunoglobulins which are ultimately transferred to the young would be sequestered within another type of phagosome currently called 'coated vesicles,' which would transfer their contents intact through transcellular transport avoiding the lysosomes and ending by exocytotic discharge in the medium, at the other side of the transferring cell (Fig. 2, route 13). This would represent another mechanism of selectivity of endocytosis, which can be distinguished from the classic ones [2, 17] in that it is based principally on differential structure and function of heterophagosomes. Certainty as to whether the same immunorelevant receptors are present on the presumably distinct zones of the plasma membrane where the two kinds of phagosome are being formed would considerably help the understanding (and thus possibly the exploitation) of the fine mechanisms of selective 'vesicular transcellular transport' (cytopempsis, diacytosis) of exogenous material; e.g., a process which is limited neither to immunological transmission nor to the placenta and the intestinal mucosa of the newborn.

Immunological receptors (C_3- and / or Fc-receptors) located on the plasma membrane of host-defense cells are also known to operate in association with nonspecific or specific humoral agents of immunity (e.g., complement derivatives and antibodies, respectively) for the endocytotic uptake of microorganisms. More recently discovered [19] is the decisive role played at a later stage by the same receptors, in the killing of the microbes within the lysosomes. Thus, in such instances at least, plasma membrane constituents conveyed to the lysosomes by the endosome membrane may be needed and operative for the performance of intralysosomal functions.

Some specialized chapters on pathology have recently been focused on endocytosis, but most often in relation to inborn or acquired dysfunctions of phagocyte lysosomes [20-22] (Thompson, chapter 15).

Extensive use is made of endocytosis in medically applied lysosomology, as a privileged procedure to convey drugs to the lysosomes (*lysosomotropic drugs* [23–25]). This is obviously impracticable in cells which are unable to endocytose and cannot be induced to do so; an intriguing example of forced endocytosis has been observed when malaria parasites (merozoite form) invade mature mammalian red blood cells [26]. Another hindrance to the use of endocytosis-dependent lysosomotropic drugs can be the absence of endosome-lysosome fusion, which can result from endocyte intoxication by a parasite or by the drug itself.

A most important notion is that 'professional phagocytes' also show an outstanding ability to exocytose lysosomal constituents; this has been observed for neutrophil [27, 28] or eosinophil [29] polymorphonuclear leukocytes, and some members of the mononuclear phagocytes family [30, 31]. That these powerful phagocytes must also be considered as powerful secretory cells not only accounts for the important role that they play in the scenario of inflammation, non-specific resistance, and specific immunity, but also raises the question as to whether endocytosis and exocytosis might not be more often associated in the same cell than is currently considered to be the case.

LYSOSOMAL APPARATUS

Within the larger framework of the concept of the vacuome (or vacuolar apparatus) conceived by the early cytologists, the lysosomal apparatus appears as a family of cytoplasmic structures — merely secretory granules and vacuoles — which usually can fuse more or less specifically with one another and with the plasma membrane. Today, however, the accent could perhaps be more usefully put on the exceptions to this rule of cytotic fusion, rather than on its generality.

The lysosomal apparatus is composed of subgroups: *phagosomes* (auto- and heterophagosomes), the *lysosomes* proper, which contain lysosomal enzymes, and *postlysosomes*, which have lost them. This apparatus, which is sketched in an oversimplified manner in Fig. 2, is involved in a huge variety of physiologic processes. As a result, it has been found to be altered in a variety of pathologic situations; sometimes, it is even the cause of the disease. More recent is the development of applied lysosomology, in which knowledge of the

155

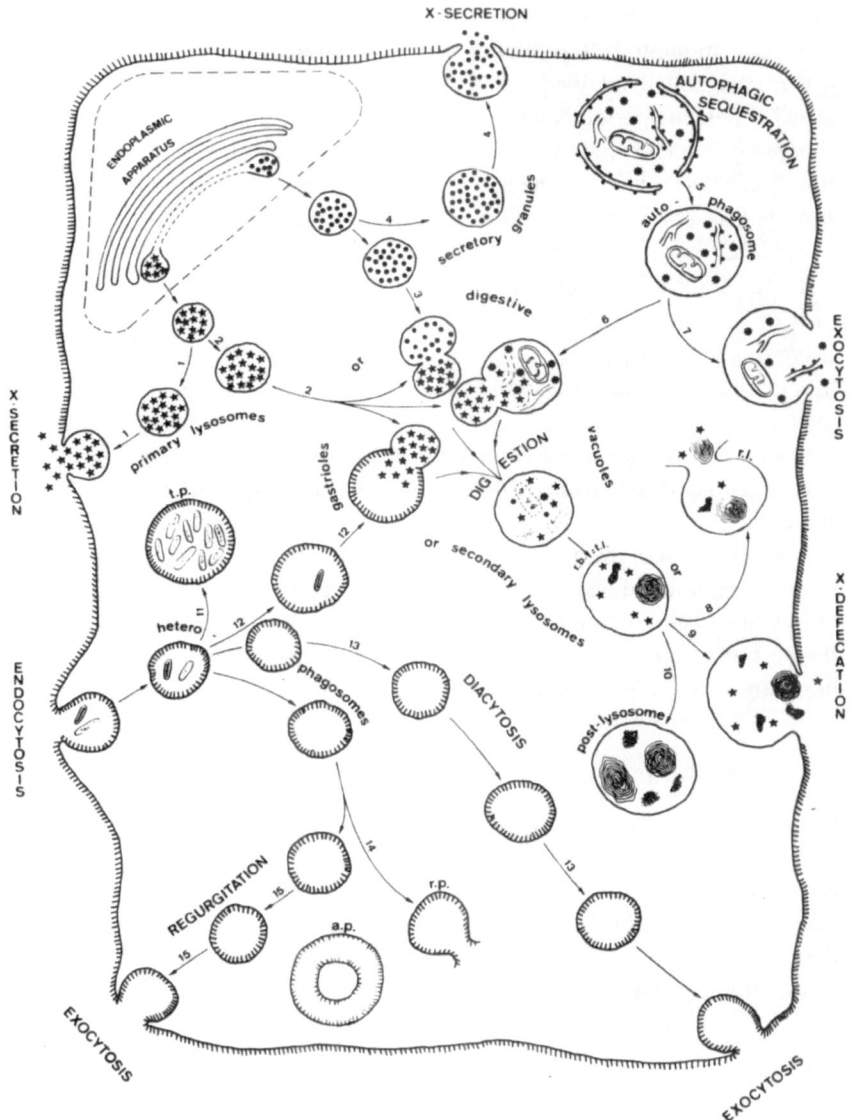

Fig. 2. Dynamics of principal cytotic exchanges in the exoplasmic apparatus: t.p., terminal phagosome; r.p., rupturing phagosome; r.l., rupturing lysosome; r.b., residual body; t.l., telolysosome; a.p., annular profile. (Simplified from Jacques, ref. 32; courtesy of *Periodicum Biologorum*.)

rules of the games played within the lysosomal machinery is exploited for the design of new approaches to the prevention or treatment of medical or other problems, or for improving preexisting procedures.

Several monographs providing a vast documentation on lysosomes in general are now available [32–37]. In addition, most aspects of this rapidly growing field are periodically reviewed in the series *Lysosomes in Biology and Pathology*, which is heroically kept up to date by Dingle. With three exceptions [38–40] centered on enzyme replacement therapy for inborn lysosomal storage diseases, information on applied lysosomology still has to be pried, paper after paper, from the ocean of current literature.

To the student starting from scratch and interested in acquiring a general view of lysosome machinery and functions, we would recommend starting by becoming familiar with the bulky story underlying Fig. 2. This means going, at a comfortable pace, through the historically important review written in 1966 by de Duve and Wattiaux [41], and then proceeding to a few complementary papers [42–53]. Acquisition of this background baggage should suffice for facing the problems of lysosomes in pathology and those of applied biology.

It is clearly out of the question to present here a general view of lysosomes in 1979, or even a full account of the recent developments in the field. What follows is rather a listing with comments, of a few important topics which, in the author's opinion, have merged in a sufficiently coherent manner to be presented as seen from a high altitude.

Cytotic phenomena

Cytotic processes are a most important and widespread property of eukaryotic cells; by no means are they the monopoly of the plasma membrane or the lysosomal apparatus (Table 1). They can be considered under two different headings: fusion (or coalescence) of cytomembranes and vesicular transport; the latter can in turn be subdivided into membrane traffic and translocation of vacuolar contents.

Membrane fusion

In the context of plasma membranes and lysosomal apparatus, the currently envisaged fusion processes are peripheral ones such as endocytosis and exocytosis and intracellular ones such as phagosome-lysosome fusion. In fact, there are many other intracellular cytotic processes of interest, especially in connection with applied lysosomology. Indeed, they have been observed occasionally to affect individual vacuoles, especially endosomes (heterophagosomes) and digestive vacuoles (secondary lysosomes). When the mem-

Table 1. Classification of cytotic processes.

	ENCYTOSIS	ECCYTOSIS
PERIPHERAL	Endocytosis (Fig. 1, process 2)	Exocytosis (Fig. 2)
	Reverse cellular budding (Fig. 1, process 3)	Cellular budding
INTRACELLULAR	Centrifugal vacuolar budding (Fig. 3, process 6)	Centripetal vacuolar budding (Fig. 3, process 10)
		Autophagic sequestration (Fig. 2)
		Cell plate formation
		Cell separation at telophase

The criterion on which the classification is based is whether the external or the internal face of the cytomembrane establishes contact prior to fusion (de Duve and Wattiaux, ref. 41); Bennett [52] called these two categories of cytotic phenomena *encytosis* and *eccytosis*, respectively.

brane of these vacuoles is in excess relative to vacuolar volume, budding in or out, or formation of annular profiles and multivesicular bodies can occur (Fig. 3).

These secondary processes are perhaps not simple curiosities; the cell does not usually waste energy in futile activities. At the very least, the increase of membrane surface area relative to contents, which accompanies budding out and the formation of daughter vacuoles (Fig. 3, process 7), should accelerate permeative exchanges across the vacuolar wall. At best, new functions might be rendered possible by these processes; thus, budding out of endosomes containing two different preys could lead to complete separation of these preys into distinct daughter-endosomes [2]; furthermore, budding in of digestive vacuoles (Fig. 3, process 10) allows the most important process of microautophagy [2, 54].

Intracellular membrane fusion thus takes place more frequently and in a more varied manner than is generally envisaged. In contrast, endosome-lysosome fusion does not invariably occur as had been thought since the days of Metchnikoff, until D'Arcy Hart [55] (D'Arcy Hart, chapter 17) established that, after phagocytosis by macrophages, some preys are not discharged into lysosomes (Fig. 2, route 12); instead, they remain confined within what might be called 'terminal phagosomes' (Fig. 2, route 11). It may not be advisable, however, to systematically designate as a terminal endosome any parasitophorous vacuole that would not fuse with lysosomes; indeed such a designation requires that endocytosis be the entry procedure of the parasite into the host cell, and that the membrane surrounding the parasitophorous vacuole

158

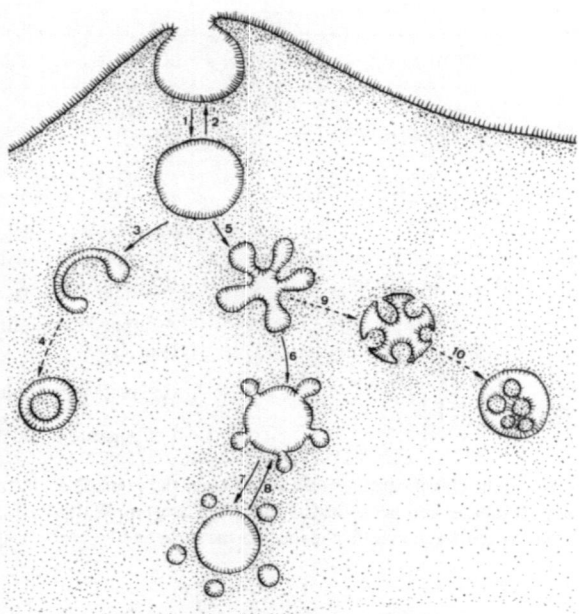

Fig. 3. Cytotic transformation of primary exoplasmic vacuoles. (Simplified from Jacques, ref. 32; courtesy of *Periodicum Biologorum.*)

still be the same one that surrounded the parasite when it was being endocytosed; these conditions are far from being universally respected, even when the host cell is a macrophage. One tempting conclusion to be drawn from D'Arcy Hart's findings is that the nature of the endosome contents might determine whether endosome-lysosome fusion will take place. The possible relationship between this hypothesis and that put forward by Wild (see section on *Endocytosis*), about 'nonfusing' coated vesicles is intriguing.

The classification of cytotic processes presented in Table 1 is based on the perhaps exaggerated importance attributed to the well-known dissymetry between the two faces of cytomembranes in general and of plasma membranes in particular. A direct consequence of this classification is that, at least from the viewpoint of membrane fusion, exocytosis should not be considered simply as 'reverse endocytosis.' The validity of this proposal seems supported by the more recent findings that endocytosis and exocytosis involve different microfilamentous contractile structures [11], that they respond in opposite ways to selected pharmacologic agents [11, 56], and that their relative intensity at a given moment of the cell's activity may be modulated by the respective concentrations, at that moment, of adenine and guanine cyclic nucleotides [57].

Undoubtedly, the elucidation of the role played by microfilaments and microtubules as energy transformers during membrane fusion represents important progress from both the fundamental and the cytopharmacologic viewpoints. However, the subsequent questions as to how the thus apposed membranes coalesce and how, after coalescence, the membrane bridges are split to open vesicles or to free them from another membrane structure, are as yet unanswered [58]. In the particular case of vacuole fusion involving a lysosome as one of the partners, a possible explanation has been proposed [35, 59]; it involves membrane-associated lysosomal enzymes, and assigns them a role in the mutual recognition of the fusing entities as well as in splitting of the membrane bridge separating (or associating) them after fusion.

According to Fig. 1 (process 3) and Table 1, the rather vague expression 'fusing liposomes,' which is used to designate liposomes coalescing with the target cell's plasma membrane as opposed to liposomes that are endocytosed unaltered, refers to the process which is called here 'reverse cellular budding.' The latter expression is not only terribly heavy to handle but is certainly also as bad a misnomer as 'reverse endocytosis.' Evidently, the help of an imaginative linguist is needed to avoid intellectual confusion and hence lack of efficiency and precision in scientific communication.

Vesicular transport

Between two fusion events, the location of the vacuole usually changes. Vacuole motion means translocation of both the container (vacuole membrane) and the contained (vacuole contents), and it seems obvious that in most instances the peregrinations and the chemical fate of container and contained cannot indefinitely remain the same.

The translocation and fate of vacuolar contents within the lysosomal apparatus has been discussed repeatedly and in detail elsewhere (e.g. [2, 3, 25, 41]); it will not be considered here.

In contrast, traffic and destiny of cytomembranes, which can be tremendously intense in cells actively engaged in endocytosis or in quantal secretion, has long remained a subject of speculation. In the mid-1950s many cytologists expressed concern about the precise mechanism(s) involved in the well-known 'regeneration' of the plasma membrane after endocytosis. Is the endosome membrane completely broken down within digestive vacuoles, so that the plasma membrane should be completely and expensively synthetized de novo? At the other extreme, is the membrane exchanged intact between the various organs of the vacuome in such a way that, under usual conditions, it would remain available everywhere in minimal if not sufficient amounts? It has been repeatedly suggested that, in endocytosis, the phagosome membrane might cyclically commute between the plasma membrane and the digestive vacuoles; a name (*emeocytosis*) was even put forward to designate this perpetual shuttle. Rather recently, abundant evidence compatible with the concept of emeocytosis was obtained in an extensive biochemical cytology study of cultured cells [60, 61]. Such studies will definitely stimulate both work and thinking. For instance, if the intracellular killing of microorganisms that necessitates plasma-membrane receptors (see section on *Endocytosis*) and/or plasma-membrane enzymes (see the following section) does take place within the digestive vacuoles, then the precise mechanism of killing by these substances and the exact timing of emeocytotic events will have to be worked out in the most refined detail.

Lysosomes of phagocytic leukocytes

To us, the most impressive progress in special lysosomology during the last decade has occurred in the particular field of phagocytic leukocytes, more precisely of mononuclear phagocytes (monocytes and macrophages) and polymorphonuclear leukocytes (neutrophils and, to a lesser extent, eosinophils). Several of the breakthroughs illustrated above indeed resulted from studies performed in one of these cell types.

These developments, which caused a real and most enriching revolution in the lysosome concept, include such unclassic findings as multiplicity of lysosome forms within a same cell, the presence of oxidative enzymes and other odd macromolecules in these lysosomes, killing as the most prominent function which can be exerted against extracellular as well as intracellular parasites (Fig. 4), and a secretory capacity as considerable as the phagocytotic power of these cells (see section on *Endocytosis*).

Also impressive is the coherence of these findings, which assuredly stems from the fact that these cells cooperate with one another (and with lymphocytes and humoral or tissue factors) in a single though highly complex, fundamental and never completed function: to defend the body against endogenous and exogenous parasites. With this particular chapter of special lysosomology, we are entering the fortress of immunity, whose major towers are named inflammation, nonspecific resistance, and specific immunity.

In this context, the functions of lysosomes are important and highly diversified, by no means restricted to killing [62]. Their complete inventory is not only a fascinating task leading to interesting improvements of fundamental knowledge; it is our conviction that it will also help the bionics-oriented drug designer to develop powerful tools for the prevention and treatment parasitic diseases.

With respect to the lysosomes, the most complete and complex of these cells is undoubtedly the neutrophil polymorphonuclear leukocyte [63]. In this cell there are several types of lysosomes which differ in enzymic equipment [64] and morphologic properties [65]. These lysosome types are formed in a

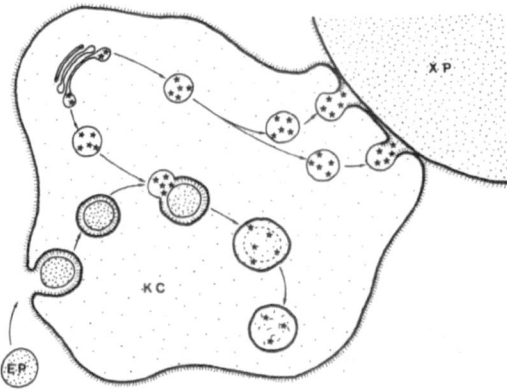

Fig. 4. Lysosomes in parasiticidal action of inflammatory cells. EP, endocytosable parasite; KC, killer cell; XP, extracellular parasite. (From Jacques and Lambert, ref. 62; courtesy of the Plenum Press.)

sequential manner during maturation of the neutrophil, and they are discharged sequentially into phagocytic vacuoles after endocytosis.

The enzymic equipment of neutrophil lysosomes of course comprises a variety of acid hydrolases as in most any cell, but the battery of hydrolases is expanded toward neutral (protease) and even alkaline (phosphatase) enzymes. The most unusual feature of the equipment of neutrophil lysosome is, however, the presence of a collection of enzymes (myeloperoxidase, lysozyme) and of nonenzymic proteins which are endowed with considerable parasiticidal power [66–68].

Myeloperoxidase deserves special attention in the latter context, not simply because an oxidase can seldom be found in the constitutive enzymic dotation of lysosomes, but also because this enzyme forms, together with a type-II oxidase (NADH- or NADPH-specific) located in the plasma membrane, an enzymic couple which is able to reduce molecular oxygen in a very stepwise manner. Among the oxygen derivatives formed during the first reaction are superoxide radical and hydrogen peroxide; others, such as electronically excited molecular (singlet) oxygen, hydroxyl radical, and hypochlorite, tend to derive more or less directly from the sequential reactions, provided that the medium composition be adequate.

All these substances, and even much more so mixtures of them are endowed with important but different cytocidal power whose spectrum of activity may be close to universal. They are also among the strongest oxidizers known to date, so that oxidative lysis of organic material resistant to the combination of hydrolases found in common lysosomes can be expected to take place within the digestive vacuoles of neutrophils and similar cells.

As shown schematically in Fig. 4, the peroxidase should meet the oxidase whenever phagocytosis occurs and is followed by phagosome-lysosome fusion, and also when lysosomes are exocytosed, as during the attacking of schistosomules by eosinophils or mononucleate phagocytes [29]. In either case, the oxidase comes into contact with the parasite before peroxidase has the opportunity to do so.

The lysosomal apparatus of monocytes, and much more so that of macrophages, is definitely simpler than that of the neutrophil. One highly significant simplification concerns the macrophage group. Daems and his associates [69, 70] have succeeded in separating the macrophages into two different categories, according to the precise intracellular location of the peroxidase. In one of these categories the enzyme was demonstrated within the lysosomes and should therefore be able to participate efficaciously in the killing of parasites. In the other subgroup the lysosomes lack the enzyme; however, the latter can be detected in the cavities of the endoplasmic apparatus, a location that disqualifies it for the usual parasiticidal activity. This duality of macrophages may reflect a differential origin during adult life, but it would probably lead to a classification of macrophages between poor killers and good killers, depending on peroxidase localization. Pathologists concerned with infectious granuloma [71] have long recognized profound differences in the ability of mononuclear phagocytes to kill the microbes, depending on in which polar form of the granuloma (e.g., tuberculoid versus lepromatous leprosy granuloma) they are considered. One may wonder whether Daems's fundamental conclusions might not help in finding a solution to that dichotomizing pathology problem.

Two inborn lysosomal diseases, i.e., chronic granulomatous disease (CGD) and myeloperoxidase deficiency, are characterized by a lack of the oxidase and the peroxidase, respectively, in the lysosomes of leukocytes. Clinically, the patients are subject to recurrent infections [72]. At the experimental level, administration of a type-I oxidase to macrophages from patients with CGD restored to a large extent the microbicidal ability of these cells [73]. Also, administration of the same oxidase together with a peroxidase to mice infected with *Mycobacterium leprae* resulted in considerable bactericidal activity and in acceleration of the intracellular biodegradation of mycobacterial remnants [74].

Applied lysosomology

Applied lysosomology is a typical example of the services that fundamental research in cell biology can offer medicine and other disciplines of applied science. Unfortunately, time and place limitations do not allow me to explain here the various approaches used in this recently growing field, or even to list its already numerous achievements. This information can, however, be gleaned from various complementary general articles [24, 25, 75–78] (Trouet, chapter 23).

As an example outside medicine, let us mention that fundamental studies on these very odd lysosomes represented by natural latex particles made it possible to considerably improve latex production by hevea trees in West Africa. In veterinary medicine, the early diagnosis of an inborn lysosomal disease of cattle, by a single enzyme determination in a blood sample, allowed secure application of eugenism and thus virtually made it possible to solve what used to be a huge economic problem for farmers and populations in Oceania and Southern Asia.

In medicine, the simple determination of the degree of lysosome preservation in biopsy specimens of livers and kidneys stored in organ banks has already made it possible to predict with the utmost accuracy whether the organ will overcome the manipulation stress during transplantation surgery.

In due course, the prophylaxis and treatment of diseases by procedures based on applied lysosomology have become much better documented. We can already list a wide variety of pathologic situations (inborn or acquired, metabolic, infectious, degenerative or carcinomatous, environmental, iatrogenic, etc.) [25, 76], which responded favorably to various applied lysosomology methods, most often in experimental models, sometimes also in clinical trials.

Among the methods used, that involving 'lysosomotropic agents' is by far the most widely applied. This term was coined [23] to designate the sending of pharmacologic agents into the lysosomes of target cells. It had long been known by students of *speicherung* (storage) that there are two major ways for exogenous material in general to reach the storage vacuoles (lysosomes): the purely cytotic pathway of Metchnikoff, involving endocytosis, and the pathway of dual permeation, i.e., successively across the plasma membrane and the lysosome membrane [79]. Progress in cell biology now allows the enumeration in most cells of almost a dozen other pathways combining endocytosis, permeation, and macro- or microautophagy [25], at least in the case of permeating micromolecules.

In most therapeutic attempts based on the use of lysosomotropic agents the purely cytotic pathway, which is obligatory for macromolecules and endocytozable particulate drug carriers [80, 81], has been preferentially exploited. This holds for the enzyme-replacement therapy of inborn lysosomal storage diseases [38–40] and the parasitic diseases studied by Trouet and his associates (Trouet, chapter 23). In view of all the recently discovered factors which can impair endocytosis or endosome-lysosome fusion at a later stage, one can only be agreeably surprised to hear that the lysosomotropic approach has worked in so many instances.

164

When applied to intracellular parasitism, this approach is confronted by another type of potential difficulty; for instance, when a directly acting antiparasitic drug must reach, via the cytotic pathway, the very vacuole where the parasite is entrenched. Would such a drug or drug complex reach the parasite (e.g., tubercle bacilli in terminal phagosomes)? Translated into the language of the cell biologist, the question becomes: would a terminal phagosome which, by definition, does not fuse with lysosomes, nevertheless succeed in fusing with a freshly formed (and drug-containing) heterophagosome? The answer to this question seems of vital importance.

Another kind of problem in the same context is the great diversity of the intracellular location(s) of obligate or facultative intracellular parasites within the host cell (Fig. 5). For one thing, not all such parasites are taken up by endocytosis, whether spontaneous or forced [26, 82, 83]. *Toxoplasma gondii* for instance has been reported to penetrate into macrophages by two con-

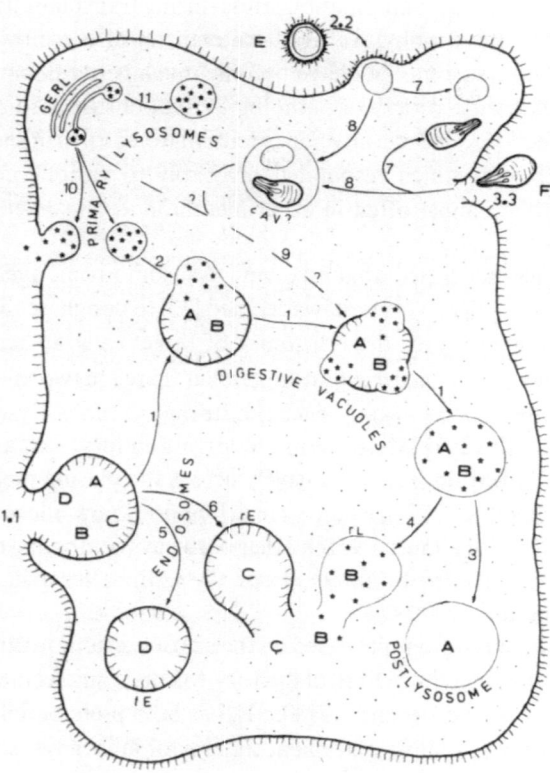

Fig. 5. Varieties of intracellular host-parasite relationships. 1.1, endocytosis; 2.2, reverse cellular budding; 3.3, membrane perforation; tE, terminal endosome; rE, rupturing endosome; rL, rupturing lysosomes; A–E, distinct parasites as discussed in text; GERL; Golgi, endoplasmic reticulum and primary lysosomes. (From Jacques et al., ref. 78; courtesy of ICRO/Unesco.)

comitant mechanisms: endocytosis and 'active penetration' (possibly membrane perforation; Fig. 1, process 1); in contrast, only the latter could be observed when toxoplasma invaded (nonphagocytic) HeLa cells [83]. What is then the cytologic significance of the 'nonfusing' vacuoles containing this parasite (Jones, chapter 18)? For parasites that have been endocytosed, the vacuole can undoubtedly be a terminal phagosome (Fig. 5, type D); but when active penetration was involved, the vacuole, if any, could only have appeared some time after entry and would have a different meaning.

The case of intracellular parasites taken up exclusively by endocytosis is not as simple as it had originally been envisaged [55, 84]. Indeed, only in a few instances (e.g., *Mycobacterium lepraemurium*, some rickettsiae), does the parasite sojourn for a prolonged period of time within lysosomes (Fig. 5, type A). But cytopathogenic viruses would rupture these vacuoles after some time (Fig. 5, type B), thus escaping into the extravacuolar cytoplasm and causing severe damage to the host cell. *Rickettsia prowazeki* is quicker at escaping from the lysosomal apparatus, which it leaves at the stage of endosomes (Fig. 5, type C), a few minutes after endocytotic uptake, thus avoiding contact with the lysosome contents. In mouse footpad macrophages, *Mycobaterium leprae* has been reported to leave the vacuoles after some time, at an unknown stage; but after remaining for some time in the extravacuolar cytoplasm, it reappeared in the vacuolar compartment.

Difficulties of higher degree of complexity, which are an even greater challenge for the drug designer, could also be described.

The object of raising these potential problems was not to discourage further work in applied lysosomology. It was rather to help make two conclusive points. One, that the lysosomologist involved in the treatment of cellular disorders can intelligently design appropriate modular drugs, only if he has at least a minimal background in general cell biology and if he knows the precise host-parasite relationship in each type of parasitized cell, at the very time in the evolution of the disease when he has decided to attack it. Two, that there is much fundamental work ahead in the field of host-parasite relationships, for the cell biologist — or would you say cellular pathologist? — who wishes to contribute his share to the development of applied lysosomology.

Acknowledgments. This work was made possible by the financial help of Belgian FRSM (contract 4580) and FRFC (contract 4542). The author holds tenure as research professor in the Fonds National de la Recherche Scientifique.

166

REFERENCES

1. Allison AC, Davies P: Mechanisms of endoctytosis and exocytosis. Symp Exp Biol 28: 419–446, 1974.
2. Jacques PJ: The endocytic uptake of macromolecules. In: Trump BJ, Arstila AU (eds) Pathobiology of cell membranes. New York, Academic Press, 1975, pp 255–279.
3. Jacques PJ: Cell biological processes involved in transport of matter across tissue membranes. In: Hemmings WA (ed) Maternofoetal transmission of immunoglobulins. Cambridge, Cambridge University Press, 1975, pp 201–217.
4. Korn ED: Biochemistry of endocytosis. In: Fox CF (ed) Biochemistry of cell walls and membranes. Baltimore, University Park Press, 1975, pp 1–26.
5. Silverstein SC, Steiman RM, Cohn ZA: Endocytosis. Annu Rev Biochem 46: 669–722, 1977.
6. Stockem W: Endocytosis. In: Jamieson GA, Robinson DM (eds) Mammalian cell membranes, vol 5. London, Butterworths, 1977, pp 151–195.
7. Stossel TP: Phagocytosis. In: Greenwalt TJ, Jamieson GA (eds) The granulocyte. Function and clinical utilization. New York, Alan Liss, 1977, pp 87–102.
8. Edelson PJ, Cohn ZA: Endocytosis: regulation of membrane interactions. In: Poste G, Nicolson GL (eds) Membrane fusion. Amsterdam, North-Holland, 1978, pp 387–405.
9. Silverstein SC, Michl J, Sung S-SJ: Phagocytosis. In: Silverstein SC (ed) Transport of macromolecules in cellular systems. Berlin, Dahlem Konferenzen, 1978, pp 245–264.
10. Oss CJ van: Phagocytosis as a surface phenomenon. Annu Rev Microbiol 32: 19–39, 1978.
11. Allison AC: The role of microfilaments and microtubules in cell movement, endocytosis and exocytosis. In: Locomotion of tissue cells, Ciba Symposium 14. Amsterdam, Excerpta Medica, 1973, pp 109–148.
12. Josefsson J-O: Studies on the mechanism of induction of pinocytosis in *Amoeba proteus*. Acta Physiol Scand Suppl 432: 1–65, 1975.
13. Weissman G, Hoffstein C, Korchak H, Smolen JE: The earliest membrane responses to phagocytosis: membrane potential changes and Ca^{++} loss in human granulocytes. Trans Am Assoc Phys 91: 90–103, 1978.
14. Gee JBL, Cross CE: Drugs affecting phagocytosis and pinocytosis. In: Dikstein S (ed) Fundamentals of cell pharmacology. Springfield, Charles Thomas, 1973, pp 349–372.
15. Brambell FWR: The transmission of immunity from mother to young. Amsterdam, North-Holland, 1970.
16. Wild AE: Transport of immunoglobulins and other proteins from mother to young. In: Dingle JT (ed) Lysosomes in biology and pathology, vol 3. Amsterdam, North-Holland, 1973, pp 169–215.
17. Jacques PJ: Endocytosis. In: Dingle JT, Fell HB (eds) Lysosomes in biology and pathology, vol 2. Amsterdam, North-Holland, 1969, pp 395–420.
18. Wild AE: Mechanism of protein transport across the rabbit yolk-sac endoderm. In: Hemmings WA (ed) Maternofoetal transmission of immunoglobulins. Cambridge, Cambridge University Press, 1976, pp 155–165.
19. Leijh PCJ, Barselaar M Th van der, Zwet Th L van, Daha MR, Furth R van; Requirement of extracellular complement and immunoglobulin for intracellular killing of microorganisms by human monocytes. J Clin Invest 63: 772–784, 1979.
20. Quie PG: Disorders of phagocyte function; biochemical aspects. In: Greenwalt TJ, Jamieson GA (eds) The granulocyte; function and clinical utilization. New York, Alan Liss, 1977, pp 157–173.
21. Douglas SD: Disorders of phagocytic function; ultrastructural aspects. In: Greenwalt TJ, Jamieson GA (eds) The granulocyte; function and clinical utilization. New York, Alan Liss, 1977, pp 141–155.
22. Güttler F, Seakins JWT, Harkness RA (eds): Inborn errors of immunity and phagocytosis. Lancaster, MTP Press, 1979.
23. Duve C de, Trouet A: Lysosomotropic drugs. In: Braun W, Ungar J (eds) Non-specific factors influencing host-resistance. Basel, Karger, 1973, pp 153–170.

24. Duve C de, Barsy T de, Poole B, Trouet A, Tulkens P, Van Hoof F: Lysosomotropic agents. Biochem Pharmacol 23: 2495–2531.
25. Jacques PJ: The selection and design of lysosomotropic drugs. In: Reichard SM, Escobar MR, Friedman HH (eds) The reticuloendothelial system in health and disease, vol A. New York, Plenum Press, 1976, pp 289–313.
26. Aikawa M, Sterling CR: Intracellular parasitic protozoa. New York, Academic Press, 1974.
27. Clark RA, Klebanoff SJ: Neutrophil-mediated tumor cell cytotoxicity; role of the peroxidase system. J Exp Med 141: 1442–1447, 1977.
28. Weissmann G, Smolen JE, Hoffstein S: Polymorphonuclear leukocytes as secretory organs of inflammation. J Invest Dermatol 71: 95–99, 1978.
29. Houba V, Butterworth AE, David JR, Sher A, Glauert AM, Sturrock FR, Vadas MA: Lysosomes in immunity of schistosomes and other helminths. In: Dingle JT, Jacques PJ, Shaw IH (eds) Lysosomes in biology and pathology, vol 6. Amsterdam, North-Holland, 1979, pp 3–29.
30. Unanue ER: Secretory function of mononuclear phagocytes. In: Furth R van (ed) Mononuclear phagocytes. Oxford, Blackwell, 1975, pp 396–417.
31. Lejeune FJ, Vercammen-Grandjean A: Secretory activity of macrophages in relation to cytotoxicity and modulation of cell function. In: Dingle JT, Jacques PJ, Shaw IH (eds) Lysosomes in biology and pathology, vol 6. Amsterdam, North-Holland, 1979, pp 425–445.
32. Jacques PJ: The concept of lysosomes; concluding remarks. Period Biol 74: A3–A5, 1972.
33. Krustev LP: Lysosomes; structure, function, pathology. Sofia, Bulgarian Academy of Sciences, 1972.
34. Pitt D: Lysosomes and cell function. London, Longman, 1975.
35. Matile P: The lytic compartment of plant cells. Vienna, Springer, 1975.
36. Pokrovsky AA, Tutelyan VA: Lysosomes. Moscow, Nauka, 1976.
37. Holtzman E: Lysosomes; a survey. Vienna, Springer, 1976.
38. Hers HG, Van Hoof F (eds): Lysosomes and storage diseases. New York, Academic Press, 1973.
39. Desnick RJ, Bernlohr RW, Krivit W (eds): Enzyme therapy in genetic diseases. Baltimore, Williams and Wilkins, 1973.
40. Tager JM, Hooghwinkel GJM, Daems WTh (eds): Enzyme therapy in lysosomal storage diseases. Amsterdam, North-Holland, 1974.
41. Duve C de, Wattiaux R: Functions of lysosomes. Annu Rev Physiol 28: 435–492, 1966.
42. Gahan PB: Lysosomes. In: Pridham JB (ed) Plant cell organelles. London, Academic Press, 1968, pp 228–238.
43. Jacques PJ: Lysosomes and homeostatic regulation. In: Wolstenholme GEW, Knight J (eds) Homeostatic regulators. London, Churchill, 1969, pp 180–196.
44. Duve C de: Lysosomes in retrospect. In: Dingle JT, Fell HB (eds) Lysosomes in biology and pathology, vol 1. Amsterdam, North-Holland, 1969, pp 3–40.
45. Cohn CA, Fedorko ME: The formation and fate of lysosomes. In: Dingle JT, Fell HB (eds) Lysosomes in biology and pathology, vol 1. Amsterdam, North-Holland, 1969, pp 43–63.
46. Daems WTh, Wisse E, Brederoo P: Electronmicroscopy of the vacuolar apparatus. In: Dingle JT, Fell HB (eds) Lysosomes in biology and pathology, vol 1. Amsterdam, North-Holland, 1969, pp 64–112.
47. Matile P: Plant lysosomes. In: Dingle JT, Fell HB (eds) Lysosomes in biology and pathology, vol 1. Amsterdam, North-Holland, 1969, pp 406–430.
48. Maggy V: Lysosomes. In: Bittar EE (ed) Cell biology in medicine. New York, Wiley, 1973, pp 215–263.
49. Gahan PB: Plant lysosomes. In: Dingle JT (ed) Lysosomes in biology and pathology, vol 3. Amsterdam, North-Holland, 1973, pp 69–85.
50. Davies P, Allison AC: The secretion of lysosomal enzymes. In: Dingle JT, Dean RT, (eds) Lysosomes in biology and pathology, vol 5. Amsterdam, North-Holland, 1976, pp 61–98.
51. Novikoff AB: Lysosomes; a personal account. In: Hers HG, Van Hoof F (eds) Lysosomes and storage diseases. New York, Academic Press, 1973, pp 1–41.
52. Bennett HS: The cell surface; movements and recombinations. In: Lima de Faria A (ed) Handbook of molecular cytology. Amsterdam, North-Holland, 1969, pp 1294–1319.

168

53. Jacques PJ: Assimilation et digestion intracellulaire; les lysosomes. Ann Anesthesiol Fr [Special] 1: 18–28, 1972.
54. Arstila AU, Jauregui HO, Chang J, Trump BF: Studies on cellular autophagocytosis; relationships between heterophagy and autophagy in HeLa cells. Lab Invest 24: 162–174, 1971.
55. Hart P d'Arcy: Phagosome-lysosome fusion in macrophages; a hinge in the intracellular fate of ingested microorganisms? In: Dingle JT, Jacques PJ, Shaw IH (eds) Lysosomes in biology and pathology, vol 6. Amsterdam, North-Holland, 1979, pp 409–423.
56. Davies P, Allison AC: Effects of cytochalasin B on endocytosis and exocytosis. In: Tanenbaum SW (ed) Cytochalasins; biological and cell biological aspects. Amsterdam, Elsevier/North-Holland, 1978, pp 143–160.
57. Weissmann G, Goldstein I, Hoffstein S, Chauvet G, Robineaux R: Yin/Yang modulation of lysosomal enzyme release from polymorphonuclear leukocytes by cyclic nucleotides. Ann NY Acad Sci 256: 222–232, 1975.
58. Poste G, Allison AC: Membrane fusion. Biochim Biophys Acta 300: 421–465, 1973.
59. Krustev L, Tutelyan VA, Kravchenko L, Tashev T, Pokrovsky A: On the mechanism of formation of secondary lysosomes. CR Acad Bulg Sci 28: 1129–1132, 1975.
60. Tulkens P: The role of lysosomes and plasma membrane in the intracellular accumulation of exogenous substances. Physiological, pharmalogical and toxicological studies in cultured cells. Academic thesis, University of Louvain, 1979.
61. Tulkens P, Schneider Y-J, Trouet A: Membrane recycling (shuttle) in endocytosis. In: Furth R van (ed) Mononuclear phagocytes. The Hague, Martinus Nijhoff, 1980.
62. Jacques PJ, Lambert F: Alterations of rat liver lysosomes after treatment with particulate β-1,3 glucan from *Saccharomyces cerevisiae*. In: Escobar MR, Friedman HH (eds) Macrophages and lymphocytes; nature, functions and interaction, part A. New York, Plenum Press, 1979, pp 225–234.
63. Klebanoff SJ, Clark RA: The neutrophil; function and clinical disorders. Amsterdam, North-Holland, 1978.
64. Avila JL: Comparative biochemical cytology of the exoplasmic apparatus in polymorphonuclear leukocytes. In: Dingle JT, Jacques PJ, Shaw IH (eds) Lysosomes in biology and pathology, vol 6. Amsterdam, North-Holland, 1979, pp 235–266.
65. Bainton DF, Nichols BA, Farquahar MG: Primary lysosomes of blood leukocytes. In: Dingle JT, Dean RT (eds) Lysosomes in biology and pathology, vol 5. Amsterdam, North-Holland, 1976, pp 3–32.
66. Klebanoff SJ: Antimicrobial mechanisms in neutrophilic polymorphonuclear leukocytes. Semin Hematol 12: 117–142, 1975.
67. Spitznagel JK: Bactericidal mechanisms of the granulocyte. In: Greenwalt TJ, Jamieson GA (eds) The granulocyte; function and clinical utilization. New York, Alan Liss, 1977, pp 103–139.
68. Sbarra AJ, Selvaraj RJ, Paul BB, Mitchell GW, Louis FJ: Myeloperoxidase and leukocyte function. In: Dingle JT, Jacques PJ, Shaw IH (eds) Lysosomes in biology and pathology, vol 6. Amsterdam, North-Holland, 1979, pp 267–285.
69. Daems WTh, Wisse E, Brederoo P, Emeis JJ: Peroxidatic activity in monocytes and macrophages. In: Furth R van (ed) Mononuclear phagocytes in immunity, infection and pathology. London, Blackwell, 1975, pp 55–77.
70. Daems WTh, Roos D, Van Berkel ThJC, Van Der Rhee HJ: The subcellular distribution and biochemical properties of peroxidase in monocytes and macrophages. In: Dingle JT, Jacques PJ, Shaw IH (eds) Lysosomes in biology and pathology, vol 6. Amsterdam, North-Holland, 1979, pp 463–514.
71. Skinsnes OK: Comparative pathogenesis of mycobacterioses. Ann NY Acad Sci 154: 19–31, 1968.
72. Quie PG, Mills EL: Lysosome deficiencies in leukocytes and infectious diseases. In: Dingle JT, Jacques PJ, Shaw IH (eds) Lysosomes in biology and pathology, vol 6. Amsterdam, North-Holland, 1979, pp 279–285.
73. Baehner RL, Nathan DG, Karnovsky ML: Correction of metabolic deficiencies in the

leukocytes of patients with chronic granulomatous disease. J Clin Invest 49: 865–870, 1970.

74. Delville J, Jacques PJ: Therapeutic action of generators of free-radicals and electronically excited molecules, on the infection of the mouse foot-pad by *Mycobacterium leprae*. In: Escobar MR, Friedman HH (eds) Macrophages and lymphocytes; nature, functions and interaction, part B. New York, Plenum Press, (in press) 1979.

75. Jacques PJ: Endocytosis, exoplasmic apparatus and rudiments of applied lysosomology. In: Ledoux L (ed) Uptake of informative molecules by living cells. Amsterdam, North-Holland, 1972, pp 277–294.

76. Jacques PJ, Demoulin-Brahy L: Lysosomotropic Triton WR-1339: one method of applied lysosomology for the therapy of exoplasmic parasitoses. In: Wagner WH, Hahn H (eds) Activation of macrophages. Amsterdam, Excerpta Medica, 1974, pp 84–96.

77. Tulkens P, Trouet A: Lysosomotropic drugs; biological and therapeutical aspects. In: Bolis L, Hoffman JF, Leaf A (eds) Membranes and diseases. New York, Raven Press, 1976, pp 131–144.

78. Jacques PJ, Delville J, Avila JL, Demoulin-Brahy L, Song M, Stadtsbaeder S, Nguyen BT, Gillet J, Convit J: Lysosomes and the medical care of infectious diseases. In: Matangka-sombut P (ed) Global impacts of applied microbiology. Bangkok, ICRO/Unesco, 1979, pp 248–254.

79. Jancsö N: Speicherung. Budapest, Akademiai Kiado, 1955.

80. Speiser PP: Non-liposomal nanocapsules; methodology and application. In: Dingle JT, Jacques PJ, Shaw IH (eds) Lysosomes in biology and pathology, vol 6. Amsterdam, North-Holland, pp 653–668.

81. Gregoriadis G (ed): Drug carriers in biology and medicine. New York, Academic Press, 1979.

82. Aikawa M, Kilejian A: Invasion procedures and intracellular localization of parasitic protozoa. In: Dingle JT, Jacques PJ, Shaw IH (eds) Lysosomes in biology and pathology, vol 6. Amsterdam, North-Holland, 1979, pp 31–48.

83. Nguyen BT: La toxoplasmose expérimentale chez la souris NMRI; thérapeutique et immunité. Doctoral thesis, University of Louvain, 1979.

84. Goren MB: Phagocyte lysosomes; interactions with infectious agents, phagosomes, and experimental perturbations in function. Annu Rev Microbiol 31: 507–533, 1977.

13. MORPHOLOGY OF ENDOCYTIC MECHANISMS

H. GLAUMANN AND L. MARZELLA

Most large molecules cannot penetrate membranes, but must be taken up by active movements of plasma membranes. This process is referred to as *endocytosis*. The term endocytosis covers two types of mechanisms, the first being *phagocytosis*, which concerns large particles (> 1 μ) such as bacteria or cell debris; and secondly *macropinocytosis* (1.0–0.5 μ) and *micropinocytosis* (< 0.5 μ), which refer to uptake of small soluble molecules by 'cell drinking.' In both cases the material is endocytosed for digestion in lysosomes or in some instances for transport through the cytoplasm and subsequent exocytosis.

PHAGOCYTOSIS

Morphological analysis of phagocytosis in Kupffer cells [1–3] has revealed that this process can be divided into two steps: (1) attachment (Fig. 1) and (2) engulfment (Fig. 2), followed by two additional phenomena, namely; (3) fusion and degradation (Fig. 3), and (4) residual-body formation (Fig. 4).

Attachment

Most foreign material, such as bacteria, attaches to the surface of macrophages. In general, this attachment is mediated by specific or nonspecific receptors on the plasma membrane. However, at the area of attachment, fusion never occurs between the plasma membrane and the particle to be taken up (Fig. 1). Instead, a gap of 300–500 Å separates the particle from the cell surface [4]. This gap corresponds to the glycocalix of the cell surface. The mere attachment of particles to the cell surface seems to initiate the next phase, called engulfment. Attachment is not energy dependent but is a prerequisite for interiorization of the particle [5].

Abbreviations: LDL, low-density lipoproteins; TCA, trichloro acetic acid; PVP, polyvinyl-pyrolydone.

W.Th. Daems et al. (eds.), Cell Biological Aspects of Disease, 171–184. All rights reserved.
Copyright © 1981 by Martinus Nijhoff Publishers bv, The Hague/Boston/London.

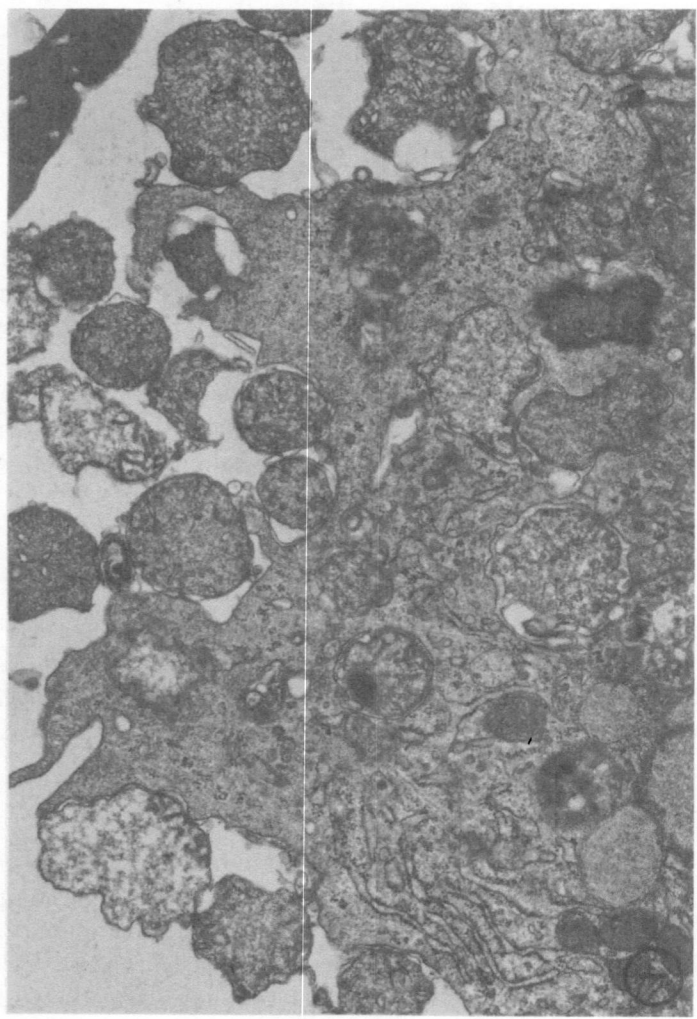

Fig. 1. Attachment of mitochondria on the surface of a Kupffer cell. Flap-like processes embrace mitochondria.

Engulfment

This process involves channels formed by indentations or 'pockets' in the cell membranes. Parallel to these egg-cup-like invaginations, flap-like cell processes are formed which seem to embrace the trapped material (Fig. 2). According to Griffin et al. [6, 7] and Silverstein et al. [5], the interaction of ligands on the surface of the particle with the receptor of the macrophage

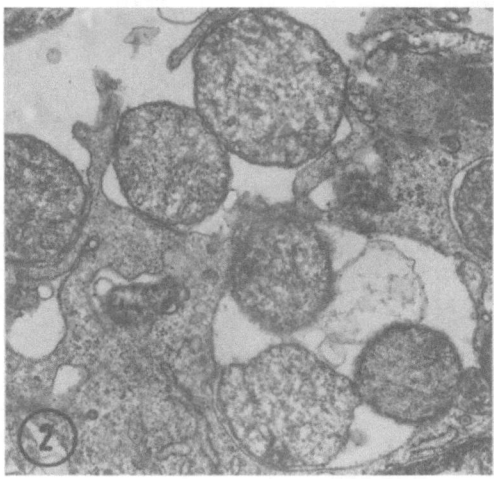

Fig. 2. Engulfment of mitochondria and formation of a phagosome.

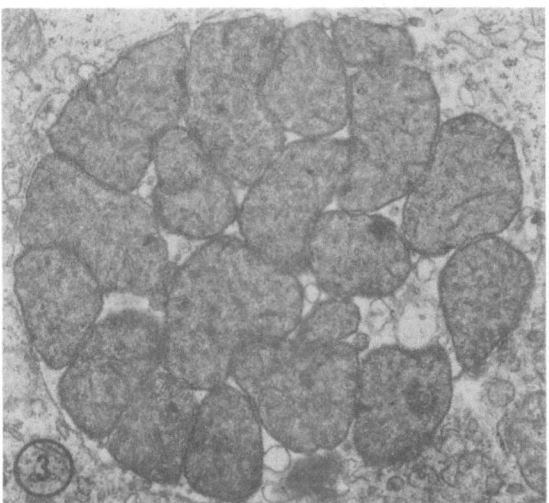

Fig. 3. A nascent phagosome is present in the cytoplasm of a Kupffer cell.

generates a signal that causes aggregation or organization of microfilamentous material in such a way that nascent pseudopodia are formed. This
formation leads to additional interaction between ligand and receptor, which
in turn is thought to continue the organization of the microfilaments. At the
end of the process the particle is enclosed by plasma membrane. This process
has been called the zipper mechanism. Griffin et al. [7] demonstrated that the

174

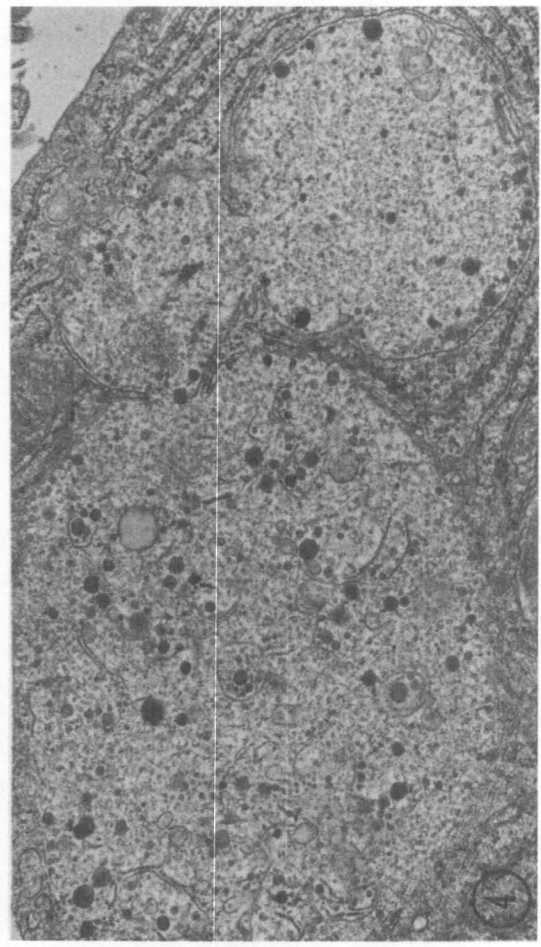

Fig. 4. Fusion between phagolysosomes and advanced degradation of engulfed mitochondria.

distribution of ligands on the particle's surface is of importance for the engulfment process. Lack of ligands on the entire surface may lead to attachment but not fusion of the plasma-membrane pseudopodia. Attachment does not seem to be energy dependent, but occurs at 4° C.

Vesicles or vacuoles derived from the cell surface by the zipper mechanism form the *endosomes* (phagosomes). As these vacuoles enter the cell, they often fuse to form a large endosome (Fig. 3). Within the cell, the endosome will in general fuse either with primary or secondary lysosomes (Fig. 4). By this mechanism the endosome acquires hydrolytic enzymes and becomes a 'phagolysosome,' and the digestion phase is initiated. Normann [8] showed that phagocytic rate of the reticuloendothelial system is proportional to the number of particles injected into the blood stream of rats. Accordingly, a Lineweaver-Burk plot of phagocytic rate measured as uptake by the liver versus the injected amount of material can be made and a K_m value calculated (Fig. 5). Another indirect measurement of phagocytosis is based on the vascular clearance after intravenous injection, as illustrated in Fig. 6. After the first

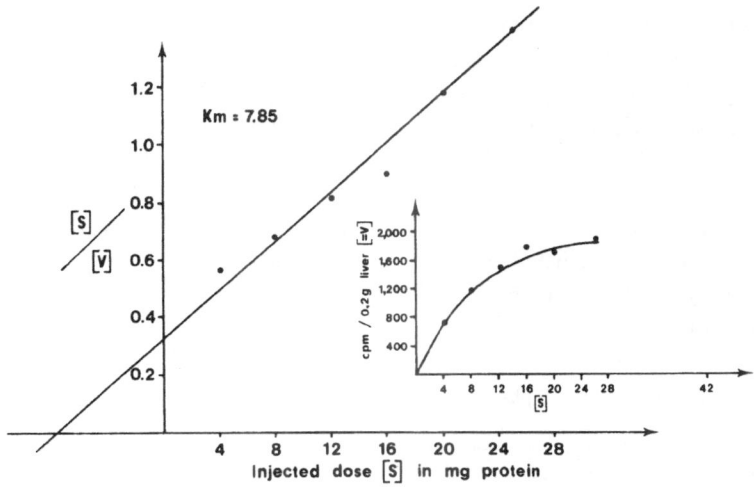

Fig. 5. Rate of phagocytosis as a function of the initial amount of injected ^{14}C-leucine-labeled microsomes. Various amounts of microsomes (5–45 mg protein per 100 g of rat) were administered via the portal vein. The phagocytic rate was measured as uptake of label per gram of liver. The animals were killed 15 min after injection. The label denotes activity recovered in the TCA precipitate.

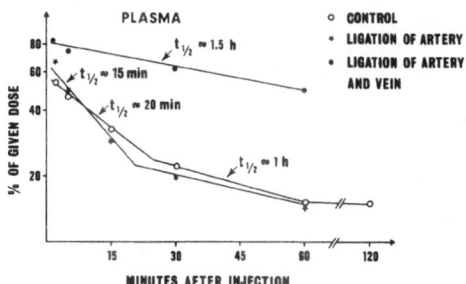

Fig. 6. Effect of ligation of the common liver artery and portal vein on the disappearance of injected ^{14}C-leucine-prelabeled microsomes from the plasma. Ligation of either the common liver artery or both the artery and the portal vein was performed 1 or 2 min before intravenous (femoral vein) administration of microsomes. Percent given dose denotes percent of injected dose recovered in the plasma after the indicated intervals.

hour, most of the radioactivity disappears from the circulation. Ligation of the portal vein and common liver artery prolongs the circulation time of the injected material significantly, thus demonstrating the predominance of the liver (Kupffer cells) in the uptake of foreign material from the circulation.

Fusion with lysosomes, degradation, and residual-body phase

Fusion between phagosomes and lysosomes is initiated shortly after engulfment of material and is in general completed with an hour or less. Most biological material, e.g., membranes, is then degraded into small molecular derivatives such as amino acids, glycerol, and fatty acids. The degradation time (half-life) differs for different membrane components. However, in general it seems as if lipids are degraded somewhat more slowly than proteins. The half-life values obtained for various membrane components introduced into lysosomes are listed in Table 1. Some proteins such as ferritin and cytochromes seem to be more resistant to hydrolytic lysosomal attack than others [9].

Table 1. Measured half-life of phagocytosed microsomal membrane components in Kupffer cell lysosomes.

Component	Isotope	Disappearance curve during interval 0–24 h	Shortest $t\frac{1}{2}$ (h)
Proteins	^{14}C-leucine	Triphasic	0.8–1.5
Hemeproteins	^{55}Fe	Biphasic	20
Phospholipids	^{32}P	Biphasic	4
Phospholipids	^{14}C-glycerol	Biphasic	6
Phospholipids	^{14}C-phosphatidylcholine [a]	Monophasic	4
Cholesterol	^{14}C-mevalonate/^{14}C-cholesterol [b]	Monophasic	9
Cholesterol esters	Cholesteryl-^{14}C-palmitate [b]	Biphasic	3
Glycoproteins	^{14}C-glucosamine	Biphasic	2
Glycoproteins	^{14}C-galactosamine	Biphasic	1.5
Ribosomes	^{14}C-orotic acid	Triphasic	0.5

These data are based on a model for the study of intralysosomal degradation of cell organelles [1–9]. Isotopically prelabeled micrsomes or mitochondria were injected intravenously into rats and phagocytosed by Kupffer cells. The disappearance of label was followed in a crude lysosomal fraction.
[a] Data from liposomes.
[b] These experiments were performed with microsomes labeled in vitro by incubation.

PINOCYTOSIS

From the morphological point of view, several profiles have been described as associated with uptake of extracellular soluble material and there are special variants in different cells. In most cells, however, three types of pinocytic profiles can be distinguished (Fig. 7).

Pinosome or macropinocytic vesicle (approx. 0.5 μ), which is sometimes characterized by a fuzzy coat on the inside of the vesicle, corresponding to the carbohydrate-rich glycocalix covering the outer surface of the plasma membrane. This fuzzy coat can be demonstrated only with special fixation and staining procedures

Bristle-coated vesicles or micropinocytic vesicles (< 0.5 μ). These vesicles seem to be formed by invagination of special areas of the plasma membrane, called coated pits, whose cytoplasmic side bears bristles. The coated area accounts for about 2% of the surface area of fibroblasts. It has been shown that the coated pits are the areas of localization of specific receptors such as receptors for LDL, complement, or immunoglobulin [10]. However, LDL receptors may be lacking, as in familial hypercholesterolemia, in spite of the presence of coated pits [11]. At present, it does not appear likely that the pinocytic receptors are distributed randomly on the plasma membrane.

Vermiform structure is another morphologic entity in pinocytic uptake. This structure is characteristic of Kupffer cells. Under optimal fixation conditions a double fuzzy layer can be demonstrated, suggesting that this appearance is the result of infolding of plasma membrane. The vermiform structures disappear after intensive phagocytosis, which indicates that they represent a means of storage of excess plasma membrane [4] utilized during endocytosis.

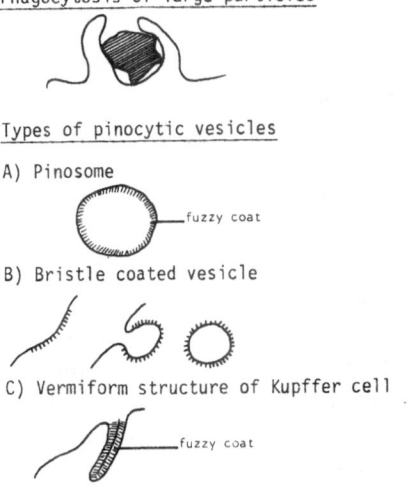

Fig. 7. Schematic illustration of phagocytosis and pinocytosis. (From ref. 24.)

MECHANISMS OF ENDOCYTOSIS

The process of pinocytosis does not differ in principle from that of phago-cytosis, although it is by definition associated with uptake of solute. If there is no adsorption of particles to the surface, the term *fluid endocytosis* is ap-plicable. Most cells generate pinocytic vesicles at a constant rate, enclosing fluid and solutes at the same concentration as found in the extracellular fluid or circulation. For the situation in which particles or solutes stick to the surface, the term *adsorptive endocytosis* has been put forward [12]. In this case the adsorbed material may be taken up several times above the concentration in the fluid phase. At the biochemical level, clear-cut differences between pinocytosis and phagocytosis have not been convincingly established. The definition of phagocytosis and pinocytosis is then mainly based on morpho-logical criteria. Energy seems to be necessary for the invagination or move-ment of the cell surface and thus for the formation of an endosome. Conse-quently, endocytosis can be blocked by inhibitors of glycolysis and/or mito-chondrial respiration, depending on the predominant energy pathway in the cell examined. The intracellular content of ATP is roughly correlated with the influence of the inhibitor. It has been postulated that ATP (energy) is nec-essary for the organization of contractile proteins (microfilaments) during the phagocytic process. The participation of microfilaments in the phagocytic process is supported by the finding that cytochalasins inhibit uptake. The rationale for this interpretation is based on the fact that cytochalasins inter-fere with actin microfilaments which appear to be of importance in various physiologic phenomena such as maintenance of cell shape and secretory and phagocytic processes. More specifically the cytochalasins destabilize the actin filament structure. Because of their inhibitory effects on microfilaments, cytochalasin B and D are often used as an experimental tool when evaluating the role of the filamentous apparatus in various cellular processes. Phago-cytosis activates several metabolic pathways, such as increase in peroxidase formation and stimulation of the hexose monophosphate shunt and oxygen consumption.

Evidence showing that the amount of certain plasma membrane carrier systems remains stable during high rates of induced endocytosis has been interpreted as indicating that the plasma membrane behaves as a mosaic [13]. Support for this proposal was recently provided by studies which showed a nonrandom interiorization of surface plasma membrane proteins during phagocytosis [14, 15]. The rate of formation of pinosomes can be stimulated by a variety of substances [16]. In certain instances the pinocytic vesicles may, after transfer across the cytoplasm, discharge their content by exocytosis at the opposite pole of the cell [17].

The mechanisms which control the intracellular traffic of pinocytic vesicles are incompletely understood. Microtubules appear to play a role. However, different results have been obtained with different experimental systems. For example, in cultured fibroblasts microtubular inhibitors depress endocytosis of low-density lipoproteins (LDL) because of interference with binding of LDL to membrane receptors; however, the uptake of sucrose seems unaffected [18]. In the same cells the degradation of glycosaminoglycans was inhibited because of impaired fusion between endocytic vesicles and lysosomes [19]. In our own studies [20], vinblastine had little effect on the endocytic uptake of albumin or microsomes by the Kupffer cells (Fig. 8). In contrast, the degradation of these substances was significantly diminished.

In general, phagocytosis is accomplished only by certain specialized cells such as macrophages. The fate of membrane material that surrounds the endocytic vesicle is not fully known. One possibility could be that the phagosome simply fuses with the preexisting lysosome and thereby adds more membrane material to the lysosomes. This would mean a continuous expansion of the lysosomal compartment. However, during induced pinocytosis there is no appreciable increase in the lysosomal compartment [21].

Based on turnover of marker enzymes for plasma membranes, it has been

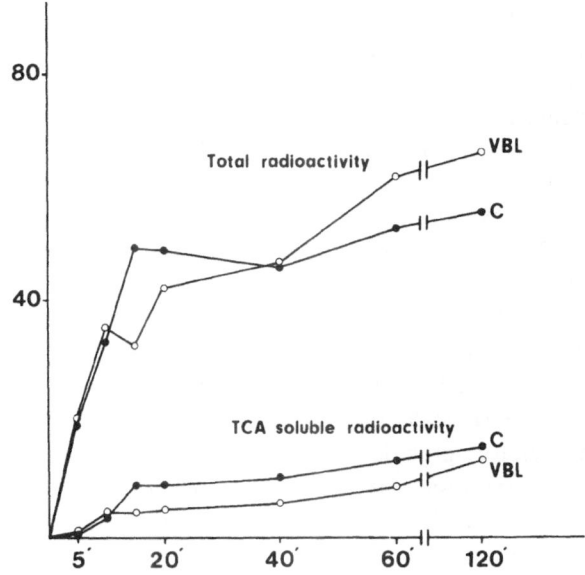

Fig. 8. Abscissa: minutes after ^{125}I-albumin injection; ordinate: CPM × 10^3/g liver. ●——● control; O——O vinblastine-treated. Phagocytic uptake of denatured ^{125}I-albumin by control and by vinblastine-treated livers. Experimental animals were pretreated with vinblastine (2 mg/100 g) 1 h before the intravenous injection of isotopically labeled denatured albumin. Livers were perfused at various intervals after the albumin injection and the radioactivity total and TCA-soluble) was determined in crude heterophagosomal fractions.

calculated that in macrophages as much as 50% of the total surface of the plasma membrane may be internalized by means of fluid endocytosis in 1 h. The uptake of plasma membrane by adsorptive endocytosis is probably even more impressive, but more difficult to evaluate. To account for this loss of plasma membrane, recycling mechanisms have been postulated [21, 22].

It is clear that in secretory cells the transport of membrane material occurs in the opposite direction to that of endocytosis; namely, to the plasma membrane by means of exocytosis. It has been postulated that endocytosis and exocytosis are coupled in a tandem process [23]. These two processes make possible the passage of particulate and soluble components between the intra- and extracellular spaces. Since the lysosomal compartment and total surface of cells are constant during the steady state, some mechanism must exist to balance exo- and endocytosis. Two mechanisms could regulate and compensate membrane loss during endocytosis, namely, (a) degradation of endocytic membranes and synthesis of new plasma membrane components, and (b) reutilization of membrane material. Since the half-life of most plasma membrane components lies in the range of one day or more, the turnover and thus synthesis is not effective enough to compensate for an internalization of 50% of the surface area per hour.

The studies by Schneider et al. [22] on the uptake of various labeled IgG molecules by fibroblasts offered an opportunity to put the recycling model to an experimental test. These authors have postulated that endocytosis involves a permanent shuttle between the cell surface and lysosomes. After temporary fusion and release of endocytosed material to the lysosome, membrane material is transported back to the plasma membrane (Fig. 9). If this model is correct, it may explain the discrepancies between the rapid endocytic rates and relatively slow turnover of plasma membranes, as measured by isotopic techniques.

In certain cells a shuttle mechanism may involve the Golgi apparatus as well as the lysosomes. Herzog and Farquhar [24] have shown that ferritin-laden endocytic vesicles fuse not only with lysosomes but also with the Golgi cisternae and in particular the most mature part of the Golgi apparatus from which the secretory granules arise. Furthermore, it has been shown that the route of incoming vesicles is dependent on the net charge of the pinocytosed marker molecule. Vesicles carrying negatively charged ferritin fuse only with elements of the lysosomal system, whereas those carrying positively charged ferritin fuse with elements along the secretory pathway, namely, Golgi cisternae and condensing or secreting granules in addition to lysosomes.

Not only the plasma membrane but also lysosomal membranes appear to undergo endocytic-like invagination in vivo [25, 26]. This process results in the interiorization of membrane vesicles into the lysosome. A mechanism for the recycling of the lysosomal membrane interiorized after the formation of

PLASMA MEMBRANE RECYCLING

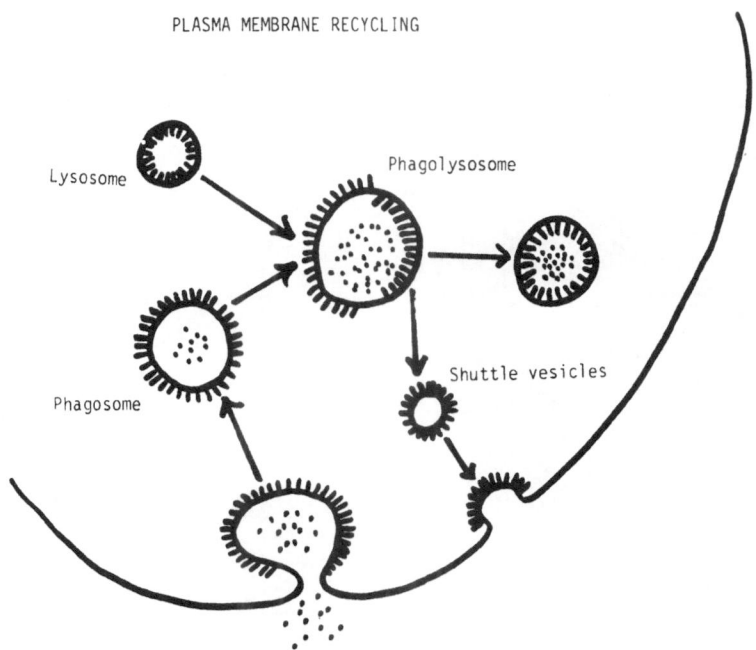

Fig. 9. Schematic model for recycling of plasma membrane. This drawing is based on the studies by Schneider et al. [22].

these endocytic-like vesicles has been proposed [25]. We have recently obtained evidence that isolated lysosomes can take up inert particles in vitro. On the basis of electron microscopy a sequence of events can be outlined, as indicated in Figs. 10–12. Lysosomal membranes seem to undergo endocytic-like changes which apparently lead to the internalization of PVP-silica (Percoll) particles into membrane-bound vacuoles. Similar particles can also be seen lying free in the lysosomes.

The relevance of these in vitro physicochemical lysosomal membrane changes for the understanding of in vivo phenomena remains to be defined. However, a similar mechanism in vivo could account for the direct uptake of soluble components into the lysosomal compartment. If this can be demonstrated, some of the controversy regarding the locus for the uptake and degradation of soluble intracellular components could be resolved.

Acknowledgment. This research has been aided by the Swedish Medical Research Council.

182

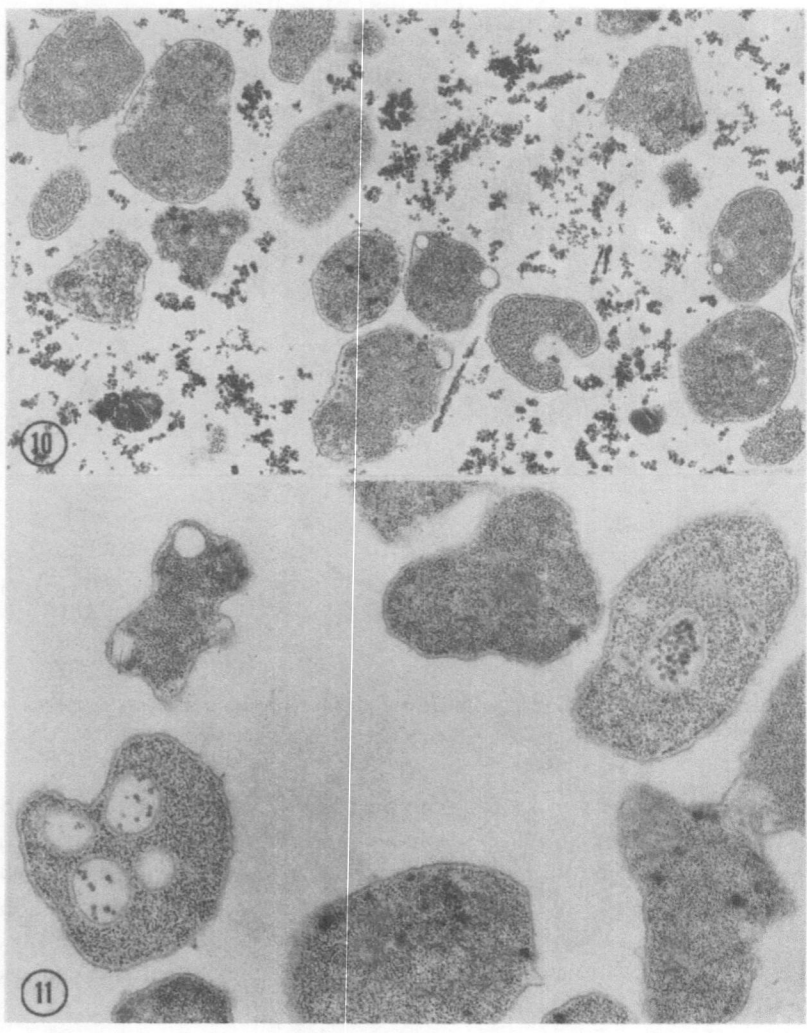

Figs. 10–12. Uptake of Percoll particles in vitro by isolated lysosomes. At early time points (Fig. 10) few particles are seen inside lysosomes. With longer incubation times (Fig. 11), particles are seen inside the lysosomes in membrane-enclosed vesicles or (Fig. 12) apparently lying free in the lysosomal matrix. This may indicate digestion of the surrounding vesicle membrane. Data taken from ref. 18.

183

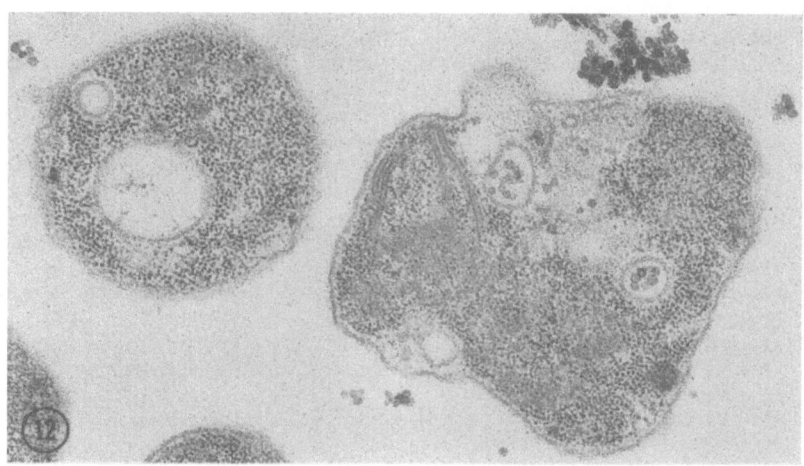

REFERENCES

1. Glaumann H, Berezesky I, Ericsson JLE, Trump BF: Lysosomal degradation of cell organelles. I. Ultrastructural analysis of uptake and digestion of intravenously injected mitochondria by Kupffer cells. Lab Invest 33: 239–251, 1975.
2. Glaumann H, Berezesky I, Ericsson JLE, Trump BF: Lysosomal degradation of cell organelles. II. Ultrastructural analysis of uptake and digestion of intravenously injected microsomes and ribosomes by Kupffer cells. Lab Invest 33: 252–261, 1975.
3. Glaumann H, Trump BF: Lysosomal degradation of cell organelles. III. Uptake and disappearance in Kupffer cells of intravenously injected isotope-labelled mitochondria and microsomes in vivo and in vitro. Lab Invest 33: 262–272, 1975.
4. Wisse E: Ultrastructure and function of Kupffer cells and other sinusoidal cells in the liver. In: Wisse E, Knook DL (eds) Kupffer cells and other liver sinusoidal cells. Amsterdam, Elsevier/North-Holland Biomedical Press, 1977, pp 33–60.
5. Silverstein SC, Steinman RM, Cohn ZA: Endocytosis. Ann Rev Biochem 46: 669–722, 1977.
6. Griffin FM Jr, Griffin JA, Leider JE, Silverstein SC: Studies on the mechanism of phagocytosis. I. Requirements for circumferential attachment of particle-bound ligands to specific receptors on the macrophage plasma membrane. J Exp Med 142: 1263–1282, 1975.
7. Griffin FM Jr, Griffin JA, Silverstein SC: Studies on the mechanism of phagocytosis. II. The interaction of macrophages with anti-immunoglobulin IgG-coated bone marrow-derived lymphocytes. J Exp Med 144: 788–809, 1976.
8. Normann SJ: Kinetics of phagocytosis. II. Analysis of in vivo clearance with demonstration of competitive inhibition between similar and dissimilar foreign particles. Lab Invest 31: 161–169, 1974.
9. Glaumann H, Marzella L: lysosomal degradation of cell organelles. Degradation of membrane components by Kupffer cells. J Cell Biol (to be published).
10. Goldstein JL, Anderson RGW, Brown MS: Coated pits, coated vesicles and receptor-mediated endocytosis. Nature 279: 679–685, 1979.
11. Anderson RGW, Goldstein JL, Brown MS: A mutation that impairs the ability of lipoprotein receptors to localize in coated pits of the cell surface of human fibroblasts. Nature 270: 695–699, 1977.
12. Jacques PJ: Endocytosis. In: Dingle JT, Fell HB (eds) Lysosomes in biology and pathology, vol 2. Amsterdam, North-Holland, 1968, pp 395–420.

184

13. Tsan MT, Berlin RD: Effect of phagocytosis on membrane transport of non-electrolytes. J Exp Med 134: 1016–1035, 1971.
14. Willinger M, Frankel FR: Fate of surface proteins of rabbit polymorphonuclear leucocytes during phagocytosis. I. Identification of surface proteins. J Cell Biol 82: 32–44, 1979.
15. Willinger M, Gonatas N, Frankel FR: Fate of surface proteins of rabbit polymorphonuclear leucocytes during phagocytosis. II. Internalization of proteins. J Cell Biol 82: 45–56, 1979.
16. Edelson PJ, Cohn ZA: Effects of concanavalin A on mouse peritoneal macrophages. II. Metabolism of endocytosed proteins and reversibility of the effects by mannose. J Exp Med 140: 1387–1403, 1974.
17. Rodewald R: Intestinal transport of antibodies in the newborn rat. J Cell Biol 58: 189–211, 1973.
18. Marzella L, Ahlberg J, Glaumann H: In vitro uptake — microautophagy — of particles by lysosomes. Exp Cell Res (to be published).
19. Figura K von, Kresse H, Meinhard V, Holtfrerich D: Effects of anti-microtubular agents on secretion and endocytosis of lysosomal hydrolases and of sulphated glycosaminoglycans. Biochem J 170: 313–320, 1978.
20. Marzella L, Sandberg PO, Glaumann H: Autophagic degradation in rat liver after vinblastine treatment. Exp Cell Res 128: 291–301, 1980.
21. Steinman RM, Brodie SE, Cohn ZA: Membrane flow during pinocytosis. A stereologic analysis. J Cell Biol 68: 665–687, 1976.
22. Schneider Y-J, Tulkens P, Duve C de, Trouet A: Fate of plasma membranes. I. Uptake and processing of antiplasma membrane and control immunoglobins by cultured fibroblasts. J Cell Biol 82: 449–465, 1979.
23. Heuser JE, Reese TS: Evidence for recycling of synaptic vesicle membrane during transmitter release at the frog neuromuscular junction. J Cell Biol 57: 315–344, 1973.
24. Herzog V, Farquhar MG: Luminal membrane retrieved after exocytosis reaches most Golgi cisternae in secretory cells. Proc Natl Acad Sci USA 74: 5073–5077, 1977.
25. Dean RT: Lysosomes and membrane recycling. A hypothesis. Biochem J 168: 603–605, 1977.
26. Saito T, Ogawa K: Lysosomal changes in rat hepatic parenchymal cells after glucagon administration. Acta Histochem Cytochem, pp 1–18, 1974.

14. THE ROLE OF RECEPTORS IN ENDOCYTOSIS

G. KAPLAN

INTRODUCTION

Endocytosis is the cellular function pertaining to transport of particles, soluble substances and fluid from the extracellular environment into intracellular vacuoles derived from the plasma membrane. On the basis of the size of the substance internalized, endocytosis has traditionally been divided into two functions (see also Glaumann and Marzella, chapter 13), i.e., phagocytosis, which involves the uptake of particulate material, and pinocytosis, the uptake of soluble substances and fluid into the cell. At the molecular and supramolecular levels the concepts 'particle' and 'soluble substance' merge, which makes an absolute division rather difficult.

However, the observation that most particles and some soluble substances bind selectively to the cell surface before being ingested suggests a more suitable criterion for the division of endocytosis. According to the involvement or lack of specific cell-surface receptors in the uptake of extracellular material, endocytosis can now be divided into receptor-mediated (phagocytosis and adsorptive pinocytosis), and non-receptor-mediated endocytosis (pinocytosis).

It is the purpose of this chapter to discuss some of the recent findings concerning the types of receptors involved and the role they play in the endocytic process. More attention will be given to phagocytic than to pinocytic receptors. For more detailed reviews, see references 1–5.

ENDOCYTIC RECEPTORS

Definitions: The term endocytic receptor evolved as an operational term describing the interaction between the ligand and the surface of the endocytic cell. Whether these receptors are actually chemical entities rather than func-

---

Abbreviations: SRBC, sheep red blood cells; FcR, Fc receptor; IgG, immunoglobulin G; E, erythrocyte; LDL, low-density lipoprotein; MW, molecular weight; EIgMC, erythrocytes coated with immunoglobulin M, and complement; C3bINA, C3b inactivator.

tional sites or areas of the endocytic cell surface has been, and still is, a controversial issue among investigators. For the purpose of this chapter an endocytic receptor is defined as a cell surface entity involved in ingestion which has the ability to interact specifically and with high affinity with the ligand, to be saturated by the ligand, and inhibited by competitive binding. In cases where these requirements are not met, the term endocytic receptor will not be used.

Clearly, endocytic receptors cannot be visualized as such. It is through their function, expressed in the presence of appropriately attached ligands, that they are recognized. By the use of rosette formation between phagocytes and particles sensitized with fresh serum components, cell surface receptors which recognize specific serum components can be identified. Membrane structures that mediate ingestion of other substances have also been described and will be discussed below.

The Fc receptors

Rosette formation between cells and sheep red blood cells (SRBC) treated with immune serum can be used to identify separate surface receptors for the Fc portion of immunoglobulin G (Fc receptors) at the level of the single cell [6]. Fc receptors (FcR) are found on a variety of cell types, but it is only on polymorphonuclear leukocytes, monocytes, and macrophages that FcRs have been shown to mediate phagocytosis [1, 4, 7, 8].

The Fc region of certain IgG subclasses is recognized by FcRs on the surface of phagocytic cells. These cells express a protease-sensitive Fc receptor (FcRI) which binds murine IgG2a [9, 10] guinea pig IgG2 [11], and human IgG1 and IgG3 [12]. These IgG subclasses bind to their FcR on the cell surface in the absence of antigen, and for this reason are called cytophilic Igs. Unkeless and Eisen [9], who studied IgG2a binding to mouse macrophages in detail, found that each cell binds $1-2 \times 10^5$ IgG2a molecules with an affinity of about 2×10^7 l/mole at 37° C.

Another FcR, distinct from the trypsin-sensitive receptor for IgG2a, has been reported for mouse macrophages [10, 13–15]. This receptor (FcRII) was found to be trypsin resistant. It mediated efficient binding of IgG-antigen complexes [16] with at least three IgG molecules clustered per complex [17]. Cells from a murine macrophage cell line have been shown to bind $5-8 \times 10^5$ soluble antigen-antibody complexes per cell at $0.7-2.4 \times 10^7$ l/mole at 37° C via the FcRII [14].

Additional evidence in favor of the presence of two independent Fc receptors on the same cells was presented by Unkeless et al. [18]. Variants of the J-774 mouse macrophage cell line were isolated. These new lines failed to bind erythrocytes (E) opsonized with IgG2b anti-E antibody, but bound monomeric IgG2a normally as compared to the parental J-774 line (Ka $4°C = \approx 1 \times 10^8 M^{-1}$, 2×10^5 sites per cell) (Fig. 1). The fact that these variants lost one FcR (the trypsin-resistant FcRII) but not the other (trypsin-sensitive FcRI) is clear evidence for the independent existence of the two FcR types on the same cells.

Recent studies have shed some light on the distribution and mechanism of FcR function. FcRs of mouse peritoneal macrophages [19, 20], rat liver macrophages [21], and rabbit alveolar macrophages [22–24] appear to be located over the entire cell surface. Macrophage subplasmalemmal micro-filaments are probably involved in the interaction of FcR and ligand. This observation is based on the fact that FcR-ligand interaction can be modu-lated by cytochalasins which specifically inhibit microfilament monomer

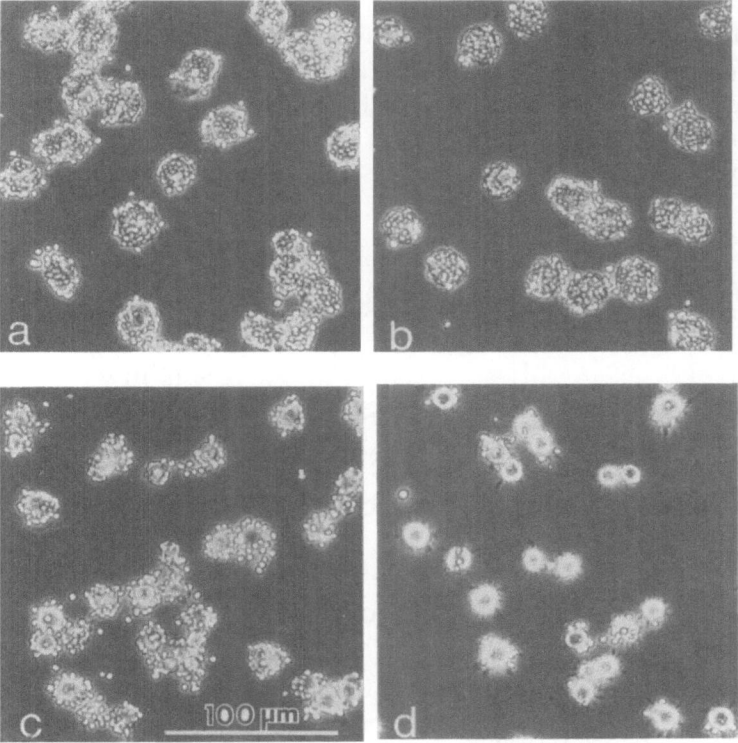

Fig. 1. Phase-contrast micrographs of rosettes formed between particles and Fc receptors (FcR) on J-774 and ICR 4.4 cells. (a) Sheep red blood cells (E) coated with rabbit anti-E IgG (EIgG) were incubated with J-774 macrophage-like cells. (b) EIgG incubated with J-774 cells first treated with 1 mg trypsin per ml medium for 15 min at 37° C (FcRI removed). (c) EIgG incubated with the variant line ICr 4.4, which lacks the trypsin-resistant Fc receptor (FcRII). (d) EIgG incubated with the variant ICR 4.4 first treated with 1 mg trypsin per ml medium for 15 min at 37° C (FcRI removed). Note the lack of EIgG binding in d.

188

polymerization [25] (see also chapter 13). Attempts to identify the domain of the IgG molecule that is actually bound by FcR have been reported by many investigators. Fragments of IgG corresponding to the third constant region of the IgG heavy chain (C_H3) domains (Fig. 2) have been prepared by peptic and tryptic digestion of human and rabbit IgG. These fragments have been shown to be the site to which the FcR binds [7]. Guinea pig FcRs have been shown in other studies to recognize the second constant region of the IgG heavy chain (C_H2) domain [26]. However, it appears that for optimal binding both C_H2 and C_H3 structures are required [27, 28]. Numerous attempts to isolate plasma-membrane FcR have yielded conflicting information concerning these structures. Peptides with apparent molecular weights (MW) ranging from 125,000 to 28,000 have been isolated by affinity chromatography on antibody-coated columns [6]. Cooper et al. [29] have reported the isolation of four proteins with MW in the same range that bind the Fc region of IgG originating from the glycoprotein extract of the plasma membrane of murine leukemia (1210) cells. This lack of general agreement on the structure and properties of the FcR will probably be resolved by the use of monoclonal antibodies with defined specificity for such analysis. In a recent paper Unkeless [30] reports on the isolation of a monoclonal antibody

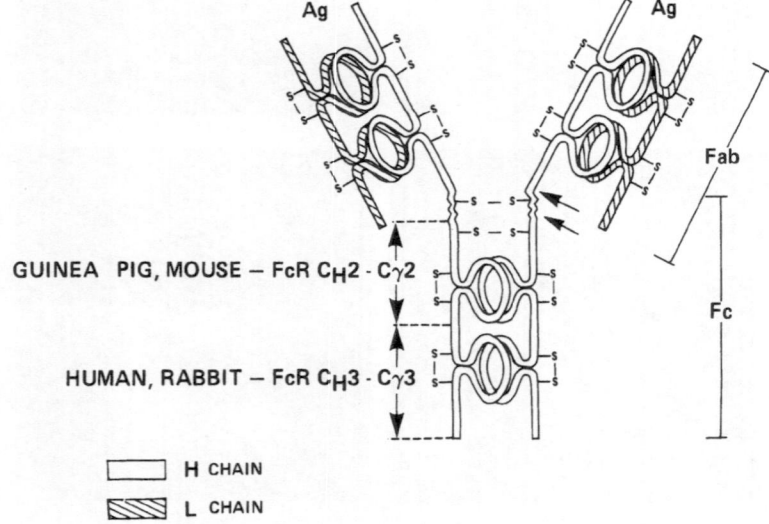

Fig. 2. Schematic structure of the immunoglobulin G (IgG) molecule in relation to its recognition by Fc receptors. Treatment of IgG with papain yields two Fab fragments (both with heavy and light chains) and the Fc fragment (residues 225–446, light chains only). Treatment of IgG with pepsin yields an F (ab′)₂ fragment and an Fc fragment (residues 335–446). The antigen binding sites (2) are at the amino terminals of the heavy and light chains. The FcR binding sites have been reported to be in the C_H3 or $C_\gamma3$ domain for man and the rabbit, and in the C_H2 or $C_\gamma2$ domain for the guinea pig and mouse.

binding selectively to the mouse macrophage trypsin-resistant Fc receptor II. The anti-FcRII antibody did not bind to variants of the J-774 macrophage-like cell line known to lack the FcRII [18]. The antigenic relatedness of mouse lymphocyte FcR to mouse macrophage FcRII was demonstrated by binding studies with the anti FcR antibody.

The C3 receptors

The existence of separate plasma-membrane receptors for complement on blood cells is well documented. These receptors are found on erythrocytes, platelets [31], lymphocytes [32], and phagocytic cells i.e., granulocytes, monocytes, and macrophages [6].

Most of the studies carried out on complement receptors utilize aggluti-nation or rosette formation between cells bearing the receptors and indicator erythrocytes coated with complement components on their surface (Fig. 3). In other studies, complement-coated zymosan, latex, radiolabeled immune complexes, and radiolabeled purified complement components and frag-ments have been used [33, 34].

Complement receptors on all cells tested are inactivated by trypsin. Mouse macrophage complement receptors require Mg^{++} ions for their function [6], whereas receptors on other cell types do not require divalent cations for binding.

Particle binding by complement receptor is temperature dependent [6, 35, 36] and is modulated by substances which disrupt microfilaments [37]. Leukocyte complement receptors bind C3 after cleavage of C3 by C3 con-vertase (C3 receptors) (Fig. 4). The particle-bound active fragment C3b loses its capacity to bind to the C3b receptor (b receptor) when treated with C3b inactivator. The binding site on the C3b molecule is located in the $\alpha_4\beta$ fragment. Its binding to the b receptor can be inhibited by fluid phase C3b, C4b, and C3c, but not C3d.

After the cleavage of C3b by its inactivator, a new fragment is generated, i.e., C3d, which is recognized by another receptor, the C3d receptor (d re-ceptor). The binding site for this receptor is located in the α_3 fragment which remains associated with the particle surface after cleavage by the inactivator (Fig. 4). Binding to the d receptor can be inhibited by fluid-phase C3b and C3d, but not C3c.

The presence of binding sites for C5 on lymphoid cells and their identity with C3 receptor has been suggested [38]. There are several indications that the C3 receptors mediate binding of particle-bound C4b too [33]. Human monocytes have been shown to bind both C3b- and C3d-coated erythrocytes [39]. Starch-elicited guinea pig macrophages also bind both forms [40], where-as C3b but not C3d binds to granulocytes [41] and mouse macrophages [33].

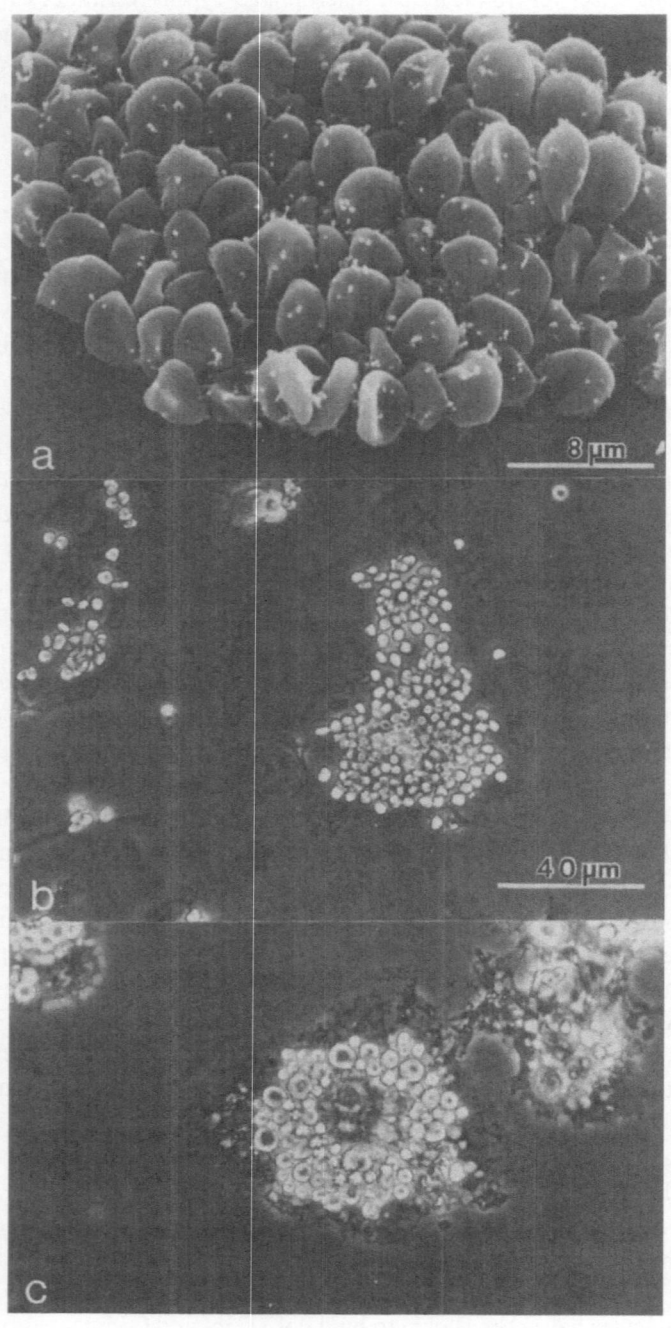

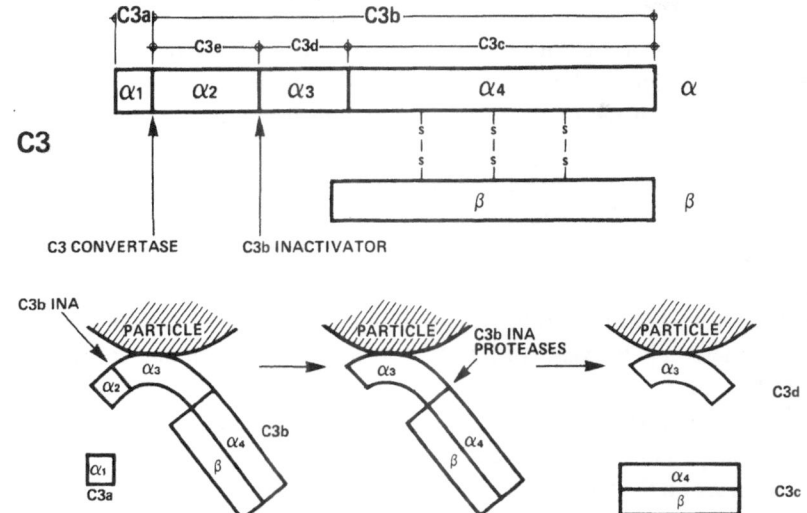

Fig. 4. Schematic representation of the structure of the C3 molecule and the fragments produced during complement activation. Activation of complement (classic and alternative pathways) induces the cleavage of C3a (left side). The fragment C3b is generated and contains a short-lived site in α3 which binds to particles. Subsequently, the C3b inactivator (C3bINA) cleaves the molecule, initially to C3b′ (center) and later to C3c (released) and C3d (particle bound) (right side). Plasma-membrane C3 receptors recognize C3b at the $\alpha_4 \beta$ fragment (b receptors) and C3d at the α_2 fragment (d receptors).

The number of complement receptors on the various cell types is not known. Their distribution on the phagocyte cell surface differs slightly from that found with Fc receptors, and receptor activity appears to be absent from the extreme periphery of the phagocytes [21, 42].

The foreign surface receptors

The presence of the Fc and C3 receptors on vertebrate leukocytes represents a highly specialized function which probably developed after the evolution of immumoglobulins and complement factors. A more primitive form of cellular recognition, found in both invertebrate and vertebrate leukocytes, is well documented [43, 44]. The ability of these cells to bind and ingest a variety of particles — such as bacteria, zymosan, latex, denatured protein aggregates,

←

Fig. 3. Micrographs showing binding and ingestion mediated by the C3 receptors of J-774 macrophage-like cells (72 h in culture). (a) Scanning electron micrograph showing binding of erythrocytes coated with IgM and complement (EIgMC) to J-774 cells. Cells were incubated with EIgMC at 20° C for 20 min. (b) Phase-contrast micrograph showing binding of EIgMC to J-774 cells. Cells were incubated with IgMC at 20° C for 20 min. (c) Phase-contrast micrograph showing ingestion of EIgMC by J-774 cells. Cells were incubated with EIgMC at 37° C for 20 min.

glutaraldehyde-treated red cells, and dead and damaged cells — without previous opsonization with serum components, is often referred to as non-specific or foreign surface receptor mediated endocytosis [1].

The role of divalent cations in the function of these receptors has been established in some cases [45], and trypsin is known to remove some types of foreign surface receptors while leaving other types intact [46].

In many cases of recognition and attachment to foreign surface receptors, the membrane component responsible and the ligands recognized have been reported to be sugars. D-Mannose residues have been shown to be involved in the receptor function during macrophage phagocytosis of certain gram-negative bacteria [47]. Aging of human erythrocytes is accompanied by a gradual loss of red cell membrane sialic acid, exposure of underlying sugar moieties, and subsequent recognition, binding, ingestion, and disposal by macrophages [48]. Here, galactose has been suggested as the target sugar [49]. Hypotheses on the role of overall surface charge and surface hydrophobicity have also been advanced, and a large number of studies have been carried out to identify the type of chemical surface modifications that render particles recognizable by phagocytes [46, 50].

Adsorptive pinocytic receptors

The specific adsorption of soluble molecules to the cell surface prior to their internalization by membrane invagination is referred to as adsorptive pinocytosis. This type of pinocytosis, distinguished by its selectively, requires the presence of specific receptors on the cell membrane. Adsorptive pinocytosis is the mechanism for the uptake of various growth factors and regulatory proteins depending on entry into cells for the exertion of their physiological functions.

The most extensive studies on this type of uptake mechanism are those on low-density lipoprotein (LDL), the major cholesterol-carrying lipoprotein of human plasma [51]. Uptake of LDL by cells is facilitated by the binding of this molecule to receptors localized in discrete regions of the plasma membrane called coated pits. The coated pits invaginate into the cell to form vesicles, thus transporting LDL and cholesterol into the cell. Some of the other systems studied are those involving the uptake of the transport protein for vitamin B_{12} by human placenta cells and fibroblasts, and the uptake of epidermal growth factor by human fibroblasts [52]. A large body of data relating specific membrane receptors to the recognition and ingestion of glycoproteins has recently been acquired. Studies by Ashwell and Morell [53] suggest a general role for terminal sialic acid residues of circulating glycoproteins. The hypothesis has been advanced that sialic acid is essential for the continued viability in the circulation of many glycoproteins. Removal of the terminal sialic acid residue from the carbohydrate chains exposes underlying galactosyl residues. This results in rapid transfer of the glycoprotein from the plasma into liver cells. A hepatic binding protein specific for galactose-terminated glycoproteins has been identified and isolated from parenchymal cells by Ashwell and Morell [53]. It is this molecule that mediates the clearance.

A similar receptor recognizing N-acetylglucosamin and/or mannose terminated glycoproteins has been found on Kupffer cells. Recent studies by Kawasaki et al. [54] have resulted in the isolation and characterization of a mannan binding protein (MW 31,000). This protein is probably the principle receptor mediating the uptake of glycoproteins with terminal N-acetylgluco-samin and/or mannose residues. Another glycoprotein recently studied is the complement fragment C5a [55]. This fragment is bound to the polymorpho-nuclear leukocyte cell surface via a specific receptor. Cellular uptake is rapid, and the rate of dissociation is extremely slow. The binding of the glycoprotein to the receptors is saturable, and the number of binding sites per cell is estimated at $1–3 \times 10^5$. Binding is inhibited by analogues, indicating a specific recognition structure.

THE ROLE OF RECEPTORS IN ENDOCYTOSIS

The wide variety and distribution of endocytic receptors reflects the importance of this process. At least three different functions can be ascribed to these receptors: (1) the recognition of ligands, which provides the specificity of the process; (2) binding of the ligands, which gives close contact between the endocytic cell and the ligand, as well as concentration of the ligand in the microenvironment of the cell; and (3) induction of the ingestion of the ligand.

The different types of receptors have been shown to function independently of each other when mediating binding and ingestion, but they have also been shown to have synergistic effects in many cases. Binding of IgG-coated particles to the Fc receptors of phagocytes directly stimulates particle ingestion. The presence of two different Fc-binding sites on the same cell makes the structure-function relationship of these receptors very difficult to interpret. Walker [56] suggested that two macrophage functions, phagocytosis and antibody-dependent cell-mediated cytotoxicity, are initiated by antibodies of different IgG subclasses operating through different FcRs. On the other hand, the use of homogeneous monoclonal antibodies led Diamond et al. [57] to a different conclusion. They have shown that naturally occurring complexes between antigen and mouse IgG2a and IgG2b antibodies are bound to mouse macrophages and phagocytosed via both of the functionally distinguishable FcRs. These observations suggest the possibility that the two types of FcR on the same cell could contribute to the efficiency, rather than to the specificity, of the phagocyte function. A synergy between the two receptor types in induction of phagocytosis is suggested.

Unlike the Fc receptors, C3 receptors mediate the binding of particles to the phagocyte very efficiently, but under normal conditions do not stimulate ingestion [39]. However, recent observations [58–60] show that C3 opsonized red cells are avidly ingested by inflammatory exudate mouse macrophages, which suggests that the function of this receptor can change with the physiological state of the cell. C3 receptor-mediated ingestion has also been found in rat Kupffer cells, where it is dependent on the presence of heat-inactivated fetal calf serum [61] and in the macrophage cell line J-774 [36]. Obvious synergy between Fc and C3 receptors can be demonstrated. Ehlenberger and Nussenzweig [39] have shown that once C3 opsonized particles have bound to the macrophage surface, a very low number of IgG molecules (60 per particle) suffice to induce ingestion of the attached particles. They further suggest that the stimulus for ingestion of the C3 opsonized red cells is mediated by the presence of low amounts of IgG or even the presence of the IgM molecules used for the fixation of C3 to the particles. They therefore conclude that complement receptors alone possibly mediate only binding and not ingestion. Whether this is indeed true has yet to be clearly established.

In many cases, foreign surface receptor mediated phagocytosis has been shown to function quite independently from that mediated by the Fc and C3 receptor [62, 63]. The binding of particles to some foreign surface receptors leads to avid ingestion [64]. This ingestion appears to be independent of immunological opsonins, but the involvement of nonimmunological opsonins [65] is not completely ruled out. Besides the large variety of particles recognized by the receptors for foreign surfaces, there are indications that heterogeneity in the function of these receptors exists. Seljelid [66] has reported the existence of two distinct morphological mechanisms of ingestion mediated by these receptors. There is also evidence that some of the substances recognized by foreign surface receptors can activate complement [67], which would permit synergy between the foreign surface and the C3 receptors. In other cases, such as the phagocytosis of senescent red cells, it has been suggested that the Fc receptor is eventually involved together with the foreign surface receptor [68].

Studies on receptor function in macrophages have suggested a role for receptor mobility along the plane of the membrane in induction of ingestion. When macrophages are seeded on immobilized ligands (culture dishes coated with antigen-antibody complexes or complement), mobile receptors are depleted from the upper surface of the cells and the function of those receptors is inhibited. This clearly holds for the macrophage Fc receptors [69, 70]. C3 receptors are affected only in activated cells [63]. This suggests an explanation for the difference in receptor function between normal and activated macrophages.

Phagocytosis is inhibited by substances which inhibit normal microfilament function [1]. Although all receptor types are affected, a difference in sensitivity, indicating a possible difference in the association of microfilaments, is found in the different receptor types [21, 42]. Ingestion of particles mediated by the Fc and C3 receptors is inhibited by 2-deoxy-D-glucose. Phagocytosis of latex and zymosan (foreign surface receptors) is not inhibited [63, 63]. The attachment of particles to the various membrane receptors is a prerequisite for internalization and leads to a localized membrane response beneath the attachment site. This is characterized by the aggregation of actin-like filaments and is associated with the formation of pseudopods that enclose the particle [1, 5]. The mechanism by which this transmembrane signal functions to induce ingestion is unknown.

The receptors involved in adsorptive pinocytosis are found on many cell types, and by no means only on phagocytic cells. These receptors provide for specificity of ligand uptake into the cells. In addition, the receptors allow for considerable concentration of the ligand on the cell surface. Thus, for the internalization of a large number of ligand molecules (found in relatively low concentrations in the extracellular fluid), only small segments of the plasma membrane must be internalized. This is achieved by the formation of coated pits and the segregation of the receptors (with ligands bound to them) to these areas prior to ingestion. In all cases studied, this mechanism of uptake appears to operate, and, as already mentioned, carbohydrates of glycoproteins and glycolipids seem to be involved in the recognition [71].

SUMMARY

The identification and characterization of functional membrane receptors are essential for an understanding of the molecular basis of the endocytic process. Endocytosis is a widespread cellular function involving the uptake of exogeneous substances, both soluble and particulate. Although most eukaryotic cells demonstrate this function, it is particularly prominent in leukocytes. Endocytic processes are involved in host defense, immunological reactions, macromolecular transport, hormone transformation, and the regulation of metabolic pathways.

Endocytic receptors are responsible for recognition of the substances to be ingested. Recognition is related to the nature of the ligand surface. Recognition is a prelude to attachment and ingestion, although attachment is not always followed by ingestion.

Rosette formation between phagocytes and particles can be used to identify separate cell surface receptors. Distinct receptors for the Fc portion of different subclasses of IgG (Fc receptors), with different trypsin sensitivity, have been reported. The Fc receptors are distributed over the entire surface of the cell, and the number of the receptors on various cell types has been quantitated. They can be inhibited, and their binding affinity has been calculated. Attempts to isolate the receptors are in progress.

Two types of trypsin-sensitive receptors for complement have been identified on the plasma membranes of phagocytic cells: b receptors, which recognize the complement fragments C3b and C4b, and d receptors, which bind C3d. Normal macrophages bind, but do not ingest, particles coated with C3b. On the other hand, activated macrophages bind and ingest opsonized particles via the b receptor. Receptor activity is temperature dependent. No information is available concerning their number, binding affinity, or structure.

Furthermore, a heterogeneous group of substances are recognized and bound by nonspecific receptors (foreign surface receptors). Divalent cations and trypsin affect some but not others. A role for hydrophobic binding has been suggested. Circulating recognition molecules, which are somehow activated and changed by foreign surfaces and are recognized by phagocytes, might be involved.

The specific adsorption of soluble molecules to the cell surface, prior to their internalization by membrane invagination, is dependent on another group of membrane receptors. These receptors (adsorptive pinocytosis receptors) regulate the uptake of various growth factors as well as regulatory proteins and glycoproteins. Depending on the receptors concerned, differences have been detected in the response of the cells to ligand binding. The different types of receptor have been shown to function independently of each other when mediating binding and ingestion, but they also have synergistic effects. Although the molecular mechanism of phagocytosis is as yet poorly understood, there are some indications that the different receptors mediate phagocytosis by different mechanisms. The pathway of biosynthesis of the receptors and the mechanisms of insertion and stabilization within the membrane are unknown.

REFERENCES

1. Silverstein SC, Steinman RM, Cohn ZA: Endocytosis. Ann Rev Biochem 46: 669–722, 1977.
2. Weir DM, Ögmundsdöttir HM: Non-specific recognition mechanisms by mononuclear phagocytes. Clin Exp Immunol 30: 323–329, 1977.
3. Stossel TP: How do phagocytes eat? Ann Intern Med 89: 398–402, 1978.
4. Walters MNI, Papadimitriou JM: Phagocytosis: a review. CRC Crit Rev Toxicol 5: 377–421, 1978.

5. Michl J, Silverstein SC: Role of macrophage receptors in the ingestion phase of phago-cytosis. Birth Defects 14: 99–117, 1978.
6. Lay WH, Nussenzweig V: Receptors for complement on leukocytes. J Exp Med 128: 991–1009, 1968.
7. Winkelhake JL: Immunoglobulin structure and effector functions. Immunochemistry 15: 645–714, 1978.
8. Dickler HB: Lymphocyte receptors for immunoglobulin. Adv Immunol 24: 167–214, 1976.
9. Unkeless JC, Eisen HN: Binding of monomeric immunoglobulins to Fc receptors of mouse macrophages. J Exp Med 142: 1520–1533, 1975.
10. Heusser CH, Anderson CL, Grey HM: Receptors for IgG: subclass specificity of receptors on different mouse cell types and the definition of two distinct receptors on a macrophage cell line. J Exp Med 145: 1316–1327, 1977.
11. Berken A, Benacerraf B: Properties of antibodies cytophilic for macrophages. J Exp Med 123: 119–144, 1966.
12. Hay D, Torrigiani A, Roitt IM: The binding of human IgG subclasses to human monocytes. Eur J Immunol 2: 257–261, 1972.
13. Walker WS: Separate Fc-receptors for immunoglobulins IgG2a and IgG2b on an estab-lished cell line of mouse macrophages. J Immunol 116: 911–914, 1976.
14. Unkeless JC: The presence of two Fc receptors on mouse macrophages: evidence from a variant cell line and differential trypsin sensitivity. J Exp Med 145: 931–947, 1977.
15. Anderson CL, Grey HM: Physiocochemical separation of two distinct Fc receptors on murine macrophage-like cell lines. J Immunol 121: 648–652, 1978.
16. Arend WP, Mannik M: In vitro adherence of soluble immune complexes to macrophages. J Exp Med 136: 514–531, 1972.
17. Mannik M, Arend WP, Hall AP, Gilliland BC: Studies on antigen-antibody complexes. I. Elimination of soluble complexes from rabbit circulation. J Exp Med 133: 713–739, 1971.
18. Unkeless JC, Kaplan G, Plutner H, Cohn ZA: Fc-receptor variants of a mouse macrophage cell line. Proc Natl Acad Sci USA 76: 1400–1404, 1979.
19. Tizard IR, Holmes WL, Parappally NP: Phagocytosis of sheep erythrocytes by macro-phages: a study of the attachment phase by scanning electron microscopy. J Reticulo-endothel Soc 15: 225–231, 1974.
20. Kaplan G, Gaudernack G, Seljelid R: Localization of receptors and early events of phago-cytosis in the macrophage. Exp Cell Res 95: 365–375, 1975.
21. Munthe-Kaas AC, Kaplan G, Seljelid R: On the mechanism of internalization of opsonized particles by rat Kupffer cells in vitro. Exp Cell Res 103: 201–212, 1976.
22. McKeever PE, Garvin AJ, Spicer SS: Immune complex receptors on cell surfaces. I. Ultra-structural demonstration on macrophages. J Histochem Cytochem 24: 948–955, 1976.
23. McKeever PE, Garvin AJ, Hardin DH, Spicer SS: Immune complexe receptors on cell surfaces. II. Cytochemical evaluation of their abundance on different cells, distribution, uptake and regeneration. Am J Pathol 84: 437–456, 1976.
24. McKeever PE, Spicer SS, Brissie NT, Garvin AJ: Immune complex receptors on cell surfaces. III. Topography of macrophage receptors demonstrated by new scanning electron microscopic peroxidase marker. J Histochem Cytochem 25: 1063–1068, 1977.
25. Atkinson JP, Parker JM: Modulation of macrophage receptor function by cytochalasin-sensitive structures. Cell Immunol 33: 353–363, 1977.
26. Alexander MD, Andrews JA, Leslie RGQ, Wood NJ: The binding of human and guinea pig IgG subclasses to homologous macrophage and monocyte Fc receptors. Immunology 35: 115–123, 1978.
27. McNabb T, Koh TY, Dorrington KJ, Painter RH: Structure and function of immuno-globulin domains. V. Binding of immumoglobulin G and fragments to placental membrane preparations. J Immunol 117: 882–888, 1976.
28. Arend WP, Webster DE: Catabolism and biologic properties of two species of rat IgG2a Fc fragments. J Immunol 118: 395–400, 1977.
29. Cooper SM, Sambray Y, Friou GJ: Isolation of separate Fc receptors for IgG complexes to antigen and native IgG from murine leukaemia. Nature 270: 253–255, 1977.

198

30. Unkeless JC: Characterization of a monoclonal antibody directed against mouse macrophage and lymphocyte Fc receptors. J Exp Med 150: 580–596, 1979.
31. Nelson DS: Immune adherence. Adv Immunol 113: 131–180, 1963.
32. Bianco C, Patrick R, Nussenzweig V: a population of lymphocytes bearing a membrane receptor for antigen-antibody-complement complexes. I. Separation and characterization. J Exp Med 132: 702–720, 1970.
33. Bianco C: Plasma membrane receptors for complement. In: Day NK, Good RA (eds) Biological amplification systems in immunity. New York, Plenum Press, 1977, pp 69–84.
34. Bianco C, Nussenzweig V: Complement receptors. In: Porter RR, Ada GL (eds) Contemporary topics in molecular immunology, vol 6. New York, Plenum Press, 1977, pp 145–176.
35. Munthe-Kaas AC, Berg T: In vitro studies on phagocytosis and lysosomal enzyme patterns in rat Kupffer cells. In: Rossi F, Patriarca PL, Romeo D (eds) Movement, metabolism and bactericidal mechanisms of phagocytes. Padua and London, Piccin Medical Books, 1977, pp 65–73.
36. Kaplan G, Mørland B: Properties of a murine monocytic tumor cell line J-774 in vitro. I. Morphology and endocytosis. Exp Cell Res 115: 53–61, 1978.
37. Atkinson JP, Michael JM, Chaplin H, Parker CW: Modulation of macrophage C3b receptor function by cytochalasin-sensitive structures. J Immunol 118: 1292–1299, 1977.
38. Landen B, Dierich MP: Identity of C3- and C5-receptors on lymphoid cells. J Immunol 122: 1015–1017, 1979.
39. Ehlenberger AG, Nussenzweig V: The role of membrane receptors for C3b and C3d in phagocytosis. J Exp Med 145: 357–371, 1977.
40. Wellek B, Hahn HH, Opterkuch W: Evidence for macrophage C3d-receptor active in phagocytosis. J Immunol 114: 1643–1645, 1975.
41. Eden A, Miller GW, Nussenzweig V: Human lymphocytes bear membrane receptors for C3b and C3d. J Clin Invest 52: 3239–3242, 1973.
42. Kaplan G: Differences in the mode of phagocytosis with Fc and C3 receptors in macrophages. Scand J Immunol 6: 797–807, 1977.
43. Anderson RS: Phagocytosis by invertebrate cells in vitro. In: Maramorsch K, Shope RE (eds) Invertebrate immunity. Mechanisms of invertebrate vector-parasite relations. New York, Academic Press, 1975, pp 153–180.
44. Rabinovitch M, Stefano MJ de: Particle recognition by cultivated macrophages. J Immunol 110: 695–701, 1973.
45. Stossel JP: Quantitative studies of phagocytosis: kinetic effects of cations and heat labile opsonins. J Cell Biol 58: 346–356, 1973.
46. Rabinovitch M: Phagocytosis: the engulfment stage. Semin Hematol 5: 134–155, 1968.
47. Bar-Shavit Z, Ofek I, Goldman R, Mirelman D, Sharon N: Mannose residues on phagocytes as receptors for the attachment of E. coli and S. typhi. Biochem Biophys Res Commun 78: 455–460, 1977.
48. Baxter A, Beeley JG: Surface carbohydrates of aged erythrocytes. Biochem Biophys Res Commun 83: 466–471, 1978.
49. Kolb H, Kolb-Bachofen V: A lectin-like receptor on mammalian macrophages. Biochem Biophys Res Commun 85: 678–683, 1978.
50. Mudd S, McCutcheon M, Lucké B: Phagocytosis. Physiol Rev 14: 210–275, 1934.
51. Goldstein JL, Brown MS: The low-density lipoprotein pathway and its relation to arteriosclerosis. Annu Rev Biochem 46: 897–930, 1977.
52. Gorden P, Carpentier JL, Cohen S, Urci L: Epidermal growth factor: morphological demonstration of binding, internalization, and lysosomal association in human fibroblasts. Proc Natl Acad Sci USA 75: 5025–5029, 1978.
53. Ashwell G, Morell AG: Membrane glycoproteins and recognition phenomena. TIBS 2: 76–78, 1977.
54. Kawasaki T, Etoh R, Yamashina I: Isolation and characterization of a mannan-binding protein from rabbit liver. Biochem Biophys Res Commun 81: 1018–1024, 1978.
55. Chenoweth DE, Hugli TE: Demonstration of specific C5a receptor on intact human poly-

morphonuclear leukocytes. Proc Natl Acad Sci USA 75: 3943–3947, 1978.

56. Walker WS: Mediation of macrophage cytolytic and phagocytic activities by antibodies of different classes and class specific Fc-receptors. J Immunol 119: 367–373, 1977.

57. Diamond B, Bloom BR, Scharff MD: The Fc receptors of primary and cultured phagocytic cells studied with homogeneous antibodies. J Immunol 121: 1329–1333, 1978.

58. Bianco C, Griffin FM, Silverstein SC: Studies on the macrophage complement receptor. Alteration of receptor function upon macrophage activation. J Exp Med 141: 1278–1290, 1975.

59. Griffin FM, Bianco C, Silverstein SC: Characterization of the macrophage receptor for complement and demonstration of its functional independence from the receptor for the Fc portion of immunoglobulin G. J Exp Med 141: 1269–1277, 1975.

60. Mørland B, Kaplan G: Macrophage activation in vivo and in vitro. Exp Cell Res 108: 270–288, 1977.

61. Munthe-Kass AC: Phagocytosis in rat Kupffer cells in vitro. Exp Cell Res 99: 319–327, 1976.

62. Michl J, Ohlbaum DJ, Silverstein SC: 2-Deoxyglucose selectively inhibits Fc and complement receptor-mediated phagocytosis in mouse peritoneal macrophages. I. Description of the inhibitory effect. J Exp Med 144: 1465–1483, 1976.

63. Michl J, Pieczonka MM, Unkeless JC, Silverstein SC: Effects of immobilized immune complexes on Fc- and complement-receptor function in resident and thioglycollate-elicited mouse peritoneal macrophages. J Exp Med 150: 607–621, 1979.

64. Kaplan G, Bertheussen K: The morphology of echinoid phagocytes and mouse peritoneal macrophages during phagocytosis in vitro. Scand J Immunol 6: 1289–1296, 1977.

65. Saba TM: Humoral control of Kupffer cell function after injury. Bull Kupffer Cell Found 1: 12–22, 1978.

66. Seljelid R: Properties of Kupffer cells. In: Van Furth R (ed) Mononuclear phagocytes, functional aspects. The Hague, Martinus Nijhoff, 1980.

67. Czop JK, Fearon DT, Austen KF: Membrane sialic acid on target particles modulates their phagocytosis by a trypsin-sensitive mechanism on human monocytes. Proc Natl Acad Sci USA 75: 3831–3835, 1978.

68. Kay MMB: Mechanisms of removal of senescent cells by human macrophages in situ. Proc Natl Acad Sci USA 72: 3521–3525, 1975.

69. Rabinovitch M, Menejias RE, Nussenzweig V: Selective phagocytic paralysis induced by immobilized immune complexes. J Exp Med 142: 827–838, 1975.

70. Kaplan G, Eskeland T, Seljelid R: Differences in the effect of immobilized ligands on the Fc and C3 receptors of mouse peritoneal macrophages in vitro. Scand J Immunol 7: 19–24, 1978.

71. Hughes RC, Sharon N: Carbohydrates recognized. Nature 27: 637–638, 1978.

15. PATHOLOGY OF ENDOCYTOSIS WITH SPECIAL REFERENCE TO LIPOPROTEINS

G.R. THOMPSON

Low-density lipoprotein (LDL) transports approximately 70% of the cholesterol in normal human plasma. Each LDL particle is 220 Å in diameter and has a pseudomicellar structure, with a surface coat of free cholesterol, phospholipid and apolipoprotein B (apoB) and an inner core of cholesterol ester and triglyceride. The arrangement and relative proportions of these constituents are illustrated in Fig. 1.

An excess of LDL is the hallmark of familial hypercholesterolaemia (FH), a dominantly inherited disorder which affects 0.2% of the population and predisposes to premature death from coronary heart disease (CHD). Homozygous FH is rare, and characterised by extreme elevation of LDL from birth and the appearance in childhood of cholesterol deposits in skin, tendons, cornea and arterial wall. Until recently, sudden death before age 30 was almost inevitable, consequent on atheromatous involvement of the aorta and coronary arteries. The great majority of subjects with FH, however, are heterozygotes in whom LDL levels are only hafl as high as in homozygotes, although two- to threefold greater than in the general population. Heterozygotes develop tendon xanthomata and coronary atheroma in their second or third decade, approximately 25% of males dying from CHD before the age of 50.

LDL
Composition and Structure

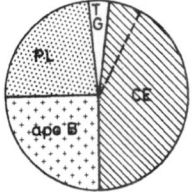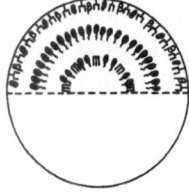

Fig. 1. Diagrammatic representation of the structure and composition of a low-density lipoprotein (LDL) particle. TG, triglyceride (∎); CE cholesterol ester (⸱); PL phospholipid (⋏); apoB apolipoprotein B (β). Unesterified or free cholesterol is delineated by the broken line in the left-hand diagram and represented by the symbol (⸱) in the right-hand diagram.

LDL BINDING IN FIBROBLASTS AND THE PATHOGENESIS OF FH

In 1973 Goldstein and Brown first reported the results of a continuing series of studies of lipoprotein metabolism in cultured skin fibroblasts [1, 2]. Their findings have greatly advanced knowledge of LDL metabolism and have helped elucidate the nature of the molecular defect in FH. These workers discovered that fibroblasts from a patient with homozygous FH had a higher level of hydroxymethylglutaryl-coenzyme A (HMG-CoA) reductase, the rate-limiting enzyme on the cholesterol-synthetic pathway, than normal fibroblasts although the latters' activity increased after prolonged incubation in a lipoprotein-deficient medium. Addition of LDL suppressed HMG-CoA reductase activity, and thus cholesterol synthesis, in normal fibroblasts but had no effect on FH cells. They went on to show that normal fibroblasts bound labelled LDL by means of a specific, high-affinity mechanism which was saturable at an LDL-apoB concentration of 20–40 μg/ml, and that this mechanism was totally absent from fibroblasts from homozygotes and partially absent from heterozygotes' fibroblasts [3]. High-affinity binding was demonstrable at both 4° and 37° C, the bound labelled LDL being displacable both by unlabelled LDL and by very low density lipoprotein (VLDL), which also contains apoB, or by the addition of heparin. LDL was also taken up by both normal and FH fibroblasts by a low-affinity, non-saturable mechanism; both types of uptake were accompanied by the subsequent degradation of LDL within fibroblasts [4]. Hydrolysis of both the apoB and cholesterol ester components was maximal at pH 4 and inhibited by chloroquine, which suggested that LDL degradation took place within lysosomes [5]. The fact that high-affinity binding of LDL by normal fibroblasts was prevented by prior exposure of the latter to pronase suggested that cell-surface receptors were involved in this process.

Subsequent studies showed that incubation of normal fibroblasts with LDL resulted in an increased rate of formation of intracellular cholesterol esters, whereas incubation in an LDL-deficient medium had the reverse effect [6, 7]. This led to the proposal that the rôle of the LDL receptor was to provide growing cells with a carefully regulated supply of free cholesterol. Absence of receptors, as in homozygous FH, resulted in a reduced influx of LDL cholesterol into the cell and thus a failure of repression of HMG-CoA reductase, although repression did occur in heterozygotes' cells if these were exposed to a sufficiently high concentration of LDL [8]. The observation that partial repression of HMG-CoA reductase by LDL was evident in the cells of some homozygotes [9] led to their sub-division into receptor-negative and receptor-defective categories [10], the latter possessing up to 20% of the normal complement of receptors and thus being intermediate between receptor-negative homozygotes, with a complete lack, and heterozygotes, with 40% of normal.

The scheme of events whereby LDL is metabolised in fibroblasts is illustrated in Fig. 2 and can be summarised as follows [11, 12]: initial high-affinity uptake by specific receptors on the cell surface of normal fibroblasts is followed by endocytosis, leading to lysosomal hydrolysis of apoB and cholesterol ester and release of free cholesterol; repression by the latter of HMG-CoA reductase inhibits cholesterol synthesis within the cell, excess free cholesterol being esterified to cholesterol oleate by acyl CoA:cholesterol acyltransferase (ACAT). FH fibroblasts lack LDL receptors, the deficit being

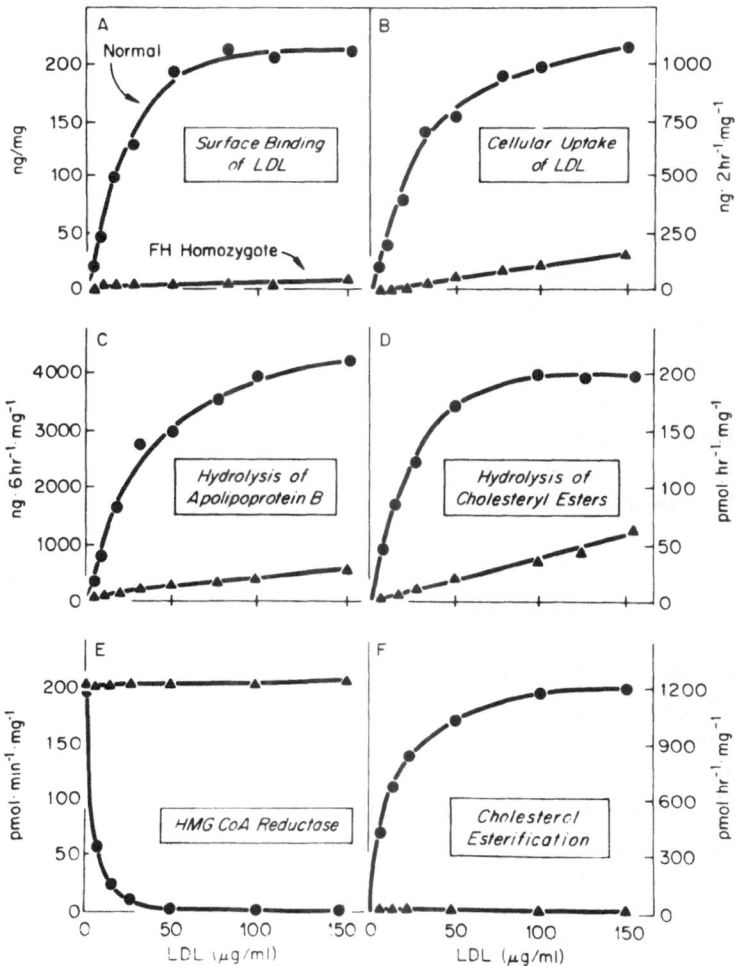

Fig. 2. Comparison of the metabolic events resulting from incubation of normal and homozygous FH fibroblasts with various concentrations of LDL. (Reproduced from Brown MS, Goldstein JL: Receptor-mediated control of cholesterol metabolism. *Science* 191: 150–154, 1976; copyright 1976 by the American Association for the Advancement of Science.)

partial in heterozygotes and total or sub-total in homozygotes; the resultant impairment of LDL binding reduces its rate of internalisation so that neither apoB nor cholesterol ester get hydrolysed normally; consequently, insufficient free cholesterol is released to inhibit HMG-CoA reductase or provide a substrate for ACAT.

LDL UPTAKE BY CELLS OTHER THAN FIBROBLASTS

Fogelman et al. [13] studied cholesterol-synthesis in human leucocytes and showed that this could be enhanced by incubating them in a lipoprotein-free medium. Freshly isolated lymphocytes take up and degrade LDL by a low-affinity, non-saturable mechanism [14] but the presence of high-affinity binding sites can be revealed in normal cells by pre-incubating them in a lipoprotein-deficient medium for 72 h; homozygotes' lymphocytes fail to respond to this stimulus [15]. Smooth muscle cells cultured from human arteries also bind and degrade LDL [16]. Binding is enhanced but degradation impaired by exposure of the cells to hypoxia [17]. Calculations based on the uptake of LDL by pig arterial smooth muscle cells in vitro suggest that all the LDL degraded in vivo could be accounted for on this basis [18]. Both rabbit and human arterial endothelial cells bind and degrade LDL, but less efficiently than fibroblasts or smooth muscle cells [19, 20]. Finally, receptor-mediated uptake of LDL has been demonstrated in cultured mouse adrenal cells, which are able to obtain over 75% of the cholesterol required steroid synthesis by this means [21].

RECEPTOR-MEDIATED ENDOCYTOSIS OF LDL

Anderson et al. [22] were the first to show that binding of LDL, labelled with ferritin, took place at specific sites on the surface of normal fibroblasts. On electron microscopy these sites appeared as indentations in the cell membrane, coated with a fuzzy material. FH fibroblasts had similar regions but these did not bind the ferritin-labelled LDL. Serial transmission electron micrographs show ferritin-labelled LDL adhering to these coated pits on the surface of normal fibroblasts at 4° C and then, after warming to 37° C, becoming incorporated into the cell within endocytic vesicles. Scanning electron micrographs of freeze-fractured normal fibroblasts incubated with un-labelled LDL also reveal shallow pits to which LDL-sized particles adhere; homozygotes' fibroblasts possess similar pits but without any adherent particles [23]. These data suggest that LDL receptors are located in coated pits on the surface of normal cells but are absent in FH, even though the pits are present.

It has been calculated that fully de-repressed, normal fibroblasts possess up to 70,000 binding sites per cell [24]. The number of LDL receptors on the cell surface and the intracellular activity of ACAT are both inversely proportional to the cholesterol content of fibroblasts [25]. Thus, exposure of fibroblasts to a constant amount of LDL initially leads to intracellular accumulation of cholesterol ester, followed by a progressive decrease in the number of receptors on the cell surface and limitation of any further high-affinity uptake of LDL.

In contrast to the classical form of receptor-deficient FH, Anderson et al. [26] recently described a patient whose fibroblasts bound LDL normally but failed to internalise the bound particles. Studies with ferritin-labelled LDL indicated the presence of receptors all over the cell surface but not in the coated pits. Thus, FH can result either from a non-functioning or malfunctioning LDL receptor, which causes a primary defect of binding and secondarily impairs endocytosis, or from a mislocated receptor, which causes a primary defect of endocytosis.

Further information regarding receptor-mediated endocytosis of LDL has been obtained by studying the effects of metabolic inhibitors on fibroblasts [27], as shown in Table 1. Addition of cytochalasin to the incubation medium enhances surface binding of LDL but reduces endocytosis and degradation; addition of colchicine reduces binding, endocytosis and degradation; and addition of chloroquine impairs degradation alone. High-affinity binding, endocytosis and degradation of LDL are also impaired by tunicamycin [28], a blocker of glycosylation. These data can be interpreted in the light of current views on receptor-mediated endocytosis [29] as follows: LDL receptors are synthesised in ribosomes and then glycosylated in the Golgi apparatus, the latter process being blocked by tunicamycin. Subsequently the receptors migrate to the surface of the cells where they cluster within coated pits; cytochalasin is thought to interfere with clustering by disrupting microfilaments, the ensuing impairment of receptor re-entry resulting in enhanced binding of LDL [27]. After remaining on the cell surface for about 10 min, LDL receptors normally re-cycle into the cell via the coated pits as endocytic

Table 1. ^{125}I-LDL metabolism in fibroblasts (after Miller and Yin [27]).

Addition to culture medium	Binding %	Endocytosis %	Degradation %
Nil	100	100	100
Cytochalasin B	262	43	26
Colchicine	35	30	17
Chloroquine	93	91	2

vesicles, together with any LDL that may have been bound. Reduction of endocytosis and degradation of LDL by colchicine suggests that microtubules play a rôle in facilitating the fusion of endocytic vesicles with lysosomes [30]. Finally, degradation of LDL is mediated within lysosomes by acid hydrolases, which are inhibited by chloroquine.

MECHANISM OF BINDING OF LDL TO RECEPTORS

Binding of LDL to its receptor has been shown to be mediated by apoB, whereas suppression of HMG-CoA reductase is dependent upon entry of LDL cholesterol esters into lysosomes and their subsequent hydrolysis to free cholesterol [31]. However, it had earlier been shown that not only LDL but also HDL_c suppress HMG-CoA reductase activity [32]. HDL_c is an abnormal high-density lipoprotein (HDL) found in the plasma of pigs fed a high-cholesterol diet. It does not contain any apoB but is rich in apolipoprotein E (apoE), which was originally known as the arginine-rich peptide. Since HDL_c binds avidly to fibroblasts, this suggests that apoE and apoB share the physico-chemical characteristics necessary for recognition by LDL 2eceptors [33, 34].

Both apoB and apoE are rich in arginine residues, which can be blocked by incubating the parent lip + protein with cyclohexanedione [35]; this markedly impairs the high-affinity binding of both LDL and HDL_c to fibroblasts and suggests that LDL uptake is determined by interaction between the positively charged arginyl residues of apoB and the LDL receptor. The nature of this interaction was explored by Filipovic et al. [36], who found that increasing the sialic acid content of LDL inhibited its high-affinity uptake by fibroblasts whereas desialisation had the reverse effect. This suggested that high-affinity binding was determined by the net charge on an LDL particle rather than by its arginine content [37]. However, alterations of charge can have other effects. For example, cationisation of LDL by dimethylpropanediamine markedly increases its non-specific uptake by both normal and FH fibroblasts [38] and smooth muscle cells [39]. The considerable accumulation of LDL cholesterol which takes place within these cells represses HMG-CoA reductase, even though their receptors have been by-passed. Conversely, anionisation of LDL by acetylation markedly enhances its uptake by macrophages in vitro [40] and by Kupffer cells in vivo [41]. These findings make one wonder whether high-affinity binding of LDL is not too specific a process to be explicable simply on the basis of ionic interaction between LDL-apoB and its receptor.

CLINICAL CONSEQUENCES OF FH

Defective catabolism of LDL in FH, which is demonstrable in vivo as well as in vitro, results in a two- to fourfold increase in plasma cholesterol concentration from birth and, as mentioned previously, leads to premature morbidity and mortality from atherosclerosis. Effective control of hypercholesterolaemia must be achieved on a lifelong basis if these consequences are to be prevented. Serum cholesterol levels can be reduced in heterozygotes by cholestyramine, a drug which enhances LDL catabolism, whereas plasma exchange is currently the most effective means to this end in homozygotes [42].

Several questions remain unanswered regarding the relevance of receptor-mediated endocytosis of LDL in vivo. Firstly, it is not clear as to whether the liver is a major site of LDL catabolism, nor whether hepatocytes possess LDL receptors. Further, the overall quantitative rôle of the receptor-mediated pathway remains to be established, especially since fibroblast receptors are fully repressed in vivo at concentrations of LDL well below those found in vivo. Using cyclohexanedione-blocked LDL, Shepherd et al. [43] recently suggested that the receptor-mediated pathway accounts for only about one-third of the LDL catabolised in vivo in normal subjects. The results of similar studies in patients with FH will be of interest both to cell biologists and to clinicians.

REFERENCES

1. Brown MS, Dana SE, Goldstein JL: Regulation of 3-hydroxy-3-methylglutaryl coenzyme A reductase activity in human fibroblasts by lipoproteins. Proc Natl Acad Sci USA 70: 2162–2166, 1973.
2. Goldstein JL, Brown MS: Familial hypercholesterolemia: identification of a defect in the regulation of 3-hydroxy-3-methylglutaryl coenzyme A reductase activity associated with overproduction of cholesterol. Proc Natl Acad Sci USA 70: 2804–2808, 1973.
3. Brown MS, Goldstein JL: Familial hypercholesterolemia: defective binding of lipoproteins to cultured fibroblasts associated with impaired regulation of 3-hydroxy-3-methylglutaryl coenzyme A reductase activity. Proc Natl Acad Sci USA 71: 788–792, 1974.
4. Goldstein JL, Brown MS: Binding and degradation of low density lipoproteins by cultured human fibroblasts. J Biol Chem 249: 5153–5162, 1974.
5. Goldstein J, Brunschede GY, Brown MS: Inhibition of the proteolytic degradation of low density lipoprotein in human fibroblasts by chloroquine, concanavalin A, and Triton WR 1339. J Biol Chem 250: 7854–7862, 1975.
6. Goldstein JL, Dana SE, Brown MS: Esterification of low density lipoprotein cholesterol in human fibroblasts and its absence in homozygous familial hypercholesterolemia. Proc Natl Acad Sci USA 71: 4288–4292, 1974.
7. Brown MS, Faust JR, Goldstein JL: Role of the low density lipoprotein receptor in regulation the content of free and esterified cholesterol in human fibroblasts. J Clin Invest 55: 783–793, 1975.

208

8. Goldstein JL, Brown MS: Familial hypercholesterolemia. A genetic regulatory defect in cholesterol metabolism. Am J Med 58: 147–150, 1975.
9. Avigan J, Bhathena SJ, Schreiner ME: Control of sterol synthesis and of hydroxy-methyl-glutaryl CoA reductase in skin fibroblasts grown from patients with homozygous type II hyperlipoproteinemia. J Lipid Res 16: 151–154, 1975.
10. Goldstein JL, Dana SE, Brunschede GY, Brown JJ: Genetic heterogeneity in familial hypercholesterolemia: evidence for two different mutations affecting functions of low-density lipoprotein receptor. Proc Natl Acad Sci USA 72: 1092–1096, 1975.
11. Brown MS, Luskey K, Bohmfalk HA, Helgeson J, Goldstein JL: Role of the LDL receptor in the regulation of cholesterol and lipoprotein metabolism. In: Greten H (ed) Lipoprotein metabolism. Berlin, Springer, 1976.
12. Brown MS, Goldstein JL: Receptor-mediated control of cholesterol metabolism. Science 191: 150–154, 1976.
13. Fogelman AM, Edmond J, Polito A, Popjak G: Control of lipid metabolism in human leukocytes. J Biol Chem 248: 6928–6929, 1973.
14. Reichl D, Postiglione A, Myant NB: Uptake and catabolism of low density lipoprotein by human lymphocytes. Nature 260: 634–635, 1976.
15. Ho YK, Brown MS, Bilheimer DW, Goldstein JL: Regulation of low density lipoprotein receptor activity in freshly isolated human lymphocytes. J Clin Invest 58: 1465–1474, 1976.
16. Bierman EL, Albers JJ: Lipoprotein uptake by cultured human arterial smooth muscle cells. Biochim Biophys Acta 388: 198–202, 1975.
17. Albers JJ, Bierman EL: The effect of hypoxia on uptake and degradation of low density lipoproteins by cultured human arterial smooth muscle cells. Biochim Biophys Acta 424: 422–429, 1976.
18. Weinstein DB, Carew TE, Steinberg D: Uptake and degradation of low density lipoprotein by swine arterial smooth muscle cells with inhibition of cholesterol synthesis. Biochim Biophys Acta 424: 404–421, 1976.
19. Reckless JPD, Weinstein DB, Steinberg D: Lipoprotein and cholesterol metabolism in rabbit arterial endothelial cells in culture. Biochim Biophys Acta 529: 475–487, 1978.
20. Stein O, Stein Y: High density lipoproteins reduce the uptake of low density lipoproteins by human endothelial cells in culture. Biochim Biophys Acta 431: 363–368, 1976.
21. Faust JR, Goldstein JL, Brown MS: Receptor-mediated uptake of low density lipoprotein and utilization of its cholesterol for steroid synthesis in cultured mouse adrenal cells. J Biol Chem 252: 4861–4871, 1977.
22. Anderson RGW, Goldstein JL, Brown MS: Localization of low density lipoprotein receptors on plasma membrane of normal human fibroblasts and their absence in cells from a familial hypercholesterolemia homozygote. Proc Natl Acad Sci USA 73: 2434–2438, 1976.
23. Orci L, Carpentier J-L, Perreley A, Anderson RGW, Goldstein JL, Brown MS: Occurrence of low density lipoprotein receptors within large pits on the surface of human fibroblasts as demonstrated by freeze-etching. Exp Cell Res 113: 1–13, 1978.
24. Goldstein JL, Brown MS: The low-density lipoprotein pathway and its relation to athero-sclerosis. Annu Rev Biochem 46: 897-930, 1977.
25. Goldstein JL, Brown MS: Atherosclerosis: the low-density lipoprotein receptor hypothesis. Metabolism 26: 1257–1275, 1977.
26. Anderson RGW, Goldstein JL, Brown MS: A mutation that impairs the ability of lipo-protein receptors to localise in coated pits on the cell surface of human fibroblasts. Nature 270: 695–699, 1977.
27. Miller NE, Yin JA: Effects of cytochalasin B on low density lipoprotein metabolism by cultured human fibroblasts. Biochim Biophys Acta 530: 145–159, 1978.
28. Chatterjee S, Kwiterovich PO, Sekerke CS: Effects of Tunicamycin on the binding and degradation of low density lipoprotein and glycoprotein synthesis in cultured human fibro-blasts. J Biol Chem 254: 3704–3707, 1979.
29. Goldstein JL, Anderson RGW, Brown MS: Coated pits, coated vesicles, and receptor-mediated endocytosis. Nature 279: 679–685, 1979.

30. Ostlund RE, Pfleger B, Schonfeld G: Role of microtubules in low density lipoprotein processing by cultured cells. J Clin Invest 63: 75–84, 1979.
31. Steinberg D, Nestel PJ, Weinstein DB, Remant-Desmetry M: Interactions of native and modified human low density lipoproteins with human skin fibroblasts. Biochim Biophys Acta 528: 199–212, 1978.
32. Assman G, Brown GB, Mahley RW: Regulation of 3-hydroxy-3-methylglutaryl coenzyme A reductase activity in cultured swine aortic smooth muscle cells by plasma lipoproteins. Biochemistry 14: 3996–4002, 1975.
33. Bersot TP, Mahley RW, Brown MS, Goldstein JL: Interaction of swine lipoproteins with the low density lipoprotein receptor in human fibroblasts. J Biol Chem 251: 2395–2398, 1976.
34. Mahley RW, Innerarity TL, Pitas RE, Weisgraber KH, Brown JH, Gross E: Inhibition of lipoprotein binding to cell surface receptors of fibroblasts following selective modification of arginyl residues in arginine-rich and B apoproteins. J Biol Chem 252: 7279–7287, 1977.
35. Innerarity TL, Mahley RW: Enhanced binding by cultured human fibroblasts of apo-E-containing lipoproteins as compared with low density lipoproteins. Biochemistry 17: 1440–1447, 1978.
36. Filipovic I, Schwartzmann G, Mraz W, Wiegandt H, Buddecke E: Sialic-acid content of low density lipoproteins controls their binding and uptake by cultured cells. Eur J Biochem 93: 51–55, 1979.
37. Filipovic I, Buddecke E: Role of net change of low density lipoproteins in high affinity binding and uptake by cultured cells. Biochem Biophys Res Commun 88: 485–490, 1979.
38. Basu SK, Goldstein JL, Anderson RGW, Brown MS: Degradation of cationized low density lipoprotein and regulation of cholesterol metabolism in homozygous familial hypercholesterolemia fibroblasts. Proc Natl Acad Sci USA 73: 3178–3182, 1976.
39. Goldstein JL, Anderson RGW, Buja LM, Basu SK, Brown MS: Overloading human aortic smooth muscle cells with low density lipoprotein-cholesteryl esters reproduces features of atherosclerosis in vitro. J Clin Invest 59: 1196–1202, 1977.
40. Goldstein JL, Ho YK, Basu SK, Brown MS: Binding site on macrophages that mediates uptake and degradation of acetylated low density lipoprotein, producing massive cholesterol deposition. Proc Natl Acad Sci USA 76: 333–337, 1979.
41. Mahley RW, Weisgraber KH, Innerarity TL, Windmueller HG: Accelerated clearance of low density and high density lipoproteins and retarded clearance of E-apoprotein-containing lipoproteins from the plasma of rats after modification of lysine residues. Proc Natl Acad Sci USA 76: 1746–1750, 1979.
42. Thompson GR: Management of familial hypercholesterolaemia and new approaches to the treatment of atherosclerosis. In: Paoletti R, Gotto AM (eds) Atherosclerosis reviews, vol 5. New York, Raven Press, 1979, pp 67–90.
43. Shepherd J, Bicker S, Packard CJ: Receptor independent low density lipoprotein catabolism in man. Eur J Clin Invest 9: 11–32, 1979.

16. VISUALIZATION AND CHARACTERIZATION OF LDL-BINDING SITES ON FIBROBLAST PLASMA MEMBRANES

W.C. DE BRUIJN AND B.J. VERMEER

Attempts to support the biochemical studies on the uptake of LDL (low-density lipoprotein) particles by human cultured skin fibroblasts by direct ultrastructural observation of the plasma membranes have so far failed to demonstrate individual LDL particles at the assumed binding sites. Ferritin conjugation to the LDL particles enabled Anderson et al. to localize ferritin particles at the plasma membrane of the fibroblast cell surface and to show that such particles were internalized by coated pits and vesicles at 37° C, but the LDL particles themselves were not visualized [1].

Vermeer et al. [2], who used unmodified LDL particles and an indirect immunoperoxidase technique with DAB/OsO_4, were able to confirm the presence of the reaction product in similar coated pits and vesicles, but they too were unable to establish the presence of LDL particles at those sites. Recently, we attempted to characterize the LDL particles on the basis of a reaction with colloidal-gold particles tagged with the same type of anti-apoprotein in combination with a contrast-enhancing post-fixation procedure, using OsO_4 plus $K_4Fe(CN)_6$. These studies resulted in the observation of vaguely contrasted LDL-sized particles decorated with small colloidal-gold particles [3]. Subsequently, the electron-scattering capacity of the individual LDL particles was enhanced by the use of tannic acid during the primary aldehyde fixation. Post-fixation was done with OsO_4 plus $K_4Fe(CN)_6$ and the lipoprotein nature of the particles was established by the attachment of a colloidal-gold-anti-apoprotein-B complex. Incubation of the fibroblast at 37°C made it possible to follow the fate of the visualized and characterized LDL particles on the cell membranes as well as to observe the internalization process.

Human foreskin fibroblasts were obtained and cultured as described by Vermeer et al. [2]. Cells were grown to confluency at 37° C on pieces of Melinex and incubated in lipoprotein-free medium with 15% (V/V) newborn calf serum for 48 h at 37° C. The cells were then cooled to 4° C for 30 min and re-incubated in fresh lipoprotein-free medium to which human LDL particles were added (protein concentration: 0.05 mg/ml serum) for 2 h at 4° C. After this incubation the cells were washed thoroughly with phosphate-buffered saline (PBS), to which 0.2% (W/V) bovine serum albumin was added to remove the aspecifically bound LDL particles and again at 4° C with PBS

W.Th. Daems et al. (eds.), Cell Biological Aspects of Disease, 211–214. All rights reserved.
Copyright © 1981 by Martinus Nijhoff Publishers bv, The Hague/Boston/London.

without bovine serum albumin to remove the excess albumin.

For the characterization, the bound LDL particles were reacted with a suspension of colloidal-gold particles (mean diameter: 10 nm) saturated with a diluted, rabbit anti-human apoprotein-B solution in saline. The LDL-loaded cells were incubated with the gold-anti-apoprotein-B complex for 30 min at 4°C, and then thoroughly washed with PBS to assure complete removal of the unattached gold-anti-apoprotein-B complex. In the experiments performed to assess internalization of the gold-tagged LDL particles, the cells were re-incubated for 5–30 min at 37°C in a lipoprotein-free medium. All cells were fixed with 2.5% (V/V) glutaraldehyde in cacodylate buffer containing 1% (W/V) tannic acid (pH 7.4) for 1 h at 4°C [4].

Post-fixation was done for 4 h at 4°C with 1% OsO_4 in the same cacodylate buffer, to which 0.05 M $K_4Fe(CN)_6$ (pH 7.5) was added [5].

After dehydration and Epon embedding, ultrathin section were cut and stained with lead citrate, and observed in a Philips EM 400 at 80 kV. To prove that the attached colloidal particles were gold, point analyses were performed in the same microscope, aided by the attached EDAX 711 X-ray microanalytical equipment and a computer.

At high magnification the outer surface of the cell membrane of the fibroblasts showed numerous contrasted particles. The morphology of these particles was rather complex, but most of them were firmly attached to the outer leaf by a type of foot process, which gradually merged into the outer leaf of the unit membrane. On these foot processes a variety of irregularly shaped particles were observed, among which two forms were recognizable, one rod-shaped without side arms, the other showing a more bolard-likeructure with (four?) side arms. In most places, several of these structures were found grouped together, forming larger aggregates in which the basic structure of the individual particles was hard to recognize. This made it difficult to assess the size accurately. The rod-like structures were about 50–60 nm high and 20–30 nm wide; the bolard-like structures were about twice that width (Fig. 1).

When the 10-nm particles were present among these structures, which was certainly not the case in all of these ultrathin sections, they were situated at the base of the bolard- or rod-shaped structures, just above theeoot process. However, in other cases with less clearly outlined structures, gold particles were situated more peripherally in the contrasted material. Free gold particles or particles not related to contrasted structures were not observed.

In the cells which were allowed to internalize the attached LDL particles tagged with the colloidal-gold-anti-apoprotein-B complex, several clathrin-coated vesicles or membrane indentations were seen in the outer plasma membrane; these contained both contrasted and attached gold particles or only the former. At some distance from the plasma membrane, inside the cell,

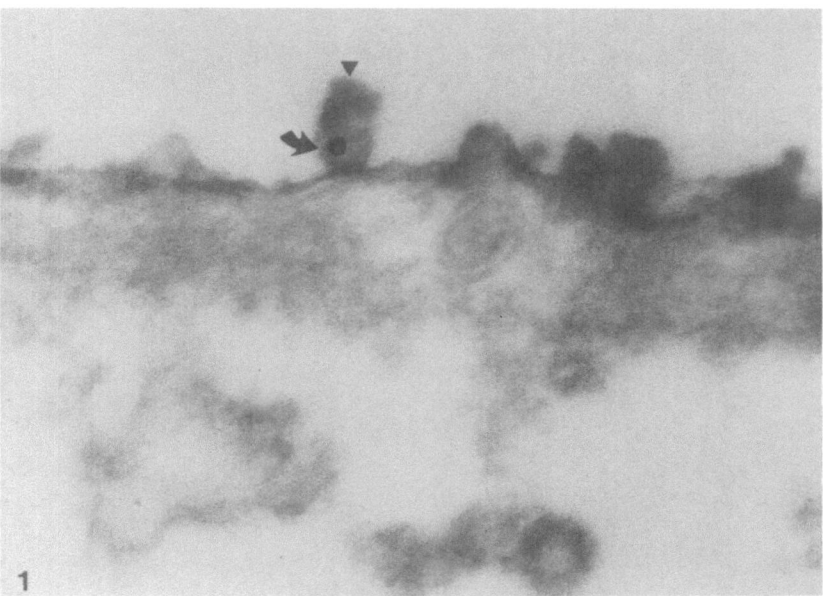

Fig. 1. Human foreskin fibroblast with contrasted rod- and bolard-shaped structures attached to the outer plasma membrane. Towards the outer leaf of the plasma membrane, foot processes merging into the unit-membrane structure can be seen. The arrow points to the single colloidal-gold particles at the base of a rod-shaped structure. In the cytoplasm, fibrillar material is present below the cell membrane; 2 h LDL at 4°C, glutaraldehyde plus tannic acid, OsO_4 plus $K_4Fe(CN)_6$, lead citrate, 80 kV. Magnification: × 106,000.

membrane-bound vesicles containing either only contrasted material or also gold particles were observed (Fig. 2). Still further inward from the plasma membrane there were vesicles containing gold particles not surrounded by contrast material from the OsO_4-$K_4Fe(CN)_6$ reaction. These vesicles are assumed to have contained the surface material internalized before the fixation of the cells by the tannic acid-glutaraldehyde fixative and which therefore had not acquired the enhanced contrast in the post-fixation procedure.

We conclude that the individual particles observed on the external surface of the cell membrane of the LDL incubated fibroblasts, which are characterized by the attached colloidal-gold-anti-apoprotein-B complexes, are the single lipoprotein particles. The internalization of such contrasted and characterized particles has been shown to occur via a mechanism described by, among others, Anderson et al. [1], Vermeer et al. [2] and de Bruijn et al. [3]. However, the total picture is not yet completely clear; for instance, the particles seen on the membranes have dimensions unlike those generally reported for LDL particles seen by negative staining or measured by ultra-centrifugation. Moreover, several non-gold-containing particles were seen on

214

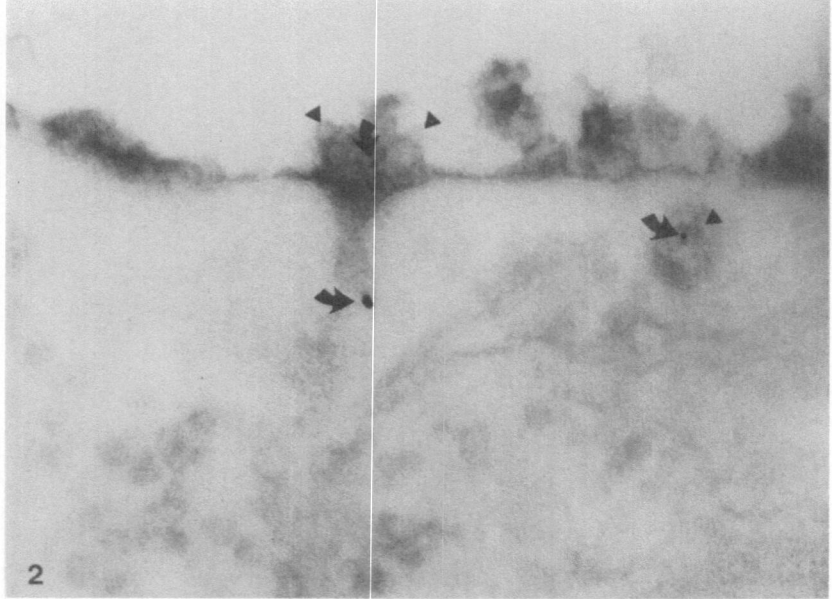

Fig. 2. Foreskin fibroblast similar to that in Fig. 1 but re-incubated at 37° C for 30 min after incubation with LDL and reaction with the gold-anti-apoprotein-B complex at 4° C. In the invaginated cell membrane, colloidal-gold particles can be seen (arrows) as well as contrasted material (arrowheads). At some distance from the plasma membrane there is a vesicle containing colloidal-gold and contrasted material. Glutaraldehyde plus tannic acid, OsO_4 plus $K_4Fe(CN)_6$, lead citrate, 80 kV. Magnification: × 106,000.

the plasma membrane too. As a working hypothesis, it is assumed that most of the contrasted material on the membrane consists of bovine serum albumin, which is attached firmly to the LDL particles and to the free surface of the cell.

REFERENCES

1. Anderson RGW, Brown MS, Goldstein JL: Role of coated endocytotic vesicle in the uptake of receptor bound low density lipoprotein in human fibroblasts. Cell 10: 351, 1977.
2. Vermeer BJ, Koster JF, Emeis JJ, Reman FC, de Bruijn WC: Binding of low-density lipoproteins to human fibroblasts, an investigation by immuno-electron microscopy. BBA 553: 169, 1979.
3. de Bruijn WC, Vermeer BJ, van den Burgh CPM, van Buitenen JMH, Reman FC: Colloidal gold of 5-nm diameter as a possible marker for the localization of LDL-receptor sites on cultured hyman fibroblasts. Ultramicroscopy 4: 123, 1979.
4. Wagner RC: The effect of tannic acid on electron images of capillary endothelial cell membranes. J Ultrastruct Res 57: 132–139, 1976.
5. de Bruijn WC: Glycogen, its chemistry and morphologic appearance in the electron microscope. I. A modified OsO_4 fixative which selectively contrasts glycogen. J Ultrastruct Res 42: 29–50, 1973.

17. SOME ASPECTS OF THE CELL BIOLOGY OF PHAGOSOME-LYSOSOME INTERACTIONS IN MACROPHAGES

P. D'ARCY HART

NATURAL SEQUELS TO INGESTION OF MICROORGANISMS BY PHAGOCYTIC CELLS

Following endocytosis of foreign bodies, including microorganisms, by leucocytes the typical lysosomal response is that the lysosomes fuse with the phagosomes (phagocytic vacuoles) to form phagolysosomes (digestive vacuoles). The targets are thus exposed to the lysosomal contents, which include a variety of digestive enzymes (Fig. 1).

In polymorphonuclear (neutrophil) leucocytes the fusion of lysosomes (as well as of other cytoplasmic granules) with the phagosomes constitutes a pivotal defense act against acute infections: lysosomal degranulation of the host cell takes place; and there is an attempt to kill the ingested microbes, and these or the leucocytes are destroyed. With macrophages the response is more varied, and so is the fate of the intracellular organisms (which are responsible, usually, for chronic infections); in some cases the invader is killed and digested, in others it resists the lysosomal attack and survives, and in still others absence or reduction of phagosome-lysosome fusion (P-LF) accompanies survival. Other variations of lysosomal response have also been observed (see T.C. Jones, chapter 18).

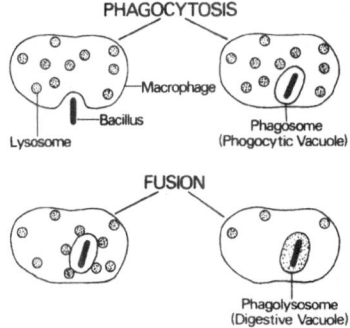

Fig. 1. Schematic simplified representation of phagosome-lysosome fusion sequence in a macrophage. Top left: bacillus being ingested. Top right: bacillus in phagosome. Bottom left: lysosomes assembling around phagosome and fusing with it. Bottom right: phagolysosome formed by the fusion.

Some of these 'natural manipulations' of macrophages by intracellular organisms are exemplified by several species of the mycobacterial genus. Thus ingestion of pathogenic *Mycobacterium tuberculosis* is associated with non-fusion, and the bacillus multiplies in its (unfused) phagosome; the mouse pathogen *Mycobacterium lepraemurium* promotes P-LF but resists the ensuing exposure to lysosomal contents and multiplies in its phagolysosome; while attenuated strains of mycobacterium, such as Bacille Calmette-Guérin (BCG) tend to die in association with the gradual onset of fusion [1–3] (Fig. 2).

THE FUSION PROCESS

Little is known about the events that occur at the apposition between phagosome and lysosome membranes when they fuse. Two current viewpoints on this process for other forms of biological membrane fusion would also apply here, namely, (a) involvement of lipid interactions, lysolecithin formation, and alteration of the fluidity of the lipid bilayers, and (b) involvement of surface proteins, these being broken down or pushed to one side. According to both viewpoints divalent cations (e.g., Ca^{2+}) are believed to participate.

CHEMICAL AGENTS THAT CAN AFFECT P-LF

Increase or decrease of P-LF by chemical agents could be expected to throw light on the basic mechanisms of this fusion phenomenon. Moreover, by mimicking the natural variations which follow infection such agents might offer a clue to the microbial substances responsible for promotion of fusion. If nonfusion represents actual inhibition and not merely 'nonpromotion,' they might also offer a clue to the substances which are responsible for this.

In much current work under this heading the model used consists of monolayer cultures of mouse peritoneal macrophages and a target of baker's yeasts (*Saccharomyces cerevisiae*) — an organism which normally promotes fusion. The lysosomes are prelabeled with acridine orange for fluorescence microscopy of living cells, or with the electron-opaque protein ferritin for transmission electron microscopy. The occurrence of fusion is assessed by the transfer of marker from lysosomes to the interior of the yeast-containing phagosomes [4].

By these means two classes of agent have been identified: one which suppresses or inhibits P-LF if administered to the cultures before ingestion of the yeasts [4–8], and the other which accelerates this process or reverses the action of an inhibitor [6, 7, 9] (Fig. 3). The first group are all negatively charged polymers (e.g., the trypanocidal drug suramin, dextran sulphate, poly-D-glutamic acid, and an amylose derivative 'COAM'). The second group are (so far) all lipophilic secondary or tertiary amines (e.g., chloroquine, tributylamine, and some local anesthetics). The polyanions enter the macrophage by endocytosis, and the amines probably by direct permeation [10]. Substances in both groups accumulate in the lysosomes; and the evidence is now strong that their activity (at least of polyanions) is initiated in these organelles [7]. The effects of these agents on P-LF can be seen not only by the degree of transfer of label from lysosome to yeast phagosome, but by the degree of lysosomal degranulation of the macrophage.

STUDY OF BASIC MECHANISMS

The use of these chemical inhibitors and enhancers of P-LF enables systems to be set up to study some basic aspects of this process. Cytochalasin B had no visible effect either on fusion or on its inhibition, as assessed by the yeast–acridine orange system, thus providing no support to the participation of microfilaments situated either below the plasma membrane or around the phagosome itself (Hart and Young, unpublished observations); nor did colchicine inhibit fusion, indicating that microtubules do not guide the lysosomes to their target [4, 11]. Another point of some interest is that when P-LF occurs in the mouse peritoneal macrophage cultures, fusion can be observed to continue (probably involving fresh as well as preexisting lysosomes) for at least one or two days, while the yeasts are being digested.

Normally the membrane of yeast phagolysosomes (as seen in electron micrographs) is close to the yeast cell wall; but prior administration of a polyanion is frequently associated with a 'looseness' of the membrane of unfused phagosomes, characterized by an obvious space between this and the yeast wall [9]. This looseness can be partially reversed to 'tightness' by chloroquine (lipophilic amine). The mechanism of these morphological changes is unclear. Electron micrographs suggest that loose phagosomes may be present also around some other intraphagosomal organisms that inhibit P-LF, e.g., toxoplasmas [9].

INFLUENCE OF FUSION-MODIFYING AGENTS ON PATHOGENIC INFECTIONS

The effects of the anionic inhibitors of P-LF in cultured macrophages, when the ingested organism is a pathogen, have been reported for two species, namely, *M. lepraemurium* [12] and *Listeria monocytogenes* [8], both of them promoters of fusion. In the first case, this fusion was moderately inhibited

218

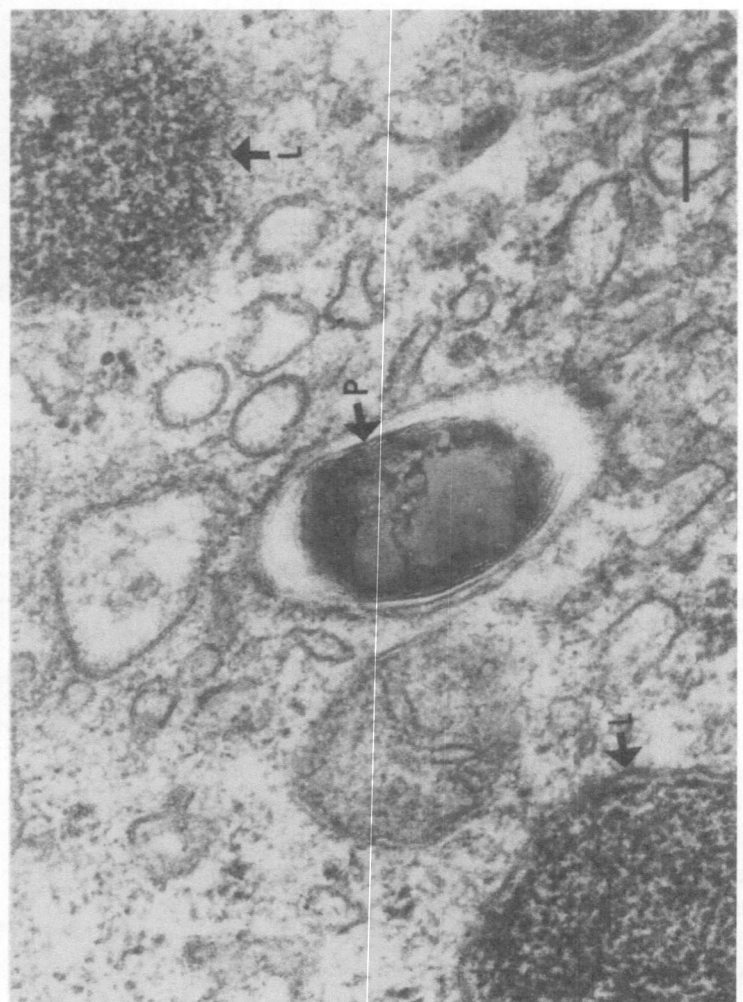

Fig. 2A. Electron micrograph of phagosome-lysosome fusion response in cultured mouse peritoneal macrophages containing mycobacteria. Secondary lysosomes were prelabeled with ferritin. *Mycobacterium tuberculosis*: ferritin marker, present in neighboring lysosomes (L), has not entered the phagosome (P), which contains an intact bacillus; nonfusion. Bar = 0.1 µM.

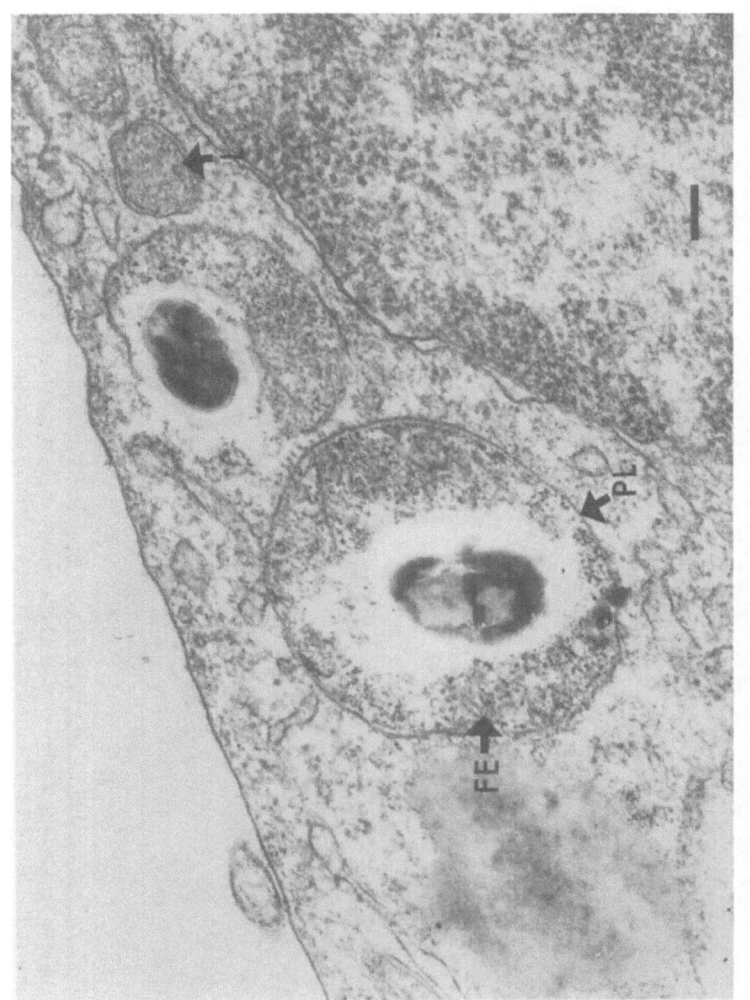

Fig. 2B. Electron micrograph of phagosome-lysosome fusion response in cultured mouse peritoneal macrophages containing mycobacteria. Secondary lysosomes were prelabeled with ferritin. *Mycobacterium lepraemurium:* ferritin is seen in lysosome (L) and also (FE) within phagolysosome (PL) surrounding an intact bacillus, indicating that phagosome-lysosome fusion has occurred. Bar = 0.1 μM.

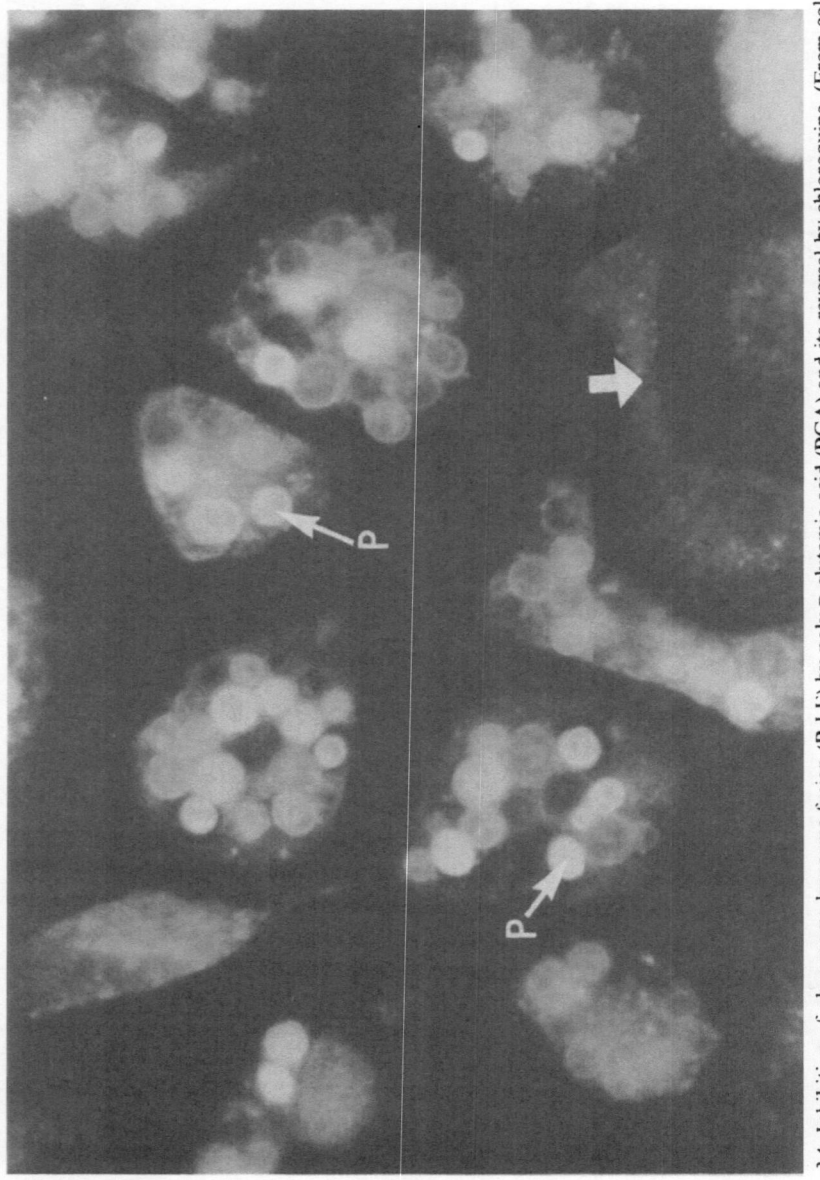

Fig. 3A. Inhibition of phagosome-lysosome fusion (P-LF) by poly-D-glutamic acid (PGA) and its reversal by chloroquine. (From color micrograph × 1350.) Living macrophages with acridine-orange-labeled lysosomes (L) after a pulse of irradiated *Saccharomyces cerevisiae* for 15 min, followed by 45 min of further incubation. The arrowed macrophage containing no yeasts shows the normal complement of lysosomes; most of the other macrophages containing yeast cells are degranulated, the lysosomal marker-dye being transferred to the phagosomes (P), and imparting an intense fluorescence (green, red, orange) to the yeasts therein. Appearance is of widespread P-LF.

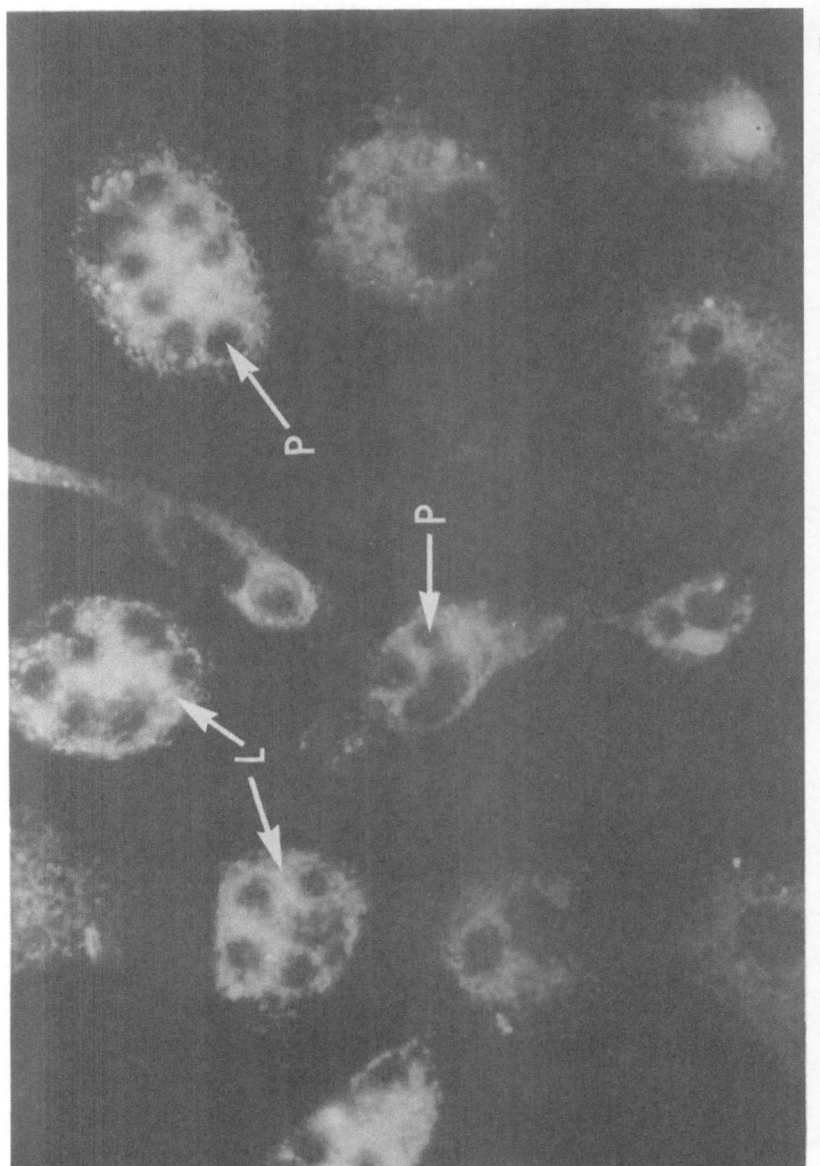

Fig. 3B. Inhibition of phagosome-lysosome fusion (P-LF) by poly-D-glutamic acid (PGA) and its reversal by chloroquine. (From color micrograph ×1350.) Conditions as in Fig. 3A. but macrophages had been pretreated for 5 days with PGA 100 μg/ml. The densely packed lysosomes (L) surround dark spaces, which indicate unstained yeasts in nonfused phagosomes (P). Appearance is of inhibited P-LF.

222

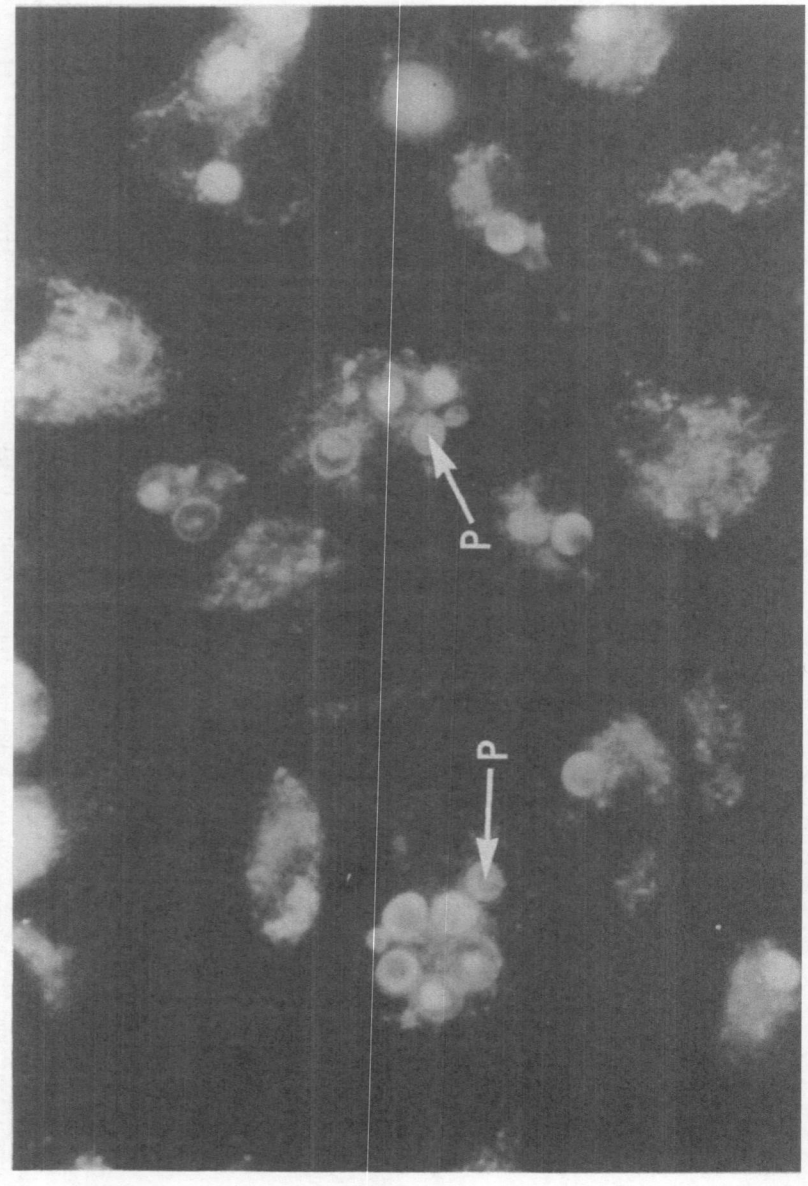

Fig. 3C. Inhibition of phagosome-lysosome fusion (P-LF) by poly-D-glutamic acid (PGA) and its reversal by chloroquine. (From color microgrph ×1350.) As Fig. 3B, but exposed, immediately after the yeast pulse, to chloroquine diphosphate 15 μg/ml for 40 min. Appearances are similar to Fig. 3A, i.e., inhibition of fusion has been reversed.

by poly-D-glutamic acid and markedly, although temporarily, by suramin, but in the second case not at all by the latter drug. Thus these effects vary with the target organism. It may be added that the fusion enhancer cloroquine reversed the usual nonfusion pattern associated with intraphagosomal *M. tuberculosis* [6].

A remarkable correlation has become evident between fusion activity of these chemical agents in the yeast system and their effects upon the progress of a virulent tuberculous infection induced in cultured macrophages. All the anionic inhibitors of P-LF in the yeast system accelerate the tuberculous infection, while all the lipophilic amines that enhance P-LF and have been tested in the tuberculous infection inhibit or suppress the latter [6, 13]. The acceleration of tuberculous infection by polyanions extends to the intact animal: suramin and COAM each markedly show this in the mouse ([14] and R.J.W. Rees, unpublished observations).

This correlation seems to be most readily shown with tuberculous infection. In vivo infection of mice by *M. lepraemurium* also is accelerated by suramin [15], but *Myobacterium leprae* is not (R.J.W. Rees, unpublished observations). *L. monocytogenes* infection in the intact mouse was unaffected by suramin, but this drug actually diminished this infection in cultured macrophages [8].

Recent evidence from our laboratories suggests that the macrophages themselves participate in both the enhancement and the inhibition of tuberculous infection brought about by these agents, i.e., that their effects are, at least in part, host-cell mediated.

RESPONSIBILITY FOR THE NATURAL INHIBITION OF P-LF
IN *M. tuberculosis* INFECTION

Since the nonfusion pattern of P-LF associated with experimental infection of macrophages by virulent *M. tuberculosis*, as well as by some other organisms (T.C. Jones, chapter 18), is an exceptional feature of intracellular invasion, its explanation should contribute to an understanding of the mechanism of fusion. So far no such explanation, including participation of polyanions produced by the microbes themselves, has been more than suggestive. Anionic sulphatides, capable of inhibiting P-LF in the yeast system [5], have been isolated from virulent *M. tuberculosis*. Another polyanion, polyglutamic acid, is present in the cell wall of this species [16] but probably not in that of *M. lepraemurium* [17]; however, it is the L form, which is inactive in the yeast system [13]. cAMP is increased within mouse peritoneal macrophages after ingestion of living *Mycobacterium microti* ('vole tubercle bacillus'), a fusion inhibitor, but not after ingestion of the fuser *M. lepraemurium* or of dead bacilli [18].

Recently the culture fluid from an established growth of *M. tuberculosis* on a simple medium has been found to inhibit P-LF in the yeast model (using either fluorescence or electron microscopy). The constituent responsible has not yet been identified, but it is not a polyanion (A.H. Gordon, M.R. Young, and P.D'Arcy Hart, in preparation).

OUTLOOK

Observations on natural behavior of microorganisms toward P-LF in macrophages, and the recent techniques by which this fusion process can be altered under defined experimental conditions (and with specified targets), have not yet progressed much beyond the descriptive stages. Hopes that the chemical fusion modifiers might alter some pathogenic infections to the advantage of the human host have been limited (e.g., lipophilic amines on tuberculous infection) by toxicity; in any case their effects on pathogens seems selective.

The agents do not necessarily indicate the type of compound responsible for the natural manipulations effected by microorganisms such as *M. tuberculosis* and *Toxoplasma gondii*, a matter of basic interest. More promising perhaps is the direct approach (mentioned above) recently commenced with a filtrate from *M. tuberculosis* cultures, which has fusion-inhibiting potency; a hitherto unsuspected type of inhibitor is suggested by preliminary study.

In spite of limitations, however, experience of manipulation of the kinetics of P-LF offers encouragement for clarification of some aspects of the mechanism of this process. Thus the labeling of one polyanion (COAM) [7] has established the location of this compound in secondary lysosomes during the time when it is blocking P-LF (and, incidentally, doing the latter without the use of a free marker, acridine orange). Even if (as is likely) the inhibition by polyanions is incomplete, 'turning them on,' and then reversing their activity by an amine, will enable basic factors to be examined under defined conditions. Isolation of macrophage lysosomes after the cultures have been treated with these fusion modifiers should also assist. With greater knowledge we should approach nearer to answering the question as to how far P-LF is important in determining the fate of intracellular pathogens (other than by digesting their dead bodies — itself not always efficient, e.g., in leprosy), and whether any deliberate alteration of the fusion process is desirable and practicable as a therapeutic measure.

REFERENCES

1. Armstrong JA, Hart P D'Arcy: Response of cultured macrophages to *Mycobacterium tuberculosis*, with observations on fusion of lysosomes with phagosomes. J Exp Med 134: 713–740, 1971.
2. Hart P D'Arcy, Armstrong JA, Brown CA, Draper P: Ultrastructural study of the behaviour of macrophages toward parasitic mycobacteria. Infect Immunol 5: 803–807, 1972.
3. Hart P D'Arcy, Armstrong JA: Strain virulence and the lysosomal response in macrophages infected with *Mycobacterium tuberculosis*. Infect Immunol 10: 742–746,1974.
4. Hart P D'Arcy, Young MR: Interference with normal phagosome-lysosome fusion response in macrophages, using ingested yeast cells and suramin. Nature (London) 256: 47–49, 1975.
5. Goren MB, Hart P D'Arcy, Young MR, Armstrong JA: Prevention of phagosome-lysosome fusion in cultured macrophages by sulfatides of *Mycobacterium tuberculosis*. Proc Natl Acad Sci USA 73: 2510–2514, 1976.
6. Hart P D'Arcy, Young MR: Manipulations of the phagosome-lysosome fusion response in cultured macrophages. Enhancement of fusion by chloroquine and other amines. Exp Cell Res 114: 486–490, 1978.
7. Geisow MJ, Beaven GH, Hart P D'Arcy, Young MR: Site of action of a polyanion inhibitor of phagosome-lysosome fusion in cultured macrophages. Exp Cell Res 126: 159–165, 1980.
8. Pesanti EL: Suramin effects on macrophage phagolysosome formation and anti-microbial activity. Infect Immunol 20: 503–511, 1978.
9. Hart P D'Arcy, Young MR: The effect of inhibitors and enhancers of phagosome-lysosome fusion in cultured macrophages on the phagosome membrane of ingested yeasts. Exp Cell Res 118: 365–375, 1979.
10. de Duve C, de Barsy T, Poole B, Trouet A, Tulkens P, van Hoof F: Lysosomotropic agents. Biochem Pharmacol 23: 2495–2531, 1974.
11. Pesanti EL, Axline SG: Colchicine effects on lysosome enzyme induction and intracellular degradation in the cultivated macrophage. J Exp Med 141: 1030–1046, 1975.
12. Draper P, Hart P D'Arcy, Young MR: Effects of anionic inhibitors of phagosome-lysosome fusion in cultured macrophages when the ingested organism is *Mycobacterium lepraemurium*. Infect Immunol 24: 558–561, 1979.
13. Hart P D'Arcy, Young MR: Manipulations of phagosome-lysosome fusion in cultured macrophages: potentialities and limitations. In: Van Furth R (ed) Mononuclear phagocytes — functional aspects. The Hague, Martinus Nijhoff, 1039–1055, 1980.
14. Rees RJW, Hart P D'Arcy: Enhancement of experimental tuberculosis in the mouse by suramin. Tubercle (London) 37: 327–332, 1956.
15. Hilson GRF, Elek SD: Intratesticular multiplication of *Mycobacterium lepraemurium* in normal and suramin-treated animals. Int J Leprosy 25: 380–391, 1957.
16. Petit J-F: Structure chimique de la paroi des mycobactéries. Ann Microbiol (Inst Pasteur) 129A: 39–48, 1978.
17. Draper P: The walls of *Mycobacterium lepraemurium*: chemistry and ultrastructure. J Gen Microbiol 69: 313–324, 1971.
18. Lowrie DB, Aber VR, Jackett PS: Phagosome-lysosome fusion and cyclic adenosine 3':5'-monophosphate in macrophages infected with *Mycobacterium microti*, *Mycobacterium bovis* BCG or *Mycobacterium lepraemurium*. J Gen Microbiol 110: 431–441, 1979.

18. PATHOLOGY OF PHAGOSOMES AND LYSOSOMES DURING MAMMALIAN CELL-MICROBE INTERACTIONS*

T.C. JONES

When microbes encounter mammalian phagocytic cells, a complex series of events determine the ultimate fate of the microbe and the destruction or the survival of the phagocytic cell. The steps include attachment of the microbe to the cell surface, recognition of the microbe leading to endocytosis, initiation of metabolic microbicidal mechanisms, fusion of lysosomes with the endocytosed phagosomal membrane, and digestion of the phagolysosomal contents [1]. These events describe the action of the phagolysosomal system. For a microbe to receive the designation of being pathogenic, it has evolved some mechanism for evading this efficient system. This review will describe the mechanisms by which microbes have successfully avoided digestion within phagolysosomes. The means which enable cells from immunized animals to control the pathologic process, in spite of a lesion of the phagolysosomal system, will be indicated.

Table 1 summarizes stages in the phagolysosomal system at which microbes subvert function of the system, thus providing for their continued survival. For certain microbes, capable of extracellular replication, avoidance of attachment to mammalian phagocytic cells is the major defense against the phagolysosomal system. The best examples of this phenomenon are demonstrated by the pneumococcus and the cryptococcus. These organisms have synthesized complex polysaccharides at the cell surface which prevent attachment of the microbe to the membrane surface of the phagocytic cell. The primary host defense against these microbes includes the production of circulating factors capable of coating these polysaccharides, rendering them susceptible to attachment, the first step of the phagocytic process. This process of opsonization allows the contact of the microbe with the phagolysosomal system. This is referred to as immunologically specified attachment and recognition. The Fc and complement receptors on the surface of macrophages mediate this immunologic attachment and recognition (see Kaplan, chapter 14) [2]. These receptors are especially important in maintaining firm attachment, and in initiating attachment which progresses to recognition stages of the ingestion of opsonized particles.

A second type of microbe-macrophage interaction is that which occurs in

* Research supported by NIH grants AI 12146 and AI 10821.

the absence of any serum factor such as antibody or complement. This has been referred to as 'non specific' because specific attachment loci on the surface of the macrophage or on the microbe have not been identified [3]. It is likely that most nonpathogenic organisms enter the phagolysosomal system by nonspecific mechanisms. Structures which resemble lectins present on the surface of microbes are one means of initiating this form of attachment and recognition. For example, certain gram-negative bacteria contain these lectin-like substances on their surface which bind with high affinity to glycoproteins containing accessible polysaccharide residues [4]. Some microbes, such as listed under 'stage 2' in Table 1, attach to the phagocytic cell surface but avoid initiation of the next step, the recognition events, which leads to endocytosis. Mycoplasma organisms and pneumocystis organisms are examples of microbes which can attach to macrophages but do not trigger the ingestion event [5, 6]. These microbes remain bound to the macrophage surface and may actually divide in this microenvironment. Both of these organisms appear to have surface proteins which interfere with the recognition stage of phagocytosis. This has been demonstrated in the case of *Myco-*

Table 1. Stages in the phagolysosomal system at which microbes subvert its function.

Stage	Organism	Action on phagolysosome system
1. Attachment	Pneumococcus and cryptococcus	Polysaccharide capsule prevents membrane attachment
2. Recognition	Mycoplasma and pneumocystis	Attaches to membrane, but endocytosis is not triggered
3. Phagosome a) Lysis	Vaccinia virus and *Trypanosoma cruzi*	Lyse phagosome after endocytosis before lysosomal fusion
b) Fusion inhibition	*Toxoplasma gondii* and *Chlamydia psittaci*	Inhibit lysosomal fusion with phagosome
4. Phagolysosome	*Mycobacteria* and *Leishmania*	Survive within phagolysosomes
	Certain viruses (ECHO)	Use lysosomal enzymes for uncoating step

plasma by the observation that treatment of surface-adherent organisms with trypsin or chymotrypsin initiates the recognition event [7]. These protease enzymes do not interfere with the ability of mycoplasma to multiply. *Pneumocystis* attachment to rodent alveolar macrophages also does not trigger ingestion unless the organisms are treated with trypsin or pronase but not with lysozyme or chymotrypsin (Masur, unpublished observations). Both of these microbes can be brought into the phagolysosomal system by opsonic immunoglobulins as described for the pneumococcus and the cryptococcus. It is of interest that another microbe, *Treponema pallidum*, which attaches to, but is not ingested by, mononuclear phagocytes cannot be opsonized to initiate immunologic recognition and phagocytosis [3]. The reason for this unusual ability to resist opsonization is unclear.

The above descriptions are of microbes which are capable of extracellular replication and, thus, they maintain survival by avoiding the intracellular environment. A third category of attachment and recognition, however, is an essential part of the life cycle of obligate intracellular microbes. Organisms such as viruses, protozoa (*Trypanosoma, Leishmania*, and *Toxoplasma*), and bacteria (*Chlamydia*) are obligate intracellular organisms. Some bacteria, such as mycobacteria and listeria, are facultative intracellular organisms. All of these organisms appear to have evolved mechanisms for utilizing the endocytic event of the phagolysosomal system but, thereafter, interrupt successful killing and digestion within the system. The mechanism of attachment, recognition, and entry of these microbes into cells has been referred to as parasite-specified phagocytosis. For example, the attachment of *Chlamydia psittaci* to cells appears to be mediated by the interaction of heat-labile components on the surface of the parasite with trypsin-sensitive components on the surface of the host cells [8]. The mechanism facilitating attachment of *Toxoplasma gondii* to cells remains unknown. Specialized protozoal structures (rhoptries) may be involved by renewing a surface coat on the toxoplasma [9]. Such a mechanism has been described for entry of *Plasmodia* into erythrocytes [10]. Most of the microbes capable of parasite-specified phagocytosis may enter both phagocytic and typically nonphagocytic cells. The addition of antibody of these microbes blocks their entry into nonphagocytic cells such as fibroblasts, which do not contain Fc receptors for antibody, but enhances their entry into phagocytic cells. This has been shown for *Chlamydia*, vaccinia virus, and *Toxoplasma*. When antibody is added to these organisms, the microbes enter the phagolysosomal system and are destroyed. This effect of antibody suggests that the process of parasite-specified phagocytosis includes, not only an attachment and entry mechanism, but techniques which avoid completion of the phagolysosomal process.

One of the first steps utilized by microbes to subvert the process is demonstrated by the vaccinia virus [11] and by *Trypanosoma cruzi* [12]. These organisms are capable of inducing lysis of the phagosomal membrane during or shortly after the entry process. The interactions responsible for this lysis remain unknown. It is clear that during trypanosome-macrophage interaction, first there is endocytosis, then there is disappearance of the phagosomal vacuolar membrane from around the protozoa, which leaves the protozoa free in the mammalian cell cytoplasm. Vaccinia virus demonstrates the same phenomenon. It is at this level, if the vaccinia virus has been coated with antibody, that the pathogenis process is interrupted, the phagosomal membrane is preserved, and phagolysosomal fusion results [11]. Following disruption of the phagosomal membrane, these microbes then replicate within the cytoplasm until their number is such that cell rupture occurs, damaging the host cell.

During parasitism by the organisms *Toxoplasma* and *Chlamydia*, a different process of subverting the phagolysosomal systems seems to occur. This includes, not only preservation of the phagosomal membrane, but marked alterations of this membrane such that it has been referred to as a parasitopherous vacuole. This new vacuolar membrane develops numerous microvillous structures in the case of toxoplasma. It then becomes surrounded by host cell endoplasmic reticulum by mitochondria and the process of fusion with primary and secondary lysosomes does not occur [13]. These morphologic changes have been seen to occur surrounding the vacuoles containing both toxoplasma and those containing *Chlamydia* [14]. At present, the functional significance of these changes remains unclear. It is clear, however, that by avoiding the process of lysosomal fusion, the organisms avoid one important host-defense mechanism. It is known, for example, that *Toxoplasma* are susceptible to the low pH of lysosomal environments and, therefore, would be susceptible to microbicidal action of this environment.

The mechanisms utilized by the microbes to initiate this impressive alteration of the phagosomal membrane remains unknown. As has been reviewed by D'Arcy Hart (chapter 17), efforts to identify the substances which may mimic this process are under way. However, in no case have definite molecules on the surface of these organisms, capable of initiating such a process, been identified. The entry of *Toxoplasma* into macrophages does initiate a number of metabolic events; for example, uptake of *Toxoplasma* increases glucose to CO_2 metabolism twofold, and it suppresses normal pinocytic activity of the cell. It does not appear to elevate levels of cyclic AMP as had been thought previously for the *Mycobacteria*. Attempts to prevent this blockade of lysosomal fusion by addition of the sugars capable of binding concanavalin A molecules have been unseccessful (Jones, unpublished observations). In some cases, *Mycobacteria* persist in phagosomes and appear to interfere with phagolysosomal fusion [15]. This process is not considered a critical stage in the survival of *Mycobacteria* since they are able to survive also within the phagolysosomes. Studies have attempted to correlate survival of these mycobacteria within cells with phagolysosomal fusion. For example, certain virulent strains of *Mycobacterium tuberculosis* appear to interfere with phagolysosomal fusion whereas strains of *Mycobacterium lepramurium* allow, or perhaps even promote, the phagolysosomal fusion [16]. Studies by Hart and colleagues have examined the substances which might inhibit the process of fusion in *M. lepramurium*. They demonstrated a temporary, but marked, inhibition of this process by suramin and poly-D-gluta-mic acid. As reported in this symposium, they have also demonstrated that filtrates of *M. tuberculosis* contain a substance or substances which promote inhibition of lysosomal fusion. The relevance of these observation to the mycobacteria model are unclear since *Mycobacteria* appear capable of surviving and replicating in fused phagolysosomes. However, the identification by their studies of molecules capable of blocking phagolysosome formation may be valuable for identifying the substances of critical importance in survival intracellularly of *Chlamydia* and *Toxoplasma*.

Some microbes, such as the Mycobacteria and *Leishmania*, and perhaps *Listeria*, appear capable of surviving within phagolysosomes. In this example, the phagolysosomal system is functioning normally, but the microbes can resist the potentially damaging enzymes, hydrogen ions, and metabolic systems. Morphologic studies have demonstrated that there is a zone surrounding certain mycobacteria which could be resistant to lysosomal enzymes [17]. In addition, in the case of *Leishmania*, Chang and Dwyer have suggested that the surface properties of that organism may render the parasite resistant to these enzymes [18]. They showed that the *Leishmania* do not appear to inactivate lysosomal enzymes since debris in the vacuole with the *Leishmania* appears to undergo digestion normally. The surface of *Leishmania* contains numerous glycoproteins, primarily polyanionic carbohydrates which provide a net negative charge on the surface [19]. Whether the composition of the surface membrane renders it protected from lysosomal enzymes remains to be further evaluated. Another alternative is that these organisms produce metabolic products which inactivate potentially lethal host metabolic products. An example of this has already been shown for the potential lethal effects of hydrogen peroxide on *Trypanosoma cruzi*, an organism which does not contain catalase [20]. *Toxoplasma gondii* and other microbes contain adequate catalase to be protected from the direct action of hydrogen peroxide [21]. In any case, at the present time, the mechanism of protection of the organisms such as *Leishmania* and *Mycobacteria* within phagolysosomes remains unknown. It is of interest that there is antigenic cross-reaction among *Leishmania* and *Mycobacteria*, suggesting the possibility that a single moiety may be common to these organisms which can survive in phagolysosomes [22].

To complete examples of the lesions of the phagolysosome system, there is one virus which actually takes advantage of the lysosomal enzymes to aid in the completion of its life cycle. The reovirus actually uses lysosomal enzymes to initiate the uncoating process — a step must precede the entry of the virus into the cytoplasma of the cell [23]. This, then, is an example of a microbe which is not only protected from lysosomal enzymes but which can utilize them for its own requirements.

In spite of the fact that the microbes under consideration in this review have effectively interfered with one important host antimicrobial system, phagocytic cells from immunized animals effectively control replication of microbes within their cytoplasm. The mechanisms of this control vary, depending on the microbe, but most depend on mechanisms which are alternatives to the phagolysosomal system. For example, when macrophages that are infected with *Toxoplasma* or *Chlamydia* are treated with the lymphocyte products from immunized animals, the *Toxoplasma* or *Chlamydia* fail to replicate within the parasitopherous vacuole [24, 25]. Electron-microscopic studies have shown that in this system there is no change in the ability of these microbes to continue inhibition of lysosomal fusion. The lymphocyte products, or lymphokines, have multiple effects on the cell which might lead to inhibition of microbe replication. For example, the cells become 'activated' and, therefore, display increased membrane activity, including increased phagocytosis, increased lysosomal-phagosomal fusion [26], enhanced metabolic activity and release of hydrogen peroxide following membrane stimulation and synthesis of proteins which are inhibitory to microbe replication [27] within the parasitopherous vacuole.

One can only speculate about which of these mechanisms are most important in the protection of cells against these microbes which have subverted the phagolysosomal system. For example, in the case of *Trypanosoma cruzi*, it seems possible that the enhanced generation of hydrogen peroxide is an important protective mechanism [20]. Similarly, enhancement of the oxygen-dependent microbicidal mechanisms may be important in the microbicidal action of these cells against *Toxoplasma* [27]. The toxoplasma-static and *Chlamydia*-inhibitory properties of such cells appear more dependent on the synthesis of microbe-inhibitory materials within the lymphokine-treated macrophage [24].

The action of the lymphokine on the macrophage, which leads to its numerous effects, remains undefined, but similarities have been noted between the structure of lymphokines and other more completely studied molecules such as cholera and diphtheria toxins. Recent studies by Possanza et al. have indicated that one lymphokine has both an attachment fragment and a fragment which may carry the active component [28]. The mechanism by which the lymphokine alters the intracellular environment, rendering it no longer ideal for microbe replication, is not known. It is clear that inhibitory materials traverse the parasitopherous vacuole, in the case of *Toxoplasma* and *Chlamydia* infection, and traverse the phagolysosomal membrane, in the case of *Leishmania* or *Mycobacteria* infections, to lead to microbe inhibition.

In summary, the mechanisms by which certain microbes evade the host phagolysosomal system have been reviewed. These mechanisms include avoidance of attachment, masking of recognition, lysis of phagosomes after endocytosis, block of lysosome-phagosome fusion and survival within the phagolysosome. Each microbe affects the system at a different point and utilizes various techniques to complete successful parasitism. The host cell, if from an immunized animal, then develops alternative mechanisms of inhibiting microbe replication. Though these mechanisms may include such features as enhanced phagocytosis and lysosomal-phagosomal fusion, direct stimulation of the phagolysosomal system does not appear the primary mechanism of host defense against these microbes. These alternative host-defense systems may simply provide microbial stasis within the phagosome or the phagolysosome or they may become microbicidal to the intracellular organism, an event which subsequently leads to digestion of the microbes within the cytoplasm of the host cell.

REFERENCES

 1. Goren MB: Phagocyte lysosomes: interactions with infectious agents, phagosomes, and experimental perturbations in function. Annu Rev Microbiol 31: 507, 1977.
 2. Silverstein SC, Steinman RM, Cohn ZA: Endocytosis. Annu Rev Biochem 46: 669–722, 1977.
 3. Jones TC, Byrne GI: Attachment and recognition factors in the interaction between microbes and mononuclear phagocytes. In: Sbarra A, Strauss R (eds) Biochemistry of the RES, vol 2. Biochemistry. New York, Plenum, (in press) 1980.
 4. Bar-Shavit Z, Ofek J, Goldman R, Mirelman D, Sharon N: Mannose residues on phagocytes as receptors for the attachment of *Escherichia coli* and *Salmonella typi*. Biochem Biophys Res Commun 78: 455, 1977.
 5. Jones TC, Hirsch JG: The interaction in vitro of *Mycoplasma pulmonis* with mouse macrophages and L-cells. J Exp Med 133: 231, 1971.
 6. Masur H, Jones TC: Interactions in vitro between Pneumocystis and rodent macrophages and L-cells. J Exp Med 147: 157–170, 1978.
 7. Jones TC, Yeh S, Hirsch JG: Studies on attachment and ingestion phases of phagocytosis of *Mycoplasma pulmonis* by mouse peritoneal macrophages. Proc Soc Med Biol Med 139: 464, 1972.
 8. Byrne GI, Moulder JW: Parasite-specified phagocytosis of *Chlamydia psittaci* and *Chlamydia trachomatis* by L and HeLa cells. Infect Immunol 19: 598, 1978.
 9. Jones TC: Entry and development of toxoplasmas in mammalian cells. In: Schlessinger D (ed) Microbiology 1979. Washington DC, Am Soc Microbiol, 1979.
10. Kilejian A: Does a histidine-rich protein from *Plasmodium lophurare* have a function in merozoite penetration? J Protozool 23: 272, 1976.
11. Silverstein SC: Macrophages and viral immunity. Hematology 7: 185, 1970.
12. Nogueira N, Cohn Z: *T. cruzi*: mechanism of entry and intracellular fate in mammalian cells. J Exp Med 143: 1402–1420, 1976.
13. Jones TC, Yeh S, Hirsch JG: The interaction between *Toxoplasma gondii* and mammalian cells. I. Mechanism of entry and intracellular fate of the parasite. JEM 136: 1157–1172, 1972.
14. Storz J, Spears P: *Chlamydiales:* properties, cycle of development, and effect on eukaryotic host cells. Curr Top Microbiol Immunol 76: 167, 1977.
15. Armstrong JA, Hart P D'Arcy: Phagosome-lysosome interactions in cultured macrophages infected with virulent tubercle bacilli. Reversal of the usual non-fusion pattern and observation on bacterial survival. J Exp Med 142: 1, 1975.
16. Draper P, Hart D'Arcy, Young MR: Effects of anionic inhibitors of phagosome-lysosome

234

fusion in cultured macrophages when the ingested organism is *Mycobacterium lepraemurium*. Infect Immunol 24: 558, 1979.

17. Draper P, Rees RJW: Electron-transparent zone of mycobacteria may be a defence system. Nature (London) 228: 860, 1970.

18. Chang KP, Dwyer DM: Multiplication of a human parasite (*Leishmania donovani*) in phagolysosomes of hamster macrophages in vitro. Science 193: 678–680, 1976.

19. Dwyer D: *Leishmania donovani:* surface membrane carbohydrates of promastigotes. Exp Parasitol 41: 341–358, 1977.

20. Nogueira N, Gordon S, Cohn Z: *T. cruzi:* modification of macrophage function during infection. J Exp Med 146: 157–171, 1977.

21. Murray HW, Cohn ZA: Macrophage oxygen-dependent antimicrobial activity. I. Susceptibility of *Toxoplasma gondii* to oxygen intermediates. J Exp Med 150: 938, 1979.

22. Smrkovski LL, Larsen CL: Antigenic cross-reactivity between Mycobacterium bovis (BCG) and *Leishmania donovani*. Infect Immunol 18: 561, 1977.

23. Silverstein SC, Astell C, Levin DH, Schonland Acs G: The mechanisms of reovirus uncoating and gene activation in vivo. Virology 47: 797, 1972.

24. Jones TC, Masur H, Len L, Fu T: Lymphocyte-macrophage interaction during control of intracellular parasitism. Am J Trop Med Hyg 26: 187–192, 1977.

25. Jones TC, Byrne GI: Interactions between macrophages and intravacuolar bacteria and protozoa. In: Van Furth R (ed) Mononuclear phagocytes. Fundamental aspects. The Hague, Martinus Nijhoff, 1980, pp 1611–1630.

26. Kielian MC, Cohn ZA: Determinants of phagosome-lysosome fusion in mouse macrophages. In: Van Furth R (ed) Mononuclear phagocytes. Fundamental aspects. The Hague, Martinus Nijhoff, 1980, pp 1077–1102.

27. Murray HW, Juangbhanich CW, Nathan CF, Cohn Z: Macrophage oxygen-dependent antimicrobial activity. II. The role of oxygen intermediates. J Exp Med 150: 950, 1979.

28. Possanza G, Cohen MD, Yoshida T, Cohen S: Human macrophage migration inhibition factor: evidence for subunit structure. Science 205: 300–301, 1979.

19. THE ROLE OF LYSOSOMES IN INTRACELLULAR DIGESTION: SYNTHESIS OF ACID HYDROLASES AND PACKAGING IN PRIMARY LYSOSOMES

J.M. TAGER, P.G. DE GROOT, M.N. HAMERS, M. HOLLEMANS, R. KALSBEEK, A. STRIJLAND, and F.P.W. TEGELAERS

INTRODUCTION

The lysosomal apparatus functions as an intracellular digestive system (for reviews see [1, 2]). Macromolecular material destined for digestion is first sequestered within phagosomes. Heterophagosomes contain extracellular material that has been taken up by endocytosis, whereas autophagosomes contain cell constituents that have ceased to function efficiently and must therefore be eliminated. Both types of phagosome fuse with primary lysosomes, which contain hydrolytic enzymes with an acid pH optimum. These enzymes bring about the breakdown of biological macromolecules to their constituent low molecular weight building blocks. Thus proteins are hydrolysed to amino acids; glycoproteins are hydrolysed to amino acids and monosaccharides; DNA and RNA are hydrolysed to nucleosides and phosphate; mucopolysaccharides are hydrolysed to monosaccharides and sulphate; neutral and acidic glycosphingolipids are hydrolysed to monosaccharides, fatty acids, sphingosine and sulphate; triglycerides are hydrolysed to fatty acids and glycerol; and glycogen is hydrolysed to glucose.

The digestion of macromolecules in the lysosomes is a stepwise process. Each step is catalysed by a specific enzyme, and the product of one reaction forms the substrate for the next reaction in the pathway. For instance, the catabolism of ceramide-3 (ceramide trihexoside) consists of the sequential removal of sugar residues by specific exoglycosidases followed by the hydrolysis of ceramide to sphingosine and a fatty acid, catalysed by ceramidase (Fig. 1). Deficiency of one of these enzymes leads to accumulation of the substrate for that enzyme in the lysosomes, and to the specific biochemical and clinical symptoms associated with a lysosomal storage disease. Thus in Fabry's disease a deficiency of α-galactosidase leads to accumulation of ceramide-3 in the kidneys and in various other tissues.

The lysosomal enzymes are contained within membrane-bound vesicles. The lysosomal membrane acts as a protective barrier and prevents extralysosomal cellular constituents from being hydrolysed by the lysosomal enzymes.

The question arises of how newly synthesized lysosomal enzymes are specifically packaged into primary lysosomes. The polypeptide moieties of the lysosomal enzymes are probably synthesized on ribosomes on the rough

W.Th. Daems et al. (eds.), Cell Biological Aspects of Disease, 235–250. All rights reserved.
Copyright © 1981 by Martinus Nijhoff Publishers bv, The Hague/Boston/London.

236

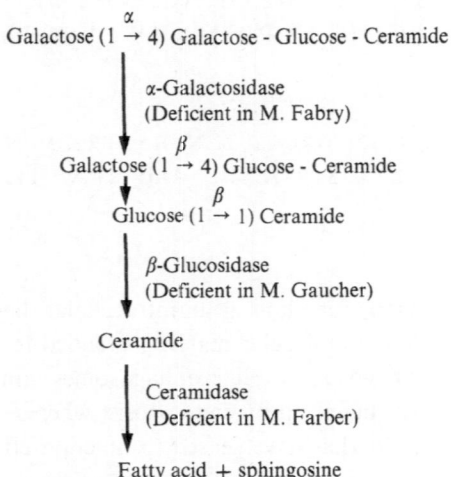

Fig. 1. Catabolism of ceramide-3 (ceramide trihexoside) in lysosomes.

endoplasmic reticulum, where, in addition, export proteins and polypeptides destined to be incorporated into the cell coat are synthesized. Thus mechanisms must exist to ensure that the various polypeptides are specifically routed to their correct destinations. This specific 'packaging' probably occurs in the Golgi apparatus [3].

Lysosomal enzymes are glycoproteins, and it is now clear that the oligosaccharide moiety plays an essential role in the routing of lysosomal enzymes to the primary lysosomes.

STRUCTURE OF LYSOSOMAL ENZYMES

Lysosomal enzymes are either monomeric or oligomeric proteins (see [4]). Cathepsin D, for instance, is a monomer. On the other hand, hexosaminidase B is composed of two identical subunits, each containing two identical polypeptide chains ($\beta_2\beta_2$), whereas hexosaminidase A contains one β_2 subunit and one α_2 subunit ($\alpha_2\beta_2$) (see [5] for a review).

The structural genes for the polypeptides in lysosomal enzymes are distributed among different chromosomes (Table 1).

All lysosomal enzymes that have been investigated so far are glycoproteins and bind to Concanavalin A (see e.g. [24–27]). The sugar composition of the oligosaccharide moieties of five human lysosomal enzymes has been determined (Table 2). All are characterized by having a high content of mannose. Furthermore, the oligosaccharide chains can be removed by treatment of the enzymes with β-N-acetylglucosaminidase H [32–34], an endoglycosidase that hydrolyses the core D-N-acetylchitobiose linkage in high-mannose, aspara-

Table 1. Localization of structural genes for lysosomal enzymes.

Enzyme	Structural gene on chromosome	References
α-Fucosidase	1	6
β-Galactosidase	3	7–9
β-Hexosaminidases (β-chain)	5	10, 11
Arylsulphatase B	5	12
β-Glucuronidase	7	13, 14
Acid phosphatase	11	15
β-Hexosaminidase A (α-chain)	15	10, 11
α-Glucosidase	17	16, 17
α-Mannosidase	19	18
DNAase	19	19
N-Acetyl-α-galactosaminidase	22	20
Arylsulphatase A	22	12
β-Galactosidase	22	9, 21
α-Galactosidase	x	22, 23

Table 2. Carbohydrate composition of human lysosomal enzymes.

Sugar	Mole/mole protein in				
	Hexosaminidase A[a]	Hexosaminidase B[a]	β-Glucuronidase[a]	Acid phosphatase[b]	α-Glucosidase[b]
Mannose	12.1	14.2	67.5	15.7	13.2
Fucose			15.2		
Galactose	2.9	2.1	12.2		
Glucose	6.2	1.9	12.7		4
N-Acetylglucosamine	6.5	6.5	18.9	4.5	8.3
N-Acetylgalactosamine			0		
Sialic acid	2.0	0.3	0		
Reference	28	28	29	30	31

[a] From placenta.
[b] From liver.

gine-linked glycopeptides [35, 36]. It has been reported [37] that bovine testicular β-galactosidase, too, contains asparagine-linked oligosaccharides of the high-mannose type.

SYNTHESIS, PROCESSING AND PACKAGING OF LYSOSOMAL ENZYMES

Key experimental observations

The following key observations have been of profound importance in unravelling the mechanisms involved in the routing of acid hydrolases to primary lysosomes in mammalian cells.

In a series of important studies beginning in 1968, Ashwell, Morell and co-workers demonstrated that glycoproteins containing galactose residues at the non-reducing ends of the oligosaccharide chains are rapidly endocytosed by mammalian liver parenchymal cells after binding to a specific receptor on the surface of the cells (see [38] for a review). The receptor has been isolated from rabbit liver and characterized [38], and its presence has been demonstrated in the livers of several other mammalian species including rat [38], mouse [39], monkey [39] and man [39]. Pricer and Ashwell [40] subsequently demonstrated that the receptor is present not only in plasma membranes but also in the Golgi apparatus, the endoplasmic reticulum and lysosomes.

Stahl, Sly and co-workers showed that a different uptake system is present in reticuloendothelial cells (see [41] for a review). In this system the lectin is specific for glycoproteins with terminal mannose or N-acetylglucosamine residues [41].

The elegant studies of Neufeld and co-workers on 'corrective factors' which prevent accumulation of mucopolysaccharides in cultured skin fibroblasts from patients with the Hurler and Hunter syndromes led to the discovery that cultured human skin fibroblasts take up exogenous lysosomal enzymes by adsorptive endocytosis (see [42] for a review). They demonstrated that fibroblasts from Hurler patients secrete a factor which prevents mucopolysaccharide accumulation in fibroblasts from Hunter patients and vice versa [42]. The 'corrective factors', which are present in secretions of normal human skin fibroblasts and also in normal urine and other materials, were subsequently identified as α-iduronidase and iduronate sulphatase; these enzymes are deficient in patients with the Hurler and Hunter syndromes, respectively [42].

It has now been demonstrated that cultured skin fibroblasts from patients with several different types of lysosomal storage diseases are able to take up the deficient enzyme when it is added to the culture medium (see [42, 43]). The uptake is saturable, suggesting that a receptor-mediated process is involved [43–47]. The demonstration by Hickman et al. [48] that 'high-uptake' and 'low-uptake' forms of lysosomal enzymes exist and that the former are converted to the latter forms by treatment with periodate suggested that carbohydrate moieties might be involved and led to the tentative identification by Sly and co-workers [46] and subsequently by others [47, 49] of mannose-6-phosphate as the specific recognition marker for the binding of lysosomal enzymes to a receptor on the surface of fibroblasts (see also [45]). The identity of the recognition marker as mannose-6-phosphate has now been established unequivocally by enzymic analyses ([33, 34]; see also [32, 37]).

Hypotheses for the packaging of lysosomal enzymes

Early morphological observations had led to the suggestion that the packaging of lysosomal enzymes to form primary lysosomes occurs either in the Golgi apparatus [3] or in a specialized region of the smooth endoplasmic reticulum closely associated with the Golgi apparatus and referred to as GERL ('associated Golgi apparatus and smooth Endoplasmic Reticulum from which Lysosomes appear to form'; see [50] for a review).

In 1972, an alternative route for the packaging of lysosomal enzymes was postulated by Hickman and Neufeld [51]. They had found that the lysosomal enzymes present in high concentrations in the medium of fibroblasts from patients with I-cell disease are of the low-uptake type [51] (Table 3). On the other hand, I-cell fibroblasts are able to take up and retain lysosomal enzymes secreted by other types of fibroblasts [51]. These observations led them to suggest that the packaging of lysosomal enzymes involves synthesis of the enzymes in a form equipped with a specific recognition marker, secretion to the exterior of the cell, binding to receptors on the cell surface via the specific recognition marker, and, finally, endocytosis and formation of pinocytic vacuoles containing the lysosomal enzymes [47, 51]. It was postulated that the mutation in I-cell disease leads to an altered recognition marker [51].

Although the 'secretion-recapture' hypothesis has been provocative and stimulating, several experimental observations are not in accordance with the hypothesis as originally formulated by Neufeld and co-workers.

Firstly, Reuser et al. [51] have carried out single-cell assays in cocultivated fibroblasts of different strains in order to test whether intercellular transfer of lysosomal hydrolases occurs; although transfer of β-hexosaminidase from normal to deficient cells was observed, no transfer of α-glucosidase or β-galactosidase could be demonstrated in analogous experiments.

Secondly, when fibroblasts are grown in the presence of mannose-6-phosphate, which inhibits the binding of the high-uptake forms of lysosomal enzymes to the receptors on the cell surface [41], there is no effect on the intracellular activity of lysosomal enzymes [41, 53–56]. Similarly, when anti-

Table 3. Uptake of secreted lysosomal enzymes by cultured human skin fibroblasts.*

Enzyme	Relative uptake of enzyme secreted from	
	Normal fibroblasts	I-cell fibroblasts
α-Iduronidase	46	7.5
β-Glucuronidase	135	11.2
β-Hexosaminidase	50	0.5

* Uptake of enzyme measured in fibroblasts deficient in that enzyme. From Hickman and Neufeld [51].

bodies to lysosomal enzymes are added to the culture medium, the intracellular activity of lysosomal enzymes is not affected [53].

Thirdly, in heterozygotes for Fabry's disease, an X-linked lysosomal disorder, inactivation of one of the X-chromosomes (the lyonization phenomenon) leads to the expression of α-galactosidase in some cells and not in others; there is no evidence for transfer of the enzyme from α-galactosidase-positive to α-galactosidase-negative cells (see discussion following [57], and [58]).

Fourthly, Hasilik and Neufeld [34, 53] have recently shown by means of pulse-labelling experiments that lysosomal enzymes are synthesized in fibroblasts in mannose-6-phosphate-containing precursor forms of higher molecular weight than the final products (Table 4). Only small amounts of the precursors are found in the medium; they persist there without being taken up [34].

The above observations suggest that the packaging of lysosomal enzymes is an intracellular process and that the secretion-recapture hypothesis must be modified. Nevertheless its most important features remain: lysosomal enzymes are synthesized as precursors containing mannose-6-phosphate as a recognition marker and binding of the recognition marker to a specific receptor (probably in the Golgi region) leads to packaging of the enzymes in primary lysosomes (see [41]). This model will be discussed in detail in the next section. Alternative models, in which binding of lysosomal enzymes to receptors prevents release of the enzymes into the extracellular space during membrane recycling [60] or during segregation of secretory proteins at the plasma membrane [41, 51] are less attractive.

Model for the synthesis and packaging of lysosomal enzymes

The stages in the synthesis, processing and packaging of lysosomal enzymes in cultured human skin fibroblasts are summarized in Table 5

Table 4. Precursors of polypeptide chains of lysosomal enzymes in cultured human skin fibroblasts.*

Polypeptide	Molecular weight of	
	Precursor	Product
Hexosaminidase (α-chain)	67,000	54,000
Hexosaminidase (β-chain)	63,000	29,000
Cathepsin D	53,000	31,000
α-Glucosidase	95,000	76,000

* The precursor forms contain mannose-6-phosphate. Experiments of Neufeld and co-workers [59].

Table 5. Stages in the synthesis, processing and packaging of lysosomal enzymes.

1) Synthesis of polypeptides.
2) Glycosylation of specific asparagine residues.
3) Modification of oligosaccharide side-chains.
4) Formation of precursor molecules with complex oligosaccharide chains containing mannose-6-phosphate.
5) Binding of precursors to mannose-6-phosphate-specific receptors in Golgi apparatus.
6) Transfer of precursors to vesicles destined to become primary lysosomes.

The synthesis of the precursor polypeptides probably occurs on ribosomes on the rough endoplasmic reticulum. In analogy with the requirement of a signal peptide in the 'pre' forms of export proteins [61, 62], it may be postulated that a hydrophobic region in the nascent polypeptide may enable it to traverse the membrane and reach the cisternae of the endoplasmic reticulum.

Next, glycosylation of the polypeptides is initiated. Asparagine residues occurring in the tripeptide sequence -Asn-X-Ser- or -Asn-X-Thr- (see [63, 64]) serve as acceptors for a complex oligosaccharide containing 2 N-acetylglucosamine, 9 mannose and 3 glucose residues which is transferred en bloc from a lipid carrier (Fig. 2) to the polypeptide chain [65]. The formation of the lipid-linked oligosaccharide is inhibited by 2-deoxyglucose [66] or tunicamycin [67].

In the third stage, processing of the oligosaccharide occurs, which involves stepwise cleavage of glucose and mannose residues and transfer of mono-

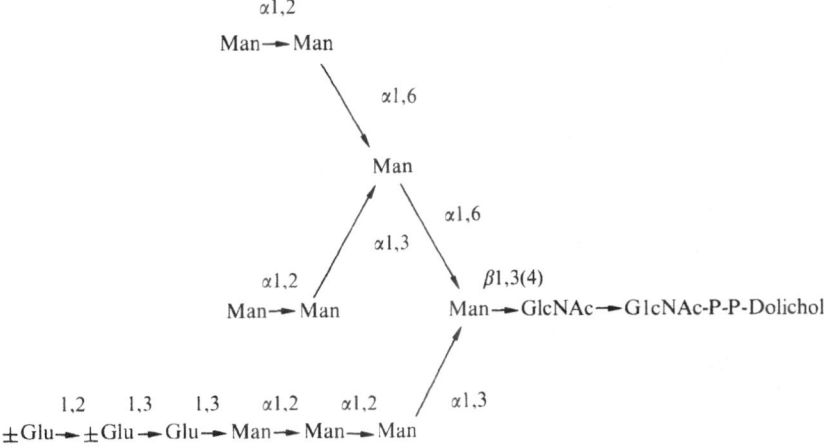

Fig. 2. Proposed structure of dolicholpyrophosphoryl oligosaccharide, the lipid-linked intermediate from which oligosaccharide is transferred to specific asparagine residues in polypeptides as the initial step in the formation of asparagine-linked oligosaccharide chains in glycoproteins. From Robbins [63].

saccharide residues to the shortened oligosaccharide chain in order to form a specific type of glycopeptide [63, 64]. In the case of lysosomal enzymes, the processing includes transfer of mannose-6-phosphate groups to the glyco-peptides so that a precursor molecule with mannose-6-phosphate-containing oligosaccharide chains is formed (Table 5, stage 4).

The fifth stage involves binding of the precursor molecule to mannose-6-phosphate-specific receptors in the Golgi apparatus.

Finally, the precursor is transferred into vesicles destined to become prim-ary lysosomes, which is accompanied by cleavage of part of the polypeptide chain. The proteolytic cleavage may occur in several steps [55]. Further processing of the oligosaccharide moieties, including removal of phosphate, occurs in the lysosomes.

Thus the enzymes and enzyme systems involved in the synthesis, process-ing and packaging of lysosomal enzymes include the protein-synthesizing machinery of the cell ($+$mRNA); the glycosyl transferases involved in the synthesis of the lipid-linked oligosaccharide; the oligosaccharide transferase responsible for the initial step in glycosylation of the polypeptide; the manno-sidases, glucosidases, glycosyl transferases and 6-phospho-mannosyl trans-ferase involved in further processing of the oligosaccharide moieties; one or more proteinases; a phosphatase; and perhaps lysosomal glycosidases.

EXPERIMENTAL APPROACHES TO THE STUDY OF THE SYNTHESIS AND
PACKAGING OF LYSOSOMAL ENZYMES

Some of the experimental approaches that can be used in the study of the synthesis, processing and packaging of lysosomal enzymes are listed in Table 6.

Table 6. Experimental approaches to the study of the synthesis, processing and packaging of lysosomal enzymes.

1) Preparation of a DNA probe by isolating mRNA and making use of recombinant DNA technology.
2) In vitro synthesis of (precursor forms of) polypeptide chains.
3) Pulse-labelling and immunoprecipitation techniques using monoclonal antibodies.
4) Stimulation or inhibition of specific steps.
5) Isolation of intermediate forms of the polypeptide chains.
6) Intracellular localization of specific steps.
7) Identification and characterization of processing enzymes.
8) In vitro processing.
9) Use of mutant human cell lines.
10) Somatic cell hybridization of human cells with mutant rodent cell lines and vice versa.
11) Complementation studies using mutant human cell lines.

The preparation of DNA probes depends on the isolation of mRNA, which will be particularly difficult technically in the case of mRNA for lysosomal enzymes since only a small percentage of total mRNA can be expected to be specific for lysosomal enzymes. If the technical difficulties can be overcome, in vitro translation of the mRNA should provide important information about the precursor forms of the polypeptide chains of lysosomal enzymes. A brief report has appeared on the in vitro synthesis of rat β-glucuronidase using polysomes isolated from liver and preputial gland [68].

The studies of Neufeld and co-workers [34, 55, 59] using elegant pulse-labelling and immunoprecipitation techniques have yielded most important information on the mechanisms involved in the processing and packaging of lysosomal enzymes. Since this approach depends on the availability of mono-specific antisera of high titre, the hybridoma technique for producing monoclonal antibodies [69] should prove particularly useful.

The use of specific inhibitors has two aims. Firstly, they can be used to ascertain whether particular reactions or types of reactions play a role in the overall proces. Thus deoxyglucose, tunicamycin or other compounds can be used as inhibitors of glycosylation [66, 67]. The role of proteolytic cleavage can be investigated by using proteinase inhibitors like antipain and leupeptin [69–71]; and tartrate can be used as an inhibitor of acid phosphatase, which may be responsible for the removal of phosphate from the mannose-6-phosphate groups in the oligosaccharide moieties of partially processed precursors of lysosomal enzymes.

Secondly, the use of inhibitors may lead to the accumulation of intermediates which can be used for analytical purposes.

Certain compounds may modify the normal pathway of synthesis and packaging of lysosomal enzymes. Thus Neufeld and co-workers [53, 59] have found that addition of chloroquine or ammonia to the culture medium of fibroblasts leads to a decrease in the amount of newly synthesized lysosomal enzymes in the cells. Concomitantly, precursor forms of the lysosomal enzymes accumulate in the medium [53, 59]. In this respect it is significant to note that chloroquine and other weak bases are accumulated in lysosomes both in vivo [72] and in vitro [73] and cause extensive vacuolization of cells [72, 74]. Furthermore, these weak bases inhibit protein degradation in lysosomes [72, 74].

Exposure of cultured fibroblasts to sucrose, a non-metabolizable sugar, causes an increase in the intracellular activity of lysosomal enzymes [75, 76]. Concomitantly, extensive vacuolization occurs [77, 78]. According to Warburton and Wynn [75], the increased activity of the enzymes is due both to an enhanced rate of synthesis and a decreased rate of breakdown of the enzymes.

In some types of cells, starvation brings about an increase in the activity of lysosomal enzymes such as proteases [80]. This effect may be related to the stimulation of proteolysis in liver by starvation [81] or more specifically by the deprivation of certain amino acids, in particular glutamine [82].

Measurement of the intracellular localization of precursor forms of lysosomal enzymes at various times after pulse-labelling is essential in order to establish the intracellular route of lysosomal enzymes during packaging. This approach can be combined with the use of processing inhibitiors in order to establish in which structures precursors and intermediates accumulate. In this respect the fractionation studies of Rome et al. [83] are of particular significance; they show that fibroblasts contain two populations of vesicles with lysosomal enzyme activity, one being associated with markers for the Golgi apparatus, the endoplasmic reticulum and plasma membranes.

The identification and characterization of processing enzymes should enable in vitro processing to be carried out, as has been done in other systems. Intriguing problems include the nature and localization of the enzyme(s) responsible for the proteolytic cleavage of the precursors of lysosomal enzymes, the role of non-lysosomal glycosidases, the identification and localization of the phosphatase that removes phosphate from mannose-6-phosphate groups in the enzymes, and the question of whether lysosomal glycosidases play a significant role in processing.

The importance of using mutant human cell lines in these studies has been stressed in the third section of this chapter. Deficiencies of lysosomal enzymes can be caused not only by mutations in structural genes, but also by mutations leading to a decreased rate of synthesis of enzyme or by a mutation in a processing gene (Table 7).

In the late-onset form of Pompe's disease, the residual acid α-glucosidase activity is indistinguishable from that in normal tissues and urine with regard to its kinetic characteristics [88–90] or reactivity with antibodies raised against acid α-glucosidase from normal liver [88, 90, 91]. Reuser et al. [90] suggested that the mutation leads to a defect in a regulatory mechanisms resulting in a decreased rate of synthesis of the enzyme or, alternatively, to a decreased rate of degradation of the enzyme. We are carrying out pulse-

Table 7. Mutations leading to deficiencies of lysosomal enzymes.

---

1) Mutation in a structural gene.
    a) Defective polypeptide synthesized.
       M. Tay-Sachs (see [5])
    b) No detectable polypeptide synthesized.
       M. Fabry [84, 85]
       M. Pompe (most cases with the infantile form) [86–88]
2) Mutation leading to decreased rate of synthesis of enzyme.
    M. Pompe (see [88–91])
3) Mutation in a processing gene.
    I-cell disease [34, 55, 59]

---

labelling studies to determine whether there is, indeed, a decreased rate of synthesis of the precursor forms of acid α-glucosidase in fibroblasts from patients with the late-onset form of Pompe's disease [92].

A similar situation exists in mice. Skudlared and Swank [93] have recently shown that in murine macrophages a precursor of β-galactosidase is synthesized with a molecular weight higher than that of the final product (82,000 and 63,000, respectively). In a mutant strain of mice in which the rate of synthesis of β-galactosidase is known to be decreased, there is a decreased rate of incorporation of [^{3}H]leucine not only into the final product but also into the precursor [93].

In man–rodent somatic cell hybrids the expression of a human gene product can be expected to be influenced by the rodent genome. For instance, the electrophoretic mobility of the bands of α-galactosidase activity in man–Chinese hamster somatic cell hybrids depends on the strain of Chinese hamster cells used [22, 94]. In hybrids derived from the a3 strain of Chinese hamster cells a two-banded pattern is observed [22], one corresponding to the Chinese hamster band in parental cells and the other containing both Chinese hamster and human gene products [23]. In contrast, a three-banded pattern is observed in hybrid cells when the E36 strain of Chinese hamster cells is used [94]; one band corresponds to the Chinese hamster parental activity, a second band has the same electrophoretic mobility as the α-galactosidase in human fibroblasts, and the third band contains both human and Chinese hamster antigenic determinants [23].

Somatic cell hybridization studies should prove to be very useful in unravelling the mAchanisms involved in the synthesis and processing of lysosomal enzymes. For instance, it would be of great interest to study (a) the expression of acid α-glucosidase in somatic cell hybrids using fibroblasts from patients with the late-onset form of Pompe's disease as the human parent, and (b) the expression of human lysosomal enzymes in somatic cell hybrids using rodent cell lines with mutations affecting the rate of synthesis of rodent lysosomal enzymes (see e.g. [95–97]). It would be of particular importance to use rodent cell lines in which the mutation affects a cluster of lysosomal enzymes (see [45]). Furthermore, suitable mutants could be selected for by the technique recently described by Robbins [98].

Finally, complementation studies using somatic cell hybrids between different mutant human cell lines have been used very successfully not only in studying genetic heterogeneity in lysosomal enzymopathies (see [99–105]), but also more recently in attempts to establish the nature of mutations involving the synthesis and processing of lysosomal enzymes (see e.g. [104]). Complementation has also been demonstrated in interspecific hybrid cells: in somatic cell hybrids between fibroblasts from a patient with I-cell disease and mouse fibroblasts, the mouse genome is able to correct the human abnormality [106].

246

CONCLUDING REMARKS

The advances that have been made in establishing some of the mechanisms involved in the synthesis and packaging of lysosomal enzymes in man have come from studies in which biochemists, cell biologists, geneticists and immunologists have cooperated closely with one another and with clinicians. Continuation of these collaborative efforts is essential. On the one hand, the clinicians provide the problems and experimental material in the form of mutant cell lines; on the other hand, the results of fundamental scientific research on the molecular nature of lysosomal enzymopathies provide the basis required for accurate diagnosis, sound genetic counselling and attempts at therapy.

Acknowledgments. The studies carried out by the authors on human lysosomal enzymes are supported by grants from the Netherlands Organization for the Advancement of Pure Research (ZWO) under the auspices of the Netherlands Foundation for Fundamental Medical Research (FUNGO), from the Prevention Fund (Praeventiefonds), and from the Princess Beatrix Fund.

REFERENCES

1. Holtzman E: The lysosomes, a survey. Vienna, Springer, 1976.
2. Dean RT, Barrett A: Lysosomes. Essays Biochem 12:1–40, 1976.
3. Cohn ZA, Fedorko ME: The formation and fate of lysosomes. In: Dingle JT, Fell HB (eds) Lysosomes in biology and pathology, vol 1. Amsterdam, North-Holland, 1969, pp 43–63.
4. Barrett AJ, Heath MF: Lysosomal enzymes. In:Dingle JT (ed) Lysosomes a laboratory handbook, 2nd ed. Amsterdam, North-Holland, 1977, pp 19–145.
5. Sandhoff K, Christomanou H: Biochemistry and genetics of gangliosidoses. Hum Genet 50: 107–143, 1979.
6. Turner BM, Smith M, Turner VS, Kucherlapati RS, Ruddle FH, Hirschhorn K: Assignment of the gene locus for human α-L-fucosidase to chromosome 1 by analysis of somatic cell hybrids. Som Cell Genet 4: 45–54, 1978.
7. Bruns GAP, Leary AC, Regina VM, Gerald PS: Lysosomal β-D-galactosidase in man-hamster somatic cell hybrids. Birth Defects Orig Artic Ser 14(4): 177–181, 1978.
8. Shows TB, Scrafford-Wolff L, Brown JA, Meisler M: Assignment of a β-galactosidase gene to chromosome 3 in man. Birth Defects Orig Artic Ser 14(4): 219–223, 1978.
9. Dewit J, Hoeksema HL, Bootsma D, Westerveld A: Assignment of structural β-galactosidase loci to human chromosomes 3 and 22. Hum Genet 51: 259–267, 1979.
10. Gilbert F, Kucherlapati R, Creagan RP, Murnane MJ, Darlington GJ, Ruddle FH: Tay-Sachs and Sandhoff's disease. The assignment of genes for hexosaminidase A and B to individual human chromosomes. Proc Natl Acad Sci USA 72: 263–267, 1975.
11. Hoeksema HL, Reuser AJJ, Hoogeveen A, Westerveld A, Braidman I, Robinson D: Characterization of β-D-N-acetylhexosaminidase isoenzymes in man-Chinese hamster somactic cell hybrids. Am J Hum Genet 29: 14–23, 1977.
12. DeLuca C, Brown JA, Shows TB: Lysosomal arylsulphatase deficiencies in human chromosomes. Chromosome assignments for arylsulphatase A and B. Proc Natl Acad Sci USA 76: 1957–1961, 1979.

13. Chern CJ, Croce CM: Assignment of the structural gene for human β-glucuronidase to chromosome 7 and tetrameric association of subunits in the enzyme molecule. Am J Hum Genet 28: 350–356, 1976.

14. Grzeschik KH: Assignment of human genes; β-glucuronidase to chromosome C7, AK-1 to C9, a second enzyme with enolase activity to C12 and mitochrondrial 1DH to D15. Birth Defects Orig Artic Ser 11(3): 142–148, 1975.

15. Bruns, GAP, Gerald PS: Human acid phosphatase in somatic cell hybrids. Science 184: 480–481, 1974.

16. Solomon E, Swallow D, Burgess S, Evans L: Assignment of the human acid α-glucosidase gene to chromosome 17 using somatic cell hybrids. Ann Hum Genet 42: 273–281, 1979.

17. D'Ancona GG, Wurm J, Croce CM: Genetics of type II glycogenosis: assignment of the human gene for acid α-glucosidase to chromosome 17. Proc Natl Acad Sci USA 76: 4526–4529, 1979.

18. Ingram PH, Bruns GAP, Regina VM, Eisenman RE, Gerald PS: Expression of α-mannosidase in man-hamster somatic cell hybrids. Biochem Genet 15: 455–476, 1977.

19. Bruns GAP, Regina VM, Gerald PS: Lysosomal DNAase and chromosome 19. J Cell Biol 83: 444A, 1979.

20. De Groot PG, Westerveld A, Meera Khan P, Tager JM: Localization of a gene for human α-galactosidase B (= N-acetyl-αD-galactosaminidase) on chromosome 22. Hum Genet 44: 305–312, 1978.

21. DeWit J, Hoeksema HL, Halley D, Hagemeijer A, Bootsma D, Westerveld, A: Regional localization of a β-galactosidase locus on human chromosome 22. Som Cell Genet 3: 351–364, 1977.

22. Grzeschik KH, Grzeschik AM, Banhof S, Romeo G, Siniscalco M, Van Someren H, Meera Khan P, Westerveld A, Bootsma D: X-linkage of human α-galactosidase. Nature [New Biol] 240: 48–50, 1972.

23. Hamers MN, Westerveld A, Meera Khan P, Tager JM: Characterization of α-galactosidase isoenzymes in human-Chinese hamster somatic cell hybrids. Hum Genet 36: 289–297, 1977.

24. Bishayee S, Bachhawat BK: Interaction between Concanavalin A and brain lysosomal acid hydrolases. Biochim Biophys Acta 334: 378–388, 1974.

25. Norden AGW, O'Brien JS: Binding of human liver β-galactosidases to plant lectins insolubilized on agarose. Biochem Biophys Res Commun 56: 193–198, 1974.

26. Beutler E, Guinto E, Kuhl W: Placental acid hydrolase purification on Concanavalin A-Sepharose. J Lab Clin Med 85: 672–677, 1975.

27. Fiddler MB, Ben-Yoseph Y, Nadler HL: Binding of human liver hydrolases by immobilized lectins. Biochem J 177: 175–180, 1979.

28. Freeze H, Geiger B, Miller AL: Carbohydrate composition of human placental N-acetyl hexosaminidase A and B. Biochem J 177: 749–752, 1979.

29. Brot FE, Bell CE Jr, Sly WS: Purification and properties of β-glucuronidase from human placenta. Biochemistry 17: 385–391, 1978.

30. Saini MS, Van Etten RL: A homogeneous isoenzyme of human liver acid phosphatase. Arch Biochem Biophys 191: 613–624, 1978.

31. Belen'ky DM, Mikhajlov VI, Rosenfeld EL: Carbohydrate content of acid α-glucosidase (γ-amylase) from human liver. Clin Chim Acta 93: 365–370, 1979.

32. Von Figura K, Klein U: Isolation and characterization of phosphorylated oligosaccharides from α-N-acetylglucosaminidase that are recognized by cell-surface receptors. Eur J Biochem 94: 347–354, 1979.

33. Natowicz MR, Chi MMY, Lowry OH, Sly WS: Enzymatic identification of mannose-6-phosphate on the recognition marker for receptor-mediated pinocytosis of β-glucuronidase by human fibroblasts. Proc Natl Acad Sci USA 76: 4322–4326, 1979.

34. Hasilik A, Neufeld ES: Biosynthesis of lysosomal enzymes in fibroblasts. II. Phosphorylation of mannose residues. J Biol Chem 255: 4946–4950, 1980.

35. Tarentino AL, Maley F: Purification and properties of an endo-βn-acetylglucosaminidase from *Streptomyces griseus*. J Biol Chem 249: 811–817. 1974.

36. Tai T, Yamashita K, Ogata-Arakawa M, Koide N, Muramatsu T, Iwashita S, Inoue Y, Kobata A: Structural studies of two ovalbumin glycopeptides in relation to the endo-β-N-acetylglucosaminidase specificity. J Biol Chem 250: 8569–8575, 1975.
37. Distler J, Hieber V, Sahagian G, Schmickel R, Jourdian GW: Identification of mannose-6-phosphate in glycoproteins that inhibit the assimilation of β-galactosidase by fibroblasts. Proc Natl Acad Sci USA 76: 4235–4239, 1979.
38. Ashwell G, Morell AG: The role of surface carbohydrates in the hepatic recognition and transport of circulating glycoproteins. Adv Enzymol 41: 99–128, 1974.
39. Kalsbeek R, Hamers MN, Tager JM: Specific binding of asialoglycoproteins by mammalian liver. In: Schauer R, Boer P, Buddecke E, Kramer MF, Vliegenthart JFG, Wiegandt H (eds) Glycoconjugates. Proceedings of the Fifth International Symposium, Kiel, September 1979. Stuttgart, Thieme, 1979, pp 498–499.
40. Pricer WE, Ashwell G: Subcellular distribution of a mammalian hepatic binding protein specific for asialoglycoproteins. J Biol Chem 251: 7539–7544, 1976.
41. Sly WS, Stahl P: Receptor-mediated uptake of lysosomal enzymes. In: Silverstein SC (ed) Transport of macromolecules in cellular systems. Berlin, Dahlem Konferenzen, 1978, pp 229–244.
42. Neufeld EF, Lim TW, Shapiro LJ: Inherited disorders of lysosomal metabolism. Annu Rev Biochem 44: 357–376, 1975.
43. Neufeld EF, Sando GN, Garvin AJ, Rome LH: The transport of lysosomal enzymes. J Supramol Struct 6: 95–101, 1977.
44. Von Figura K, Kresse H: Quantitative aspects of pinocytosis and the intracellular fate of N-acetyl-α-D-glucosaminidase in Sanfilippo B fibroblasts. J Clin Invest 53: 85–90, 1974.
45. Hieber V, Distler J, Myerowitz R, Schmickel RD, Jourdian GW: The role of glycosidically bound mannose in the assimilation of β-galactosidase by generalized gangliosidosis fibroblasts. Biochem Biophys Res Commun 73: 710–717, 1976.
46. Kaplan A, Achord DT, Sly WS: Phosphohexosyl components of a lysosomal enzyme are recognized by pinocytosis receptors on human fibroblasts. Proc Natl Acad Sci USA 74: 2026–2030, 1977.
47. Sando G, Neufeld EF: Recognition and receptor-mediated uptake of a lysosomal enzyme, α-L-iduronidase, by cultured human fibroblasts. Cell 12: 619–627, 1977.
48. Hickman S, Shapiro LJ, Neufeld EF: A recognition marker required for uptake of a lysosomal enzyme by cultured fibroblasts. Biochem Biophys Res Commun 57: 55–61, 1974.
49. Ullrich K, Mersmann G, Weber E, Von Figura K: Evidence for lysosomal enzyme recognition by human fibroblasts via a phosphorylated carbohydrate moiety. Biochem J 170: 643–650, 1978.
50. Novikoff AB: Lysosomes: a personal account. In: Hers HG, Van Hoof F (eds) Lysosomes and storage diseases. New York, Academic Press, 1973, pp 2–41.
51. Hickman S, Neufeld EF: A hypothesis for I-cell disease: defective hydrolases that do not enter lysosomes. Biochem Biophys Res Commun 49: 992–999, 1972.
52. Reuser A, Halley D, De Wit-Verbeek H, Hoogeveen A, Van der Kamp M, Mulder M, Galjaard H: Intracellular exchange of lysosomal enzymes: enzyme assays in single human fibroblasts after co-cultivation. Biochem Biophys Res Commun 69: 311–318, 1976.
53. Von Figura K, Weber E: An alternative hypothesis of cellular transport of lysosomal enzymes in fibroblasts. Biochem J 176: 943–950, 1978.
54. Vladutiu GD, Rattazzi MC: Excretion-reuptake route of β-hexosaminidase in normal and I-cell disease cultured fibroblasts. J Clin Invest 63: 595–601, 1979.
55. Hasilik A, Neufeld EF: Biosynthesis of lysosomal enzymes in fibroblasts. I. Synthesis as precursors of higher molecular weight. J Biol Chem 255: 4937–4945, 1980.
56. De Groot PG, Kalsbeek R, Strijland A: Unpublished observations.
57. Desnick RJ: Allotransplantation in genetic diseases. In: Tager JM, Hooghwinkel GJM, Daems WTh (eds) Enzyme therapy in lysosomal storage diseases. Amsterdam, North-Holland, 1974, pp 292–301.
58. Beutler E: Nature's transplant in Fabry's disease. Lancet 2: 199, 1979.
59. Neufeld EF, Hasilik A, Rome LH: Processing and recognition of lysosomal enzymes. In:

Schauer R, Boer P, Buddecke E, Kramer MF, Vliegenhart JFG, Wiegandt H (eds) Glycoconjugates. Proceedings of the Fifth International Symposium, Kiel, September 1979. Stuttgart, Thieme, 1979, pp 320–321.

60. Lloyd JB: Cellular transport of lysosomal enzymes. An alternative hypothesis. Biochem J 164: 281-282, 1977.

61. Blobel G, Dobberstein B: Transfer of proteins across membranes. I. Presence of proteolytically processed and unprocessed nascent Ig light chains on membrane-bound ribosomes of murine-myeloma. J Cell Biol 67: 835–851, 1975.

62. Blobel G, Dobberstein B: Transfer of proteins across membranes. II. Reconstitution of functional rough microsomes from heterologous components. J Cell Biol 67: 852–862, 1975.

63. Robbins PW: Glycolysation of viral glycoproteins by host animal cells. Biochem Soc Trans 7: 320–322, 1979.

64. Parodi AJ, Leloir LF: The role of lipid intermediates in the glycosylation of proteins in the eucaryotic cell. Biochim Biophys Acta 559: 1–37, 1979.

65. Li E, Tabas I, Kornfeld S: The synthesis of complex-type oligosaccharides. I. Structure of the lipid-linked precursor of the complex-type oligosaccharides of the vesicular stomatitis virus G protein. J Biol Chem 253: 7762–7770, 1978.

66. Datema R, Schwarz RT: Formation of 2-deoxyglucose-containing lipid-linked oligosaccharides. Eur J Biochem 90: 505–514, 1978.

67. Takatsuki A, Kohn K, Tamura G: Inhibition of biosynthesis of polyisoprenol sugars in chick embryo microsomes by tunicamycin. Agric Biol Chem 39: 2089–2091, 1975.

68. Popov P, Alterman L, Sabatini D, Kreibach G: In vitro synthesis of β-glucuronidase by rat liver and preputial gland membrane-bound ribosomes. J Cell Biol 79: 364A, 1978.

69. Melchers F, Potter M, Warner NL (eds): Lymphocyte hybridosomes. Curr Top Microbiol Immunol 81, 1978.

70. Edwards K, Nagashima M, Drybrugh H, Wykes A, Schreiber G: Secretion of proteins from liver cells is suppressed by the proteinase inhibitor N-α-tosyl-L-lysyl chloromethane, but not by tunicamycin, an inhibitor of glycosylation. FEBS Lett 100: 269–272, 1979.

71. Algranati ID, Sabatini DD: Effect of protease inhibitors on albumin secretion in hepatoma cells. Biochem Biophys Res Commun 90: 220–226, 1979.

72. Wibo M, Poole B: Protein degradation in cultured cells. II. The uptake of chloroquine by rat fibroblasts and the inhibition of cellular protein degradation and cathepsin B_1. J Cell Biol 63: 430–440, 1974.

73. Reijngoud DJ, Tager JM: The permeability properties of the lysosomal membrane. Biochim Biophys Acta 472: 419–449, 1977.

74. Seglen PO, Reith A: Ammonia inhibition of protein degradation in isolated rat hepatocytes. Exp Cell Res 100: 276–280, 1976.

75. Warburton MJ, Wynn CH: The effect of intralysosomal sucrose storage on the turnover of hamster fibroblast lysosomal and Golgi-apparatus enzymes. Biochem J 158: 401–407, 1976.

76. De Groot PG, Strijland A: Unpublished observations.

77. Nyberg E, Dingle JT: Endocytosis of sucrose and other sugars by cells in culture. Exp Cell Res 63: 43-52, 1970.

78. Wildenthal K, Dees JH, Bujal M: Cardiac lysosomal derangements after long-term exposure to non-metabolizable sugars. Circ Res 40: 26–35, 1977.

79. Le Marshall J, Fraser JRE, Muirden KD: Lysosomal activation by neutral saccharides in cell cultures of synosium. Ann Rheum Dis 36: 130–138, 1977.

80. Lockwood TD, Shier WT: Regulation of acid proteases during growth, quiescence and starvation in normal and transformed cells. Nature 267: 252–254, 1977.

81. Mortimore GE, Ward WF: Behaviour of the lysosomal system during organ perfusion. An enquiry into the mechanism of hepatic proteolysis. In: Dingle JT, Dean RT (eds) Lysosomes in biology and pathology, vol 5. Amsterdam, North-Holland, 1976, pp 157–184.

82. Schworer CM, Mortimore GE: Glucagon-induced autophagy and proteolysis in rat liver: mediation by selective deprivation of intracellular amino acids. Proc Natl Acad Sci USA 76: 3169–3173, 1979.

250

83. Rome LH, Garvin AJ, Allietta MM, Neufeld EF: Two species of lysosomal organelles in cultured human fibroblasts. Cell 17: 143–153, 1979.
84. Beutler E, Kuhl W: Relationship between human α-galactosidase isoenzymes. Nature [New Biol] 239: 207–208, 1972.
85. Rietra PJGM, Molenaar JL, Hamers MN, Tager JM, Borst P: Investigation of the α-galactosidase deficiency in Fabry's disease using antibodies against the purified enzyme. Eur J Biochem 46: 89–98, 1974.
86. De Barsy T, Jacquemin P, De Vos P, Hers HG: Rodent and human α-glucosidase. Purification, properties and inhibition by antibodies. Investigation in type II glycogenesis. Eur J Biochem 31: 156–165, 1972.
87. Koster JD, Slee RG: Some properties of human acid α-glucosidase. Biochim Biophys Acta 482: 89–97, 1977.
88. Schram AW, Brouwer-Kelder B, Donker-Koopman WE, Loonen C, Hamers MN, Tager JM: Use of immobilized antibodies in investigating acid α-glucosidase in urine in relation to Pompe's disease. Biochim Biophys Acta 567: 370–383, 1979.
89. Mehler M, DiMauro S: Residual acid maltase activity in late-onset acid maltase deficiency. Neurology 27: 178–184, 1977.
90. Reuser AJJ, Koster JF, Hoogeveen A, Galjaard H: Biochemical, immunological and cell genetic studies in glycogenesis type II. Am J Hum Genet 30: 132–143, 1978.
91. Beratis NG, Labadie GU, Hirschhorn K: Characterization of the molecular defect in infantile and adult acid α-glucosidase deficiency fibroblasts. J Clin Invest 62: 1264–1274, 1978.
92. Hasilik A, Kalsbeek R, De Groot PG, Von Figura K, Tager JM: Unpublished observations.
93. Skudlarek MD, Swank RT: Biosynthesis of two lysosomal enzymes in macrophages. Evidence for a precursor of β-galactosidase. J Biol Chem 254: 9939–9942, 1979.
94. Meera Khan P, Westerveld A, Würzer-Figurelli EM, Bootsma D: Alpha-galactosidase in man-Chinese hamster somatic cell hybrids. Birth Defects Orig Artic Ser 11: 205–210, 1975.
95. Håkansson EM, Lundin LG: Effect of a coat colour locus on kidney lysosomal glycosidases in the house mouse. Biochem Genet 15: 75–85, 1977.
96. Dizik M, Elliott RW: A gene apparently determining the extent of sialylation of lysosomal α-mannosidase in mouse liver. Biochem Genet 15: 31–46. 1977.
97. Berger FG, Paigen K, Meisler MH: Regulation of the rate of β-galactosidase synthesis by the Bgs and Bgt loci in the mouse. J Biol Chem 253: 5280–5282, 1978.
98. Robbins AR: Isolation of α-mannosidase mutants of Chinese hamster ovary cells. Proc Natl Acad Sci USA 76: 1911–1915, 1979.
99. Thomas GH, Taylor HA, Miller CS, Axelman J, Migeon BR: Genetic complementation after fusion of Tay-Sachs and Sandhoff cells. Nature 250: 580–582, 1974.
100. Galjaard H, Hoogeveen A, De Wit-Verbeek HA, Reuser AJJ, Keijzer W, Westerveld A, Bootsma D: Tay-Sachs' and Sandhoff's disease. Intergenic complementation after somatic cell hybridization. Exp Cell Res 87: 444–448, 1974.
101. Galjaard H, Hoogeveen A, De Wit-Verbeek HA, Reuser AJJ, Ho MW, Robinson D: Genetic heterogeneity in G_{M1}-gangliosidosis. Nature 257: 60–62, 1975.
102. Okada S, Kato T, Yabuchi H, Okada Y: The complementation of β-galactosidase in fused cells of mucolipidosis II with another variant of β-galactosidase deficiency using new single cell enzyme assay. Biochem Biophys Res Commun 88: 559–562, 1979.
103. Hoeksema HL: The genetic defects in ganglioside storage diseases. PhD thesis, Erasmus University, Rotterdam, 1979.
104. D'Azzo A, Halley DJJ, Hoogeveen A, Galjaard H: Gene mutation in I-cell disease studied by somatic cell hybridization. Birth Defect Orig Artic Ser (in press) 1980.
105. Kato T, Okada S, Yutaka T, Inui K, Yabauchi H, Chiyo H, Furuyama J, Okada Y: Beta-galactosidase deficient-type mucolipidosis: a complementation study of neuraminidase in somatic cell hybrids. Biochem Biophys Res Commun 91: 114–117, 1979.
106. Champion MJ, Shows TB: Correction of human mucolipidosis II enzyme abnormalities in somatic cell hybrids. Nature 270: 64–66, 1977.

20. PATHOLOGY OF LYSOSOMAL DIGESTION

K. SANDHOFF AND E. CONZELMANN

Final degradation of complex carbohydrates, lipids, proteins and nucleic acids takes place in lysosomes, which are intracellular digestive vesicles. The degradation is catalyzed by acid hydrolases whose specificities are directed toward certain types of bonds rather than to individual substrates. For many of these enzymes, recessively inherited deficiencies leading to storage diseases are known. Among them the infantile lipid storage diseases are especially severe, and usually lethal. They are caused by almost complete deficiency of sphingolipid hydrolases [1], as a consequence of which the lipids that cannot be degraded further accumulate in the affected organs. Due to their low solubility in water, these lipids cannot be exported from the cells where they are biosynthesized, but instead precipitate intracellularly.

SPHINGOLIPIDS

As shown in Fig. 1, sphingolipids contain a hydrophobic portion, ceramide (N-acylsphingosine: in general, N-acylsphingoid), and a hydrophilic component. The latter may be phosphorylcholine as in sphingomyelin, the most abundant sphingolipid, or a sugar residue as in the glycosphingolipids. This sugar residue may be derived from glucose or galactose as in the cerebrosides, from galactose-3-sulphate as in the sulphatides, and from oligosaccharides

---

Abbreviations:

Cer	$=$ ceramide $= N$-acylsphingosine
Gal	$=$ D-galactose
GalNAc	$=$ 2-acetamido-2-deoxy-D-galactopyranose
G_{A2}	$=$ glycosphingolipid G_{A2}(GgOse3Cer $=$ GalNAc $\beta 1 \rightarrow 4$ Gal $1 \beta 1 \rightarrow 4$ Glc $\beta 1 \rightarrow 1$ Cer)
Glc	$=$ glucose
Globoside	$=$ GalNAc $\beta 1 \rightarrow 3$ Gal $1 \alpha 1 \rightarrow 4$ Gal $1 \beta 1 \rightarrow 4$ Glc $\beta 1 \rightarrow 1$ Cer
G_{M2}	$=$ ganglioside G_{M2}(11^3NeuAc-GgOse3Cer $=$ GalNAc $\beta 1 \rightarrow 4$ Gal $(3 \leftarrow 2$ NeuAc) $\beta 1 \rightarrow 4$ Glc $\beta 1 \rightarrow 1$ Cer
NeuAc	$= N$-acetylneuraminic acid
Variant AB	$=$ variant AB of infantile G_{M2} gangliosidosis
Variant B	$=$ variant B of infantile G_{M2} gangliosidosis (Tay-Sachs disease)
Variant O	$=$ variant O of infantile G_{M2} gangliosidosis (Sandhoff disease or Sandhoff-Jatzkewitz disease)

W.Th. Daems et al. (eds.), Cell Biological Aspects of Disease, 251–257. All rights reserved.
Copyright © 1981 by Martinus Nijhoff Publishers bv, The Hague/Boston/London.

252

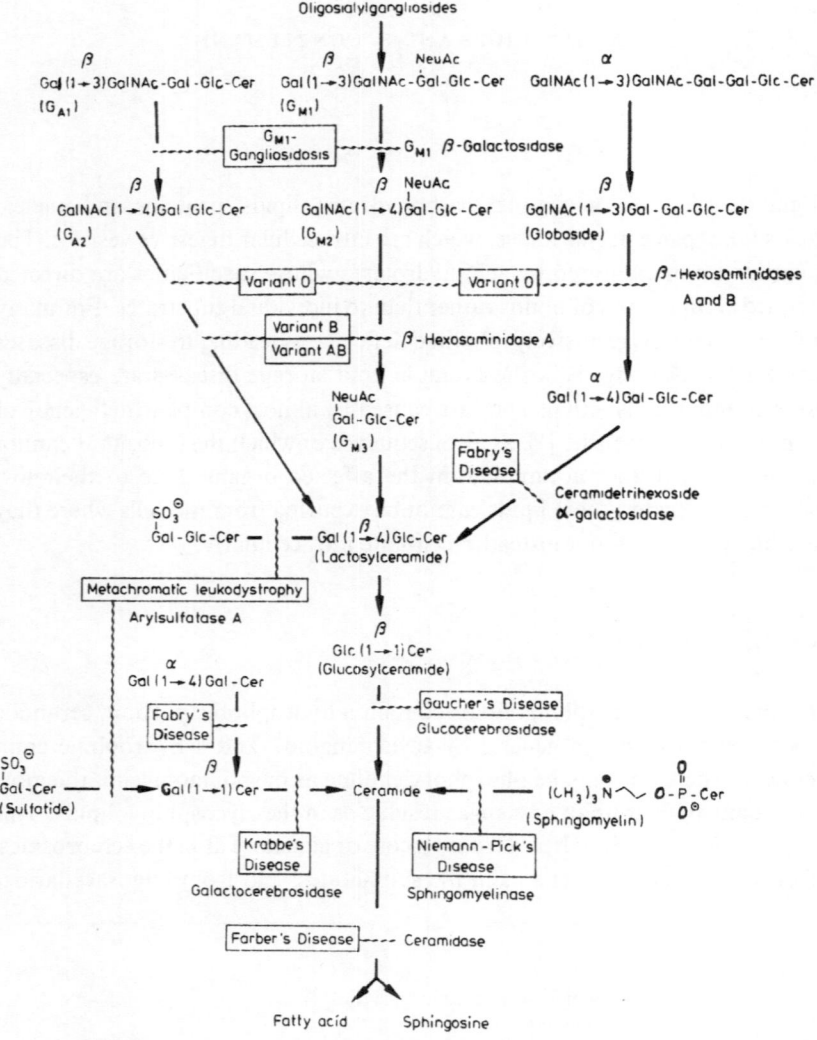

Fig. 1. Schematic representation of postulated degradation of sphingolipids with indication of metabolic blocks of known diseases [13].

which in the case of gangliosides contain sialic acid (*N*-acylneuraminic acid) as a characteristic unit.

The physiological role of glycolipids is not yet understood in detail, but their sugar residues as well as those of the glycoproteins influence the properties of the cell surface, which is important for cell-cell recognition and the expression of different cell types [2]. Gangliosides have also been shown to serve as binding sites for toxins and hormones on the cell surface [3].

ACTIVATOR PROTEINS FOR THE DEGRADATION OF GLYCOSPHINGO-
LIPIDS

In order to understand the accumulation of lipids as a consequence of a
particular deficiency, many sphingolipid hydrolases have been purified and
their substrate specificity has been analyzed. However, the attempt to study
the degradation of sphingolipids by water-soluble lysosomal hydrolases in
vitro encountered a principal problem in lipid enzymology: glycolipids are
amphiphilic molecules and form larger aggregates, called micelles, when
dispersed in water (Fig. 2). In these micelles the monomers are so tightly
packed that they are inaccessible to the enzymes, which means that virtually
no degradation is measured. The enzymic degradation can however, be
enormously stimulated by the addition of suitable detergents, such as bile
acids, in appropriate concentrations [4]. With these detergents the glycolipids
form small mixed micelles from which their oligosaccharide chains protrude
far enough to be attacked by the hydrolases.

In the lysosomes of the living cell the glycolipids are, of course, not present
as micelles but are incorporated into the membranes, where they are similarly
hidden from the enzymes. Lysosomes, however, do not contain bile acids or
other detergents. Therefore, the question arises as to how water-soluble
hydrolases gain access to their lipid substrates in vivo. Recent experiments
suggest that this is accomplished by a number of non enzymic proteins, which
are called activators [5].

The concept of the activator protein was developed by Jatzkewitz and co-
workers [6–8], who isolated the activator required for the degradation of
sulphatides by arylsulphatase A. This activator protein is heat stable, has an

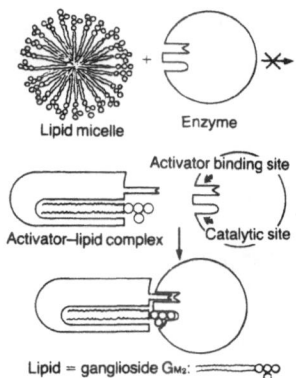

Lipid micelle   Enzyme

Activator binding site

Activator–lipid complex   Catalytic site

Lipid = ganglioside G$_{M2}$:

Fig. 2. Model for the activation of enzymic glycolipid hydrolysis by an activator protein [11].
For the system considered in this paper it is assumed that hexosaminidase A possesses a binding
site for the activator-lipid complex, whereas hexosaminidase B does not (lipid = ganglioside
G$_{M2}$:).

apparent molecular weight of 23,000 D and an isoelectric point of 4.3. With the lipid substrate it forms a 1:1 complex which is the true substrate for the degrading enzyme. Subcellular fractionation studies showed this activator to be localized in the soluble fraction of lysosomes, together with a number of other low molecular weight activators of the hydrolysis of other sphingo-lipids, such as cerebrosides, sphingomyelin, and glycolipid G_{A2}, by the re-spective enzymes [9]. Recently, such an activator for the degradation of glycolipids G_{M2} and G_{A2} by lysosomal hexosaminidase was recognized and isolated from human tissues [10, 11]. This activator is heat stable up to 60°C, labile to protease digestion, has an isoelectric point of 4.8 and an apparent molecular weight of 25,000 D, and is highly isoenzyme specific.

Human lysosomes contain mainly two hexosaminidases, A and B. In the presence of a detergent such as sodium taurodeoxycholate, both of them split off the terminal N-acetylgalactosamine residues from glycolipids G_{M2} and G_{A2} [12]. If, however, this activator protein replaces the detergent, the glyco-lipids are degraded almost exclusively by hexosaminidase A, the isoenzyme B being almost inactive [11]. Thus, the substrate specificities of the isoenzymes are obviously determined by the properties of this activator protein which specifically recognizes only hexosaminidase A.

The mechanism by which this activator stimulates glycolipid breakdown seems to be analogous to the model described by Jatzkewitz and Fischer [7] for the activation of sulphatide hydrolysis by arylsulphatase A. In accordance with this model, the turnover of water-soluble artificial substrates such as 4-methylumbelliferyl glycosides is not at all affected by the activator protein (Table 1). The kinetics of the interaction of the enzyme with both the lipid and the activator in various concentrations support the conception that the acti-vator does not act directly on the enzyme but rather binds to lipid monomers to give a soluble complex which is specifically recognized as substrate by the enzyme (Fig. 2) [11]. This complex formation could be demonstrated directly by gelelectrophoresis [11].

THE BIOCHEMICAL VARIANTS OF INFANTILE G_{M2} GANGLIOSIDOSIS

The discovery of the activator proteins and the knowledge of their properties were not only essential to explain the in vivo degradation of sphingolipids but also to understand the molecular pathology of lipid storage diseases. One of the first described and best studied lipidoses is infantile G_{M2} gangliosidosis. Patients with this disease show the accumulation in nervous tissue of large amounts of ganglioside G_{M2}, an intermediate of ganglioside catabolism occurring only in traces in the normal brain. Enzymatically, three variants of this disease can be distinguished (Fig. 3) (cf. [13]), two of which are caused by

Table 1. Degradation of glycosphingolipids by hexosaminidases A and B in the presence and absence of stimulating factors [11].

Substrate	Hexosaminidase	Additions		
		None	Sodium taurodeoxy-cholate (2mM)[a]	Activator[b]
			Degradation rate in μmol/h mg	
Ganglioside G_{M2}	A	0.009	0.40	0.97
	B	0.001	0.07	0.005
Glycolipid G_{A2}	A	0.008	6.3	2.48
	B	0.001	30.7	0.072
Globoside	A	0.004	14.4	0.42
	B	0.005	24.0	0.005
4-Methylumbelliferyl-β-	A	675	350	680
D-N-acetylgalactos-aminide	B	1350	850	1390

[a] Since this concentration of detergent leads to a time-dependent inactivation of the enzyme, the measured degradation rate depends strongly on the incubation time. Values were obtained with short incubation times (0.5 h). (For methodology, see [11].)
[b] In the presence of a partially purified activator preparation [11], the reaction rate depends on the amount of activator protein, which under the conditions used was still not at saturation level.

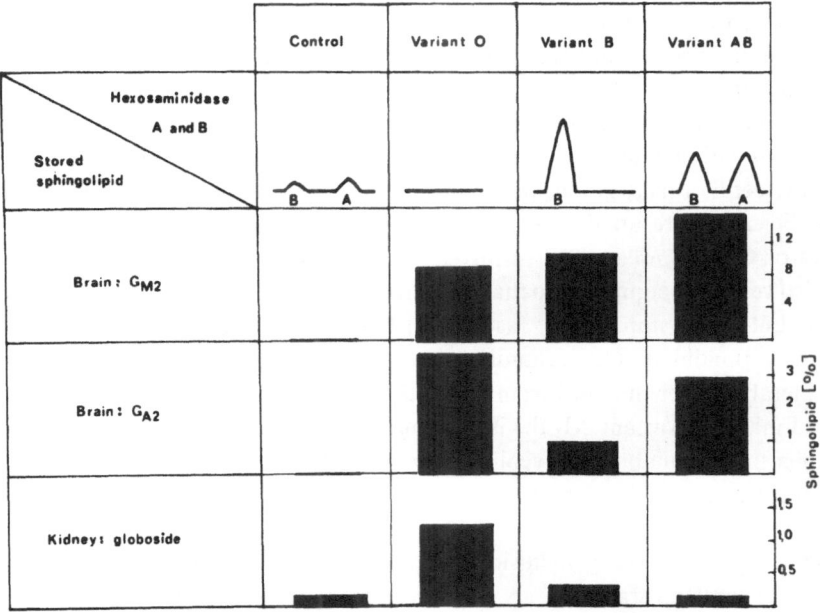

Fig. 3. Storage pattern of glycolipids and hexosaminidase in infantile G_{M2}-gangliosidosis. Hexosaminidase activity was measured with synthetic substrates after the isoelectric separation of isoenzymes A and B. Quantities of stored sphingolipids are given as percentage of the dry weight of the storage organ [13].

isoenzyme defects: in variant B (Tay-Sachs disease), only one of the two major hexosaminidase isoenzymes, hexosaminidase A, is deficient, whereas patients with variant O lack both of the major hexosaminidases (A and B), probably due to the defect of the common subunit β.

In the third variant, termed AB, no enzyme defect could be found. These patients accumulate ganglioside G_{M2} and its asialo residue G_{A2} in brain tissue at the same rate as patients with the O and B variants do, and show almost identical clinical symptoms and course of the disease, but have normal or even elevated levels of hexosaminidase A and B. These enzymes are biochemically and immunologically indistinguishable from normal ones [14]. Recently, it was shown that the AB variant is caused by a defect in the activator protein necessary for the degradation of the glycolipids G_{M2} and G_{A2} [10]. Thus, this variant not only expands the known range of biochemical variation in inherited diseases, but also illustrates the physiological significance of the activator protein. For the turnover of membrane components by soluble enzymes, this activator is as important as the enzymes themselves.

The pattern of the glycolipids stored in patients suffering from the rare AB variant confirms the specificity of the activator established in vitro. The knowledge about activator specificity is in turn very helpful in attempts to explain the storage patterns observed in the other variants of G_{M2} gangliosidosis, i.e., in terms of deficiency of the relevant isoenzyme. Unlike the reaction rates measured in the presence of detergents, the velocities obtained in the presence of the activator fully account for these patterns (Table 1): the deficiency of both hexosaminidase isoenzymes in variant O leads to the accumulation of all their substrates, including glycolipids G_{A2} and G_{M2} and in visceral organs, globoside. In variant B, where only hexosaminidase A is deficient, the residual hexosaminidase B is unable to interact with the activator-G_{M2} complex. The turnover of glycolipid G_{A2} by this isoenzyme is also very slow compared to that of the reactions catalysed by hexosaminidase A, but is still appreciably faster than that of other glycolipids substrates. Correspondingly, the accumulation of glycolipids G_{A2} in variant B is considerably lower than in variants O or AB.

Finally, in variant AB the isoenzymes are both present but cannot reach their membrane-bound glycolipid substrates, because the activator effecting this interaction is missing.

Thus, infantile G_{M2} gangliosidosis is a well-studied example of how several rather similar variants of an inherited disease are caused by different biochemical lesions. This principle can certainly be extended to other inborn errors of glycolipid metabolism. For instance, evidence has been presented recently that in one patient with metachromatic leucodystrophy, the cause of this disease is not a defect of arylsulphatase A but rather deficiency of the activator protein necessary for the degradation of sulphatides by this enzyme [15].

REFERENCES

1. Stanbury JB, Wyngaarden JB, Fredrickson DS: The metabolic basis of inherited disease. New York, McGraw-Hill, 1978.
2. Hakomori SI: Structures and organization of cell surface. Glycolipid dependency on cell growth and maligment transformation. Biochim Biophys Acta 417: 55–89, 1975.
3. Yamakawa T, Nagai Y: Glycolipids at the cell surface and their biological functions. Trends Biol Sci 3: 128–131, 1978.
4. Glew RH, Peters SP: Practical enzymology of the sphingolipidoses. New York, AR Liss, 1977.
5. Sandhoff K, Conzelmann E: Activation of lysosomal hydrolysis of complex glycolipids by non-enzymic proteins. Trends Biochem Sci 4: 231–233, 1979.
6. Mehl E, Jatzkewitz H: Eine Cerebrosidsulfatase aus Schweinenieren. Hoppe-Seylers Z Physiol Chem 339: 260–276, 1964.
7. Fischer G, Jatzkewitz H: The activator of cerebroside sulphatase. A model of the activation. Biochim Biophys Acta 528: 69–76, 1978.
8. Fischer G, Jatzkewitz H: The activator of cerebroside sulphatase. Binding studies with enzyme and substrate demonstrating the detergent function of the activator protein. Biochim Biophys Acta 481: 561–572, 1977.
9. Mraz W, Fischer G, Jatzkewitz H: Low molecular weight proteins in secondary lysosomes as activators of different sphingolipidhydrolases. FEBS Lett 67: 104–109, 1976.
10. Conzelmann E, Sandhoff K: AB variant of infantile G_{M2}-gangliosidosis: deficiency of a factor necessary for stimulation of hexosaminidase A-catalyzed degradation of ganglioside G_{M2} and glycolipid G_{A2}. Proc Natl Acad Sci USA 75: 3979–3983, 1978.
11. Conzelman E, Sandhoff K: Purification and characterization of an activator protein for the degradation of glycolipids G_{M2} and G_{A2} by hexosaminidase A. Hoppe-Seylers Z Physiol Chem 360: 1837–1849, 1979.
12. Sandhoff K, Conzelmann E, Nehrkorn H: Specificity of human liver hexosaminidases A and B against glycosphingolipids G_{M2} and G_{A2}. Purification of the enzymes by affinity chromatography employing specific elution. Hoppe-Seylers Z Physiol Chem 358: 779–787, 1977.
13. Sandhoff K, Christomanou H: Biochemistry and genetics of gangliosidoses. Hum Genet 50: 107–143, 1979.
14. Conzelmann E, Sandhoff K, Nehrkorn H, Geiger B, Arnon R: Purification, biochemical and immunological characterisation of hexosaminidase A from variant AB of infantile G_{M2}-gangliosidosis. Eur J Biochem 84: 27–33, 1978.
15. Stevens RL, Fluharty AL, Kihara H, Kaback MM, Shapiro LI, Sandhoff K, Fischer G: Metachromatic leucodystrophy — variant with apparent cerebroside sulfatase activator deficiency. Clin Res 27: A104, 1979.

21. LIPOSOMES: INTERACTION WITH THE BIOLOGICAL MILIEU AND IMPLICATIONS FOR THEIR USE IN BIOLOGY AND MEDICINE

G. GREGORIADIS, C. KIRBY, E. MANESIS, J. CLARKE, C. DAVIS, AND D. NEERUNJUN

INTRODUCTION

The use of carrier systems for the transport of drugs to target tissues, cells or subcellular organelles is now recognized as a useful method of improving drug selectivity. Carrier systems that have been proposed to date include macromolecules, cell, viruses and synthetic particles [1]. Most of these are, however, limited in the range and quantity of drugs they can incorporate. Further, they often lack an ability to prevent contact of the drug moiety with the normal biological environment or to promote its entrance to areas in need of drug action. Other limitations relate to the toxicity of the carrier's components, the availability of the latter and to technical difficulties such as, for instance, the preparation of the drug-carrier complex. Extensive efforts have therefore been made in developing the ideal drug-carrier [1, 2]. As discussed elsewhere [2] such a carrier should be capable of delivering a large variety of agents selectively into the site of action within the biological entity and at the same time provoke no ill effects. During the last decade it has become apparent that liposomes possess many of the properties expected from a multifunctional carrier and successes in applying these to membrane research have now been extended to biology and medicine [3, 4].

Liposomes, a family of artificial phospholipid vesicles, are made of one or more lipid bilayers alternating with aqueous compartments [5] and can be charged by the incorporation of a negatively or positively charged amphiphile. Using appropriate methods, water soluble and lipid soluble drugs are entrapped within the aqueous and lipid phase of liposomes, respectively. The permeability of liposomal membranes to ions or their stability can be adjusted accordingly by the incorporation of sterols or other lipid components. Preparation of liposomes with or without entrapped solutes is carried out by a variety of methods which give the classic multilamellar structures as well as small or large unilamellar or oligolamellar vesicles. Each of these types of liposomes is intended to suit particular needs in biology or pharmacology (for

---

Abbreviations: 6CF, 6-carboxyfluorescein; PC, egg phosphatidylcholine; CHOL, cholesterol; PA, phosphatidic acid.

W.Th. Daems et al. (eds.), Cell Biological Aspects of Disease, 259–280. All rights reserved.
Copyright © 1981 by Martinus Nijhoff Publishers bv, The Hague/Boston/London.

a comprehensive list of agents that have been associated with liposomes, see ref. 2).

Initial work [6–8] on the fate of protein-containing liposomes injected intravenously into rats has already established some of the principles underlying liposomal behaviour in vivo. For instance, latency of liposomal enzymes was found to be largely retained in the blood circulation, suggesting maintenance of the structural integrity of liposomes in the intravascular space. Furthermore, examination of a number of tissues showed that liposomes and their contents are taken up mostly by the liver and spleen through endocytosis to end up in the lysosomes. Such findings indicated that the system was attractive as a means of delivering drugs into the intracellular environment, particularly the lysosomes, from where drugs could subsequently enter other cell compartments [9]. In addition to being localized within specific areas of the cell, liposomal agents were also found capable of action, subsequent to their liberation from the carrier [10]. Further work from this laboratory and from many others has now revealed an intriguing variety of aspects related to the transport potential of liposomes [11]. Attempts will be made to summarize some of the basic facets of the interaction of liposomes with living systems and discuss possibilities and problems relevant to selective drug action and its applications in biological systems [11].

INTERACTION OF LIPOSOMES WITH CELLS IN VITRO

Transport of enzymes and other agents by liposomes into the lysosomes of cells [7, 8] raised the question as to whether agents transported into these organelles could free themselves from their carrier and survive in an active form in the intralysosomal environment. In work carried out to show that liposomes could control cell metabolism [10] we found that cultured cells deficient in a specific enzyme were capable of taking up liposomes, the contents of which (in this case the missing enzyme) were delivered into the lysosomes where after the disintegration of the carrier, they were set free to act. Uptake of liposomes by cells, localization in lysosomes and their subsequent disruption were expected to occur not only because a similar fate of liposomes had been already observed in vivo [7, 8], but also because most cells are expected to endocytose soluble or particulate matter when exposed to it. Obviously, with 'professional' endocytosers, uptake will be more rapid than with other cells (e.g. fibroblasts). The fate and effect of liposomal agents entering lysosomes by endocytosis of the carrier depend on the physical characteristics of such agents [1]. Thus, those which are stable in the lysosomal milieu can act within it (e.g. hydrolic enzymes, metal chelating agents, certain antimicrobial drugs) or cross lysosomal membranes to reach, and act in, other cellular sites (Fig. 1).

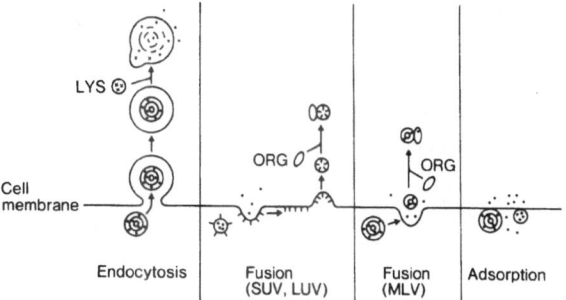

LYS

Cell
membrane

ORG

ORG

Endocytosis | Fusion (SUV, LUV) | Fusion (MLV) | Adsorption

Fig. 1. Possible mechanisms for cell-liposome interaction. Endocytosis of the multilamellar (or monolamellar) liposome is followed by fusion of the endocytic vacuole containing the liposome with a lysosome (LYS). Lysosomal phospholipases or other factors (crosses) disrupt the lipid bilayers of liposomes and free the entrapped agent (dots) which can then act either within the lysosome or, after its diffusion, in other cell compartments.

Fusion of a monolamellar liposome with the cellular membrane is followed by the entrance of water-soluble agents (dots) into the cell's cytoplasm from which they can reach other organelles. Agents incorporated in the lipid bilayers of the liposome (rods) are transferred onto the membrane of the cell. The latter agents can be internalized by the process of endocytosis. Endocytic vacuoles thus formed can interact with other organelles (ORG).

Fusion of a multilamellar liposome with the cellular membrane is followed by the entrance of agents (dots) in the outer aqueous space of the liposome and of the inner core into the cell's cytoplasm. Free agents and the core can then interact with other organelles (ORG).

Adsorption of a multilamellar or monolamellar liposome onto the cellular membrane can be of no consequence or induce changes in the permeability of both liposomal and cellular membranes. Agents (dots) diffusing from liposomes can thus penetrate the cell's interior. From Gregoriadis [2].

An alternative mechanism of cell-liposome interaction, namely fusion of the respective membranes, has been suggested by a number of workers (see review by G. Poste in ref. 11). This has opened the possibility for a method of introducing agents entrapped in the aqueous space of liposomes directly into extralysosomal areas. On the other hand, agents incorporated into the lipid phase of liposomes could, according to this mechanism, incorporate themselves into the cellular membrane (Fig. 1). Although there has been a considerable amount of indirect experimental data to support fusion [11, 12] doubts still exist as to its actual occurrence. Indeed, there is at least one mechanism which could provide an alternative explanation for such results: interaction of liposomes with cells may lead to the destabilization of the membranes of both entities with entrapped agents escaping from leaky liposomes to enter equally leaky cells at the points of contact (Fig. 1).

BEHAVIOUR OF LIPOSOMES IN VIVO

Information amassed during the last decade on the interaction of liposomes with biological entities in vivo has been reviewed extensively [3, 4, 12–14]. One of the initial observations was that following intravenous injection of unilamellar or multilamellar liposomes containing radiolabels in both their lipid and aqueous phase, the ratio of the two labels in the blood often remained similar to that in the injected preparation. It was inferred from this that the carrier retains its structural integrity in the circulation. Retention of liposomal integrity is an important prerequisite for effective drug delivery since it not only will warrant quantitative transport of drugs to target areas, but it will also protect drugs (e.g. certain drugs in cancer chemotherapy, enzymes in replacement therapy, nucleic acids in genetic engineering) from inactivation in the blood or prevent their premature loss through excretion. However, it is possible that a drug can form a complex with the lipid marker and circulate in the blood as such, even after liposomal disintegration. On the other hand, the variety of paired markers used and which include cholesterol and albumin [7], dipalmitoyl phosphatidylcholine and albumin [15], cholesterol and bleomycin [16], cholesterol and methotrexate [17], renders such a possibility unlikely. It is nevertheless true that liposomes of certain lipid compositions become permeable to entrapped solutes of small molecular weight in the presence of plasma [18] or in vivo in the circulating blood [19, 20].

Recent work [21–23] from this laboratory has shown that liposomal stability in vivo (blood circulation) and in vitro (in the presence of serum, plasma or whole blood) is dependent on the cholesterol content of liposomes relative to that of phospholipid. In the systems we have used, integrity of liposomes can be measured directly, by monitoring the extent to which the latency of a given agent entrapped in the aqueous phase of liposomes changes within a biological milieu [21–23]. Latency is defined here as the amount of the agent (% of the total) which cannot be measured unless liposomes are disrupted with a detergent. When, for instance, the latency of a liposomal enzyme after coming into contact with, say, blood is equal to that recorded in the preparation before use, it can be assumed that the integrity of the preparation has not been altered as a result of contact with blood, at least in terms of substrate penetration through the lipid bilayers. Figure 2A shows that in rats injected intravenously with invertase-containing small multilamellar liposomes, stability of the latter in the blood (measured by the extent to which sucrose permeates the liposomal membranes to reach the enzyme) is proportional to the amount of cholesterol incorporated into the liposomal structure. With cholesterol-rich liposomes (7:5 phospholipid to cholesterol molar ratio) stability is nearly equal to that observed in the preparation before injection. As the proportion of cholesterol decreases, liposomal stability is reduced accordingly (almost immediately after injection) to reach low values with liposomes devoid of cholesterol. Similar results are obtained with such liposomes exposed to whole blood in vitro (Fig. 2B) but loss of stability in the

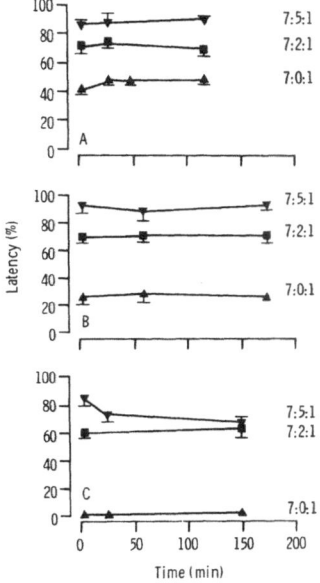

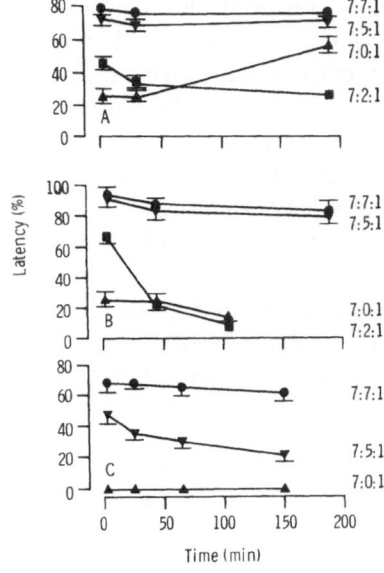

Fig. 2. The effect of cholesterol content of liposomes on the latency of entrapped β-fructofuranosidase. Liposomes containing β-fructofuranosidase and composed PC, CHOL and PA at the molar ratios shown were injected intravenously into rats (A) or incubated with rat whole blood (B) or rat serum (C). Latent β-fructofuranosidase in blood or serum is expressed as % ± SD of the latent enzyme in the injected preparation. Each point represents values from 4–7 animals (A) or fire pooled experiments (B and C).

Fig. 3. The effect of cholesterol content of liposomes on the latency of entrapped 6-CF. Liposomes containing 6-CF and composed as in Fig. 2 were injected intravenously into rats (A) or incubated with rat whole blood (B) or rat serum (C). Latent 6-CF in blood or serum is expressed as % ± SD of the latent dye in the injected preparation. Each point represents values from 4–9 animals (A) or nine (B) and six (C) pooled experiments. From Gregoriadis and Davis [22].

presence of serum is more pronounced and becomes total in the case of cholesterol-free liposomes (Fig. 2C). The dependence of liposomal stability on cholesterol content was also shown in rats injected with small multilamellar liposomes containing 0.25 M 6-carboxyfluorescein (6-CF) (Fig. 3). At this concentration the dye is quenched but when, for any reason, the dye escapes into the medium, ensuing dilution enables it to fluoresce. As with the invertase-containing liposomes, the presence of a sufficient amount of cholesterol (e.g. 7:7 or 7:5 phospholipid to cholesterol molar ratio) was instrumental in maintaining their stability (in terms of dye leakage) after liposomes came into contact with blood in vivo (Fig. 3A) and also in vitro in the presence of whole blood (Fig. 3B) or serum (Fig. 3C). Further, work with 6-CF-containing unilamellar liposomes indicated that a 7:7 phospholipid to cholesterol ratio leads to total (100%) retention of liposomal stability in the blood of injected

264

mice (Fig. 4) or in the presence of whole blood or plasma [23]. Even after exposure to serum, stability loss in such liposomes is only minor [23]. Full stability retention in cholesterol-rich unilamellar liposomes is also indicated from monitoring the ratio of ^{14}C-cholesteryl oleate incorporated into the liposomal lamellae and of 6-CF entrapped in the aqueous phase (Table 1). For up to 150 min after intravenous injection, the ratio is retained at almost its initial level of unity, the implication being that the two labels (i.e. aqueous and lipid phase of the carrier) are cleared from the circulation at nearly identical rates.

Preservation of liposomal stability with the help of cholesterol is probably related to the fact that the latter's presence in phospholipid bilayers leads to the packing of phospholipid molecules and to the reduction in the permeability to entrapped small molecules [24]. Our data [21–23] show that in the

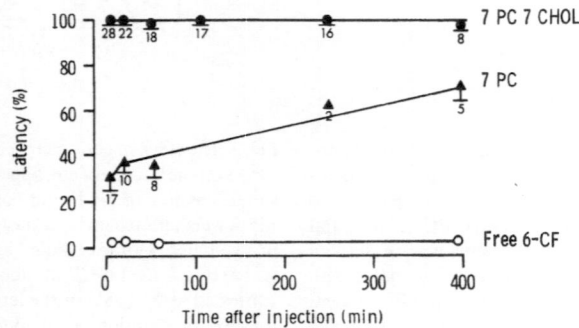

Fig. 4. Latency of liposomal 6-CF in the blood of injected mice. Mice were injected intravenously with 6-CF, free or entrapped in unilamellar liposomes. 6-CF latency values in blood at time intervals are % ± SD of latencies in the respective injected preparations. ○, free 6-CF; ▲, cholesterol-free liposomes; ●, cholesterol-rich liposomes. From Kirby et al. [23].

Table 1. ^{14}C:6-carboxyfluorescein ratios in the blood of mice injected with 6-carboxyfluorescein entrapped in ^{14}C-labelled liposomes.

Treatment		^{14}C:6-carboxyfluorescein ratio ± SD				
		2 min	20 min	110 min	150 min	450 min
Intravenous	A	1.09±08 (6)	1.09±0.09 (6)	1.05±0.0 (3)	1.02±0.0 (4)	ND
	B	2.1, 2.3	5.5 ±0.8 (3)		9.2 ±3.1 (3)	
	C	3.4, 6.0	11.5±4.8 (3)		14.3, 18.3	
Intra-peritoneal	A	ND	1.01±0.0 (4)	1.05±0.1 (4)	1.06±0.0 (4)	0.97±0.0 (4)

Mice were injected intravenously or intraperitoneally with 6-carboxyfluorescein entrapped in cholesterol-rich (A), cholesterol-poor (B), and cholesterol-free (C) small unilamellar liposomes labelled with ^{14}C-cholesteryl oleate ($3.9 \times 10^4 - 4.1 \times 10^5$ d.p.m.). The ratio of ^{14}C:6-carboxyfluorescein in the injected preparations was taken as unity. Numbers in parentheses denote animals used. ND, not determined. From Kirby et al. [23].

absence of serum, loss of 6-CF from cholesterol-free liposomes is relatively slow but it becomes almost instantaneous in its presence. Other workers [25] have suggested that such loss of entrapped solutes results from the destruction of liposomes because of liposomal phospholipid transfer to high-density lipoproteins. Our present findings (Figs. 2–4 and Table 1) tempt us to speculate that in the presence of blood or serum, cholesterol, by its imposition of molecular packing, not only retards ion diffusion, but also prevents phospholipid molecules from being transferred to lipoproteins. Very recent work has now confirmed this supposition: using cholesterol-rich unilamellar liposomes, there is very little transfer of radiolabelled egg phosphatidylcholine to high-density lipoproteins when liposomes are incubated in the presence of serum [26]. As the action of cholesterol in promoting liposomal stability in whole blood (Figs. 1A and B; 2A and B; 3) is more efficient than in serum alone (Figs. 1C and 2C) it can be assumed that blood cells in vitro and in vivo minimize the detrimental effect of serum. It is known that blood cells interact with high-density lipoproteins in terms of phospholipid movement [27] and it is possible that when both liposomes and erythrocytes are present, such movement between liposomes and lipoproteins diminishes or becomes nonexistent. Regardless of the way by which cholesterol and blood cells protect liposomal stability, it is encouraging that liposomes are now available which, depending on their cholesterol content, can release entrapped agents in vivo at specific rates. For instance, we have found that this applies to a number of drugs related to cancer (e.g. vincristine, melphalan, bleomycin) and antimicrobial (chloroquine, primaquine) therapy (C. Kirby J. Clarke D. Neerunjun and G. Gregoriadis, unpublished data). From the practical point of view it is of importance that cholesterol-rich liposomes retain their stability for several weeks and that their in vivo behaviour after prolonged storage remains unaffected [23].

In vivo leakage of liposomal contents may also be prevented by incorporating these into the lipid framework of the carrier, by the use of drugs which can interact electrostatically with liposomal lipid components or by linking drugs with macromolecules or appropriate acceptors which are already entrapped. Thus, when actinomycin D is accommodated into the lipid phase of liposomes, its rate of clearance from the blood of injected animals is very similar to that of the carrier [19] and the same applies to the lipid soluble colchicine [15] and daunomycin or vinblastine [28]. In the 'second carrier' approach [29], polyglutamic acid is incorporated into liposomes which are then allowed to interact with melphalan or methotrexate in the presence of carbodiimide. This leads to the formation of a polyglutamic acid-drug complex, and escape of the drug from liposomes in the circulation following their injection into rats is then prevented. Similar results are obtained when entrapped DNA is the second carrier for daunomycin or actinomycin D [29].

Among other factors, liposomal size and charge control the rate of elimination of liposomes from the blood: large liposomes are removed more rapidly than those of small size (and this is reflected in the biphasic rate of clearance of liposomes of mixed sizes [7]) and negatively charged liposomes are again removed more rapidly than neutral or positively charged ones [15, 23, 30]. This may be related to the fact that liposomes, regardless of their initial surface charge, become negatively charged upon contact with blood plasma [31]. However, the way by which such charge modulates rates of elimination is not known although it is possible that the surface charge originally present in liposomes controls the extent to which, or even the fashion by which, plasma components associate with liposomes to cause their uptake by cells in vivo.

Cells responsible for the uptake of liposomes are those of the reticulo-endothelial system, namely hepatic Kupffer cells and spleen macrophages [32, 33], and participation of the two tissues per unit weight is roughly similar [7, 16]. Even with liposomes prepared under identical conditions and expected to transport entrapped substances to tissues at comparable rates, apparent total uptake by tissues often differs. The explanation is that agents, depending on their nature, will behave differently once intracellularly. For example, some agents will tend to leak out while others will be degraded or metabolized with the products being released extracellularly. Whether hepatic parenchymal cells participate in the uptake of liposomes is still doubtful in spite of extensive investigation [32–34]. It is, however, conceivable that liposomes smaller than 100 nm (diameter) can reach parenchymal cells and be subsequently interiorized by them. It is also not certain whether liposomes, even at their smallest size (about 15 nm), succeed in undergoing transcapillary passage to enter the extravascular space. Liposomes are, nonetheless, known to cross membranes lining the peritoneal cavity: when small or large liposomes containing ^{125}I-labelled polyvinylpyrrolidone are injected intraperitoneally, radioactivity is recovered in the blood and liver to an extent far above that known to occur with the free polymer [35]. It can thus be assumed that transport of most of the radioactivity in these tissues is effected via liposomes. Recent experiments have shown beyond reasonable doubt that liposomes can cross the peritoneum membranes. When mice were injected intraperitoneally with small unilamellar liposomes containing 0.25 M 6-carboxyfluorescein [23] the dye was found to penetrate the blood circulation in a fully quenched form supporting passage of intact liposomes (Fig. 5). Support for liposome transport through membranes has also come from studies in which the rat testicle was injected with radiolabelled albumin or actinomycin D [36]. In contrast to large liposomes which remained and disintegrated at the site of injection, small liposomes and entrapped agents were transported either to the lymph nodes draining the injected tissue or into the blood. However, it is not known whether entrance in the blood occurred after direct crossing of the capillaries,

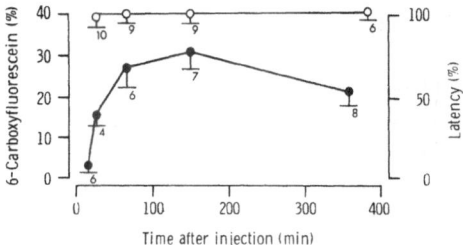

Fig. 5. Latency and levels of liposomal 6-CF in the blood of injected mice. Mice were injected intraperitoneally with 6-CF entrapped in unilamellar cholesterol-rich liposomes. 6-CF latency (O) and concentration (●) in total blood are expressed as % ± SD of the latency and the amount of the dye respectively in the injected preparation. From Kirby et al. [23].

via the lymphatic circulation, or both.

Transcapillary passage of small liposomes by the intravenous route is suggested from experiments with tumour-bearing rodents designed to investigate parameters related to the effect of size of the liposomal carrier on its localization in malignant tissues. We found [16, 35] that when small liposomes were used (about 80 nm average diameter) uptake of the liposomal radioactivity (^{111}In-labelled bleomycin) by Meth 'A', 6C3HED and Lewis lung carcinoma cells implanted in a variety of mouse strains and by Novikoff hepatoma in Wistar rats, was several-fold greater (up to about 7% ot the dose per gram tumour tissue) than that obtained with liposomes of larger size. Because of a parallel reduction in the uptake of the marker by the liver and spleen, it was proposed that extended circulation of small liposomes in the blood enabled them to cross capillaries and reach tumour cells. This has been recently confirmed in rats implanted with Walker 256 carcinoma [37]. It should be pointed out, however, that there are at least three alternative explanations for such findings: as small liposomes circulate in the blood for longer periods of time, radioactivity may be released slowly to reach the extravascular space more effectively. In addition, liposomes or their radioactive contents may interact in some way with the capillary walls, without actually crossing them. Again, by virtue of the longer survival of small liposomes in the circulation, interaction between such liposomes and capillaries would be more efficient. It is also possible that some liposomes are engulfed by macrophages which subsequently infiltrate tumours.

At the subcellular level, there is now considerable evidence that, in vivo, liposomes and their contents cross cellular membranes via endocytosis to end up in the lysosomes [7–9, 33, 34, 38, 39]. Indeed, lysosomal localization of liposomes is far from being an unusual finding. Fixed macrophages of the liver and spleen endocytose avidly macromolecules and particulate matter in the circulating blood and there is no reason to expect that liposomes would be an exception. Even stronger, although indirect, evidence for lysosomal localization of liposomes is the finding that in rats injected with liposomal radio-labelled albumin, the radioactivity content of the liver increases to high levels soon after injection but declines rapidly afterwards. This is compatible with albumin degradation and release of iodinated fragments into the circulation [8, 30]. Similar observations have been made with liposomes containing enzymes [7, 8, 30, 39] but not with liposomal polyvinylpyrrolidone or ^{111}In, which cannot be degraded or otherwise metabolized [16, 35]. In the latter cases, radioactivity in the liver reaches a plateau which is maintained for over 24 h [16].

Interaction of cells with liposomes in vivo through fusion of the respective membranes would allow the introduction of agents directly into the cell's cytoplasm, but is unlikely to occur to any significant extent: (a) although various morphological studies in vivo have provided ample evidence for endocytosis, they have failed to reveal liposome-entrapped material in the cytoplasm, unequivocally not surrounded by membranes; (b) erythrocytes and other blood cells which come into close contact for several hours with intravenously injected liposomes do not incorporate any measurable proportion of liposomal agents.

DIRECTION OF LIPOSOMES TO TARGET SITES

Unmodified liposomes present in blood circulation are, as already discussed, taken up mostly by the cells of the reticuloendothelial system and also by the hepatic parenchymal and endothelial cells. In situations where biologically active agents need introduction into these cells (e.g. lysosomal storage diseases and microbial infections) such localization can find good use. There are several instances, however, in which uptake of liposomes by alternative targets is deemed essential and, therefore, some versatility of the carrier's tissue distribution is required. This does not necessarily imply total avoidance of non-target areas, especially in cases where drugs can be tolerated or inactivated by such areas. In the treatment of some enzyme deficiencies, for instance, with exogenous enzymes or of microbial diseases with certain antibiotics, participation of non-diseased cells is unlikely to be detrimental to their well-being. However, a reasonably selective uptake of cytotoxic drugs would be essential for successful targeting (e.g. cancer chemotherapy).

Liposome-target interaction is known to be influenced not only by variables pertaining to the carrier itself (e.g. size, surface charge, fluidity) but also by other parameters. These have been tentatively classified [40] into two main categories, namely those related to the biological space travelled by the carrier (e.g. blood, various membranes) or to the target itself (e.g. cell membrane composition, endocytic capacity, receptors). Appropriate consideration of such factors may provide guidelines for the rationalization of targeting and also for the design of the overall carrier unit. Thus, there are a number of cases in which simple modifications of the liposomal carrier have been sufficient for its effective association with target areas. For instance, imposition of a negative or positive charge on the surface of ^{99}Tc-containing liposomes led to a greater degree of radioactivity localization in infarcted myocarial regions of injected dogs [41]. Furthermore, in treating diabetic rats by the intragastric route with liposomal insulin, the choice of specific phospholipids which are less likely to be attacked by pancreatic phospholipases at 37°C or disrupted efficiently by bile salts helped us to improve the glucose-lowering effect of the hormone [42]. Liposomal phospholipid choice has also been crucial in attempts to target liposomal agents at the subcellular level [43–45]. An example of modifying the non-target environment so as to improve localization of liposomal agents in specific tissues is the administration of excess 'empty' (buffer-loaded) liposomes of large average diameter together with smaller drug-carrying liposomes. As large vesicles can compete successfully for the liver [30] with those of smaller size, the latter will circulate in the blood for longer periods of time and thus be able to reach less accessible areas in the body. In experiments with tumour-bearing mice, for instance, large liposomes given at about the same time with small ones allowed these to localize their drug content in tumour tissues [16].

Although such modifications may, in certain cases, optimize drug action, there will be instances where a more sophisticated approach is needed. Towards this end we have proposed [46] coating of the liposomal surface with molecules possessing a specific affinity for the target. It was anticipated that these molecules would, by attaching themselves onto the relevant receptors of, say, cells, mediate (cellular) association of the liposomal moiety and its drug contents. This concept was originally tested in this laboratory [46, 47] using anti-tumour cell antibodies or desialylated fetuin which, along with other desialylated glycoproteins [48], binds specifically to the hepatic parenchymal cells. Proteins were associated with liposomes in a way that the Fab regions of antibodies responsible for the recognition of the relevant antigens and the terminal galactose molecules of desialylated fetuin responsible for the recognition of specific receptors on the hepatocytes [48] become available at the liposomal surface. We found that both types of macromolecules were capable of mediating uptake of liposomal agents by the respective receptor-carrying targets (i.e., tumour cells in vitro and hepatic parenchymal cells in vivo). Unfortunately, application of the antibody-coated liposome system in vivo in tumour-bearing mice was not as successful [16]. It appeared that antibodies raised against a variety of tumour cell-surface antigens (whole cells were used for the production of antiserum), also shared by liver and spleen cells, were targeting liposomes to these cells as well. Cell selectivity of liposomes coated with antibodies has recently found application in the specific stimulation or killing of cells [49]. It was shown that, in vitro, liposomes containing anti-line-10 hepatocarcinoma cells immune RNA and coated with antilymphocyte antibodies were able to stimulate lymphocytes which then became specifically cytotoxic to line-10 tumour cells. In addition, actinomycin-D-containing liposomes coated with anti-line-10 hepatocarcinoma cell antibodies were found highly cytotoxic to such cells. It has been recently suggested [50] that selective uptake of liposomal agents by cells may not always be followed by the interiorization of the carrier. Obviously interiorization will depend on the endocytic capacity of individual cell types.

Additional approaches for targeting include (a) coating of liposomes with isologous aggregated immunoglobulins which were found [51, 52] to mediate (through their Fc regions) association of liposome-entrapped horseradish peroxidase and hexosaminidase A with phagocytes from *Mustelus canis* and from a Tay-Sachs disease patient respectively; (b) incorporation into the liposome lipid structure of a sialoglycoprotein extracted from the membrane of erythrocytes which could, in the presence of lectins, facilitate binding of such liposomes to the cells in vitro [53]; (c) ganglioside GM_1 incorporated in liposomes which was shown to mediate selective uptake of the liposome moiety by receptors on the surface of hepatic parenchymal cells [54].

APPLICATIONS IN BIOLOGY

The use of drugs for the elucidation or the control of cell behaviour and metabolic processes is often handicapped by problems related to the inability of drugs to enter cells or reach specific intracellular organelles. The variety of ways by which liposomes associate with, or penetrate, cells offers a unique system for the transport of agents into otherwise inaccessible cellular regions both in vivo and in vitro. Some of the biological applications include studies of the role of fluid state of the cell membrane in cellular regulatory mechanisms [55], the introduction of new antigenic determinants into the surface of cells [56], investigations on the nature of restrictions imposed by the cell membrane to certain drugs [57, 58], induction of interferon in vivo [59, 60] and in vitro [61], production of rabbit globin by cells exposed to liposome-entrapped rabbit mRNA coding for the globin [62, 63] and gene transfer by using liposomes containing metaphase chromosomes [64]. For extensive discussions on the biological applications of liposomes see references 1–4, 11–14, 40, 65, and 66.

APPLICATIONS IN MEDICINE

The increasing use of liposomes in medical research is the outcome of efforts to harness drug action by means of appropriate drug carriers [1, 2]. There is now a wide range of conditions in therapeutic and preventive medicine where liposomes hold promise. These include the treatment of diseases involving the lysosomal apparatus, cancer chemotherapy, diabetes [42] and a number of bacterial and viral diseases for which liposomes could serve as immunological adjuvants to vaccines. Some of the applications in medicine investigated in this laboratory are discussed below.

Lysosomal storage diseases

The transport of active agents by liposomes into the cell's lysosomes offers the opportunity to test this carrier system in the treatment of lysosomal storage diseases [3, 4]. These are characterized by the partial or total absence of a specific lysosomal hydrolase as a result of which substances, normally serving as substrates to the enzyme, are deposited within the lysosomes of tissues [46]. It is now widely accepted that liposomes containing appropriate 'corrective' enzymes can be effective in degrading accumulated materials in the lysosomes of model lysosomal storage conditions [67]. However, extrapolation of successes obtained in model systems, mainly in vitro, to the efficacy of the liposome approach in vivo, especially in patients, could be meaningless. For example, in dealing with animals there are difficulties related to the voyage of the carrier to diseased areas. Indeed, liposomes must retain their enzyme content during the period of their circulation in the blood and should, therefore, be designed appropriately. In storage diseases in which tissues other than those of the reticuloendothelial system are involved, liposomes must be capable of crossing membranes to reach and enter target cells. This will require adjustment of the carrier's size and surface characteristics [14]. Size reduction will also ensure less interference by the liver and spleen although these two tissues are also expected to be enzyme-deficient and, therefore, likely to profit from participation in excessive enzyme uptake. Among other factors which should be considered, possible toxicity of the liposomal lipid components and increased immunogenicity of the entrapped enzyme [68] are prominent. Even so, carriage of enzymes via liposomes into target cells and degradation of the stored materials may not lead to the return of a normal function in the diseased organ [67].

Adult Gaucher's disease is one of the few lysosomal storage diseases which could serve as a test for the liposome approach. This disease is characterized by a deficiency of glucocerebroside:β-glucosidase and the tissues afflicted are predominantly those of the reticuloendothelial system. For over three years we have treated an adult Gaucher's disease splenectomized patient with numerous intravenous injections of liposome-associated glucocerebroside: β-glucosidase partially purified from human placentas [69]. Several months after treatment began there was some clinical improvement in terms of liver size and pressure symptoms in the abdomen and of the function of the reticuloendothelial system in clearing colloids from the circulation [69]. Owing to the patients's tendency to bleed, the anticipated variability in the glycolipid content of the liver [70] and the small amount of enzyme given, glucocerebroside and β-glucosidase levels of serial liver biopsies were not measured. However, a number of tests pertaining to the possible toxicity of the treatment were carried out [71]. Blood samples obtained before treatment began and after 4 (three treatments) and 30 months (twenty treatments) were analysed for antibodies against the β-glucosidase-rich preparation (using a positive control from mice immunized with the same preparation) and found negative. Furthermore, a variety of routine clinical and biochemical tests carried out during the three-year period were negative as well. The haemostatic function of the patient was also examined before and after the administration of the liposomal enzyme (about 100 mg of liposomal lipid per treatment) and all variables measured (clotting factors, fibrinolytic activity, platelet aggregability and α_2-macroglobulin) were found unchanged [71]. In spite of its modest benefits to the patient, treatment as applied in this study [71] cannot be considered successful, at least to the extent anticipated on the basis of preliminary experimentation in model systems. Assuming that liposomes were, after each injection, capable of delivering the enzyme into the patient's liver, presumably into the lysosomes of the Kupffer cells, a number of reasons could account for our failure to reduce liver size significantly: (a) enzyme was delivered into young lysosomes which, however, because of the diseased state of cells, could not fuse with the older glycolipid-loaded lysosomes; (b) the enzyme was reaching glycolipid-loaded lysosomes but its action on the substrate was insignificant either because of a short half-life and/or the need of co-factors for in situ action, or because the physical state of the substrate is such that enzyme cannot act upon it effectively; (c) the enzyme was acting on the substrate but diminution of the latter's concentration was not associated with the shrinking of the container cells and of the organ as a whole. This could be due either to an irreversible nature of the events leading to organ enlargement or to de novo storage of material in quantities enough to replace that which is hydrolysed.

Some of these possibilities could be investigated in animal models. Distribution of the liposomal enzyme and its survival in the relevant subcellular sites could, for instance, be studied by exposing Kupffer cells or liver biopsies as obtained from the diseased liver to the liposomal enzyme. Both methods would probably give useful information regarding biochemistry and morphology of the cells before and after treatment. On the other hand, the question of reversibility of liver enlargement and the extent to which de novo storage masks net glycolipid hydrolysis by the enzyme can only be answered by the use of animal models of the disease.

Antimicrobial therapy

Our early findings of the localization of liposomes in the tissues of the reticuloendothelial system prompted us to suggest [19] their use in the treatment of certain parasitic diseases in which microorganisms reside within the fixed macrophages. Thus, penicillin-containing liposomes were found to prolong the circulation of the drug in the blood and also favour its distribution in the phagocytic cells of the liver and spleen [19]. It has now been shown [12] that dehydrostreptomycin, which is unable to kill *Staphylococcus aureus* in the lysosomes of cultured macrophages, can do so if presented to the cells in its liposome form (Table 2).

The possibility of treating parasitic diseases with liposome-entrapped drugs has been recently promoted by workers [73, 74] who applied the system in the treatment of visceral leishmaniasis, a disease in which the parasites reside chronically in vacuoles within the Kupffer cells of the liver. Antimonial and arsenical drugs used in the management of leishmaniasis are limited in effectiveness because of severe systemic toxicity. Inoculation of mice with *Leishmania donovani* and subsequent administration of liposomal antimonials reduced the number of parasites in the liver to a much greater extent than the free drugs. In addition, doses of the entrapped drugs, which were ineffective when given in the free form, cleared the liver completely. Such improved action was concomitant to a more pronounced localization of the drugs in the liver [73].

Table 2. Fate of phagocytized *S. aureus* within macrophages treated with DHS, DHS liposomes and empty liposomes.

Time of incubation (h)	No. of staphylococci after treatment of macrophage cultures			
	Lysostaphin (control)	DHS liposomes	Empty liposomes	Free DHS
0	2.0×10^6	2.0×10^6	2.0×10^6	2.0×10^6
2.5			1.0×10^6	1.1×10^6
6.0		1.0×10^4		1.0×10^5
16.0		5.0×10^2	2.0×10^4	2.0×10^4

All macrophage monolayers (3×10^6 cells per dish) were treated with lysostaphin to establish intracellular viable staphylococci at the initiation of the experiments. Therefore, values at zero time are identical since they represent the base-line values for all groups. Values are the means of four separate experiments. From Bonventre and Gregoriadis [72].

Trypanosomiasis and malaria are two other possible candidates for treatment with liposomal drugs. With both diseases, mass therapy is impracticable. In addition, drugs used can be toxic and also ineffective, often because of drug-resistance development. It would be of interest to see whether liposomes given intravenously can help in speeding up therapy and in circumventing drug resistance, especially the type associated with changes in the permeability of cell membranes to drugs. In the case of trypanosomiasis, liposomes containing the appropriate drug should be capable of interacting with trypanosomes in intravascular and, to some extent, extravascular areas. It has been found [75] that the non-pathogenic insect trypanosome *Crithidia fasciculata* can take up in vitro considerable amounts of liposomes and their contents, mainly by endocytosis. With liposomes containing colchicine, such uptake was 15 times greater than when the drug was presented to the cells in its free form [75]. However, work is needed to show that pathogenic trypanosomes also interact with liposomes, especially in the presence of blood. Other bacterial, viral and fungal infections of which treatment can be improved by the use of liposomes include brucellosis, leprosy, trachoma, typhoid and psittacosis as well as some viral infections associated with the herpes species [76]. In the case of brucellosis, treatment requires daily oral administration of large doses of antibiotics over an extended period of time. Many antibiotics are not suitable for older patients with renal disease and it could be that liposomes given by the intravenous route will improve the uptake of the drug by the phagocytic cells harbouring the microbes and decrease both the amount of drug required and the period of treatment.

Cancer chemotherapy

One of the first suggestions made regarding the drug-carrier potential of liposomes in medicine was their use in cancer chemotherapy [19]. It was anticipated that transport of cytotoxic agents to tumour tissues would not only circumvent undesirable reactions due to drug action on normal tissues but also prevent drugs from being inactivated or otherwise wasted. Initially, there were indications of drug leakage from the carrier during its circulation in the blood but methods now exist by which drug retention can be improved [16, 21, 23, 29]. Liposomes capable of retaining their drug contents not only influence the rate of clearance of their cytotoxic contents from the blood and protect them from inactivation [17], but they also determine their fate in the body. Although liver and spleen take up significant portions of the injected dose (reflecting their major participation in liposome uptake), localization of the entrapped drugs in tissues such as the intestinal mucosa, skeletal and cardiac muscle, lungs and kidney, is usually less pronounced than that of the free agents [14].

As already mentioned, when small liposomes are injected in tumour-bearing rodents [16], uptake of the liposomal drug by tumours is considerably greater than that obtained with large liposomes. These results are consistent with a variety of reports pointing to the usefulness of liposomes as carriers of drugs in experimental cancer chemotherapy. In most related studies entrapped drugs have been found to prolong the mean survival time of tumour-bearing rodents more than the corresponding free drugs (for a discussion on the subject see ref. 14). However, application of the liposomal system in cancer patients is anticipated to be problematic. Among the difficulties expected are interference by the liver and spleen and poor transport of liposomal drugs through the blood capillaries. Presumably, these can be avoided to some extent by the use of liposomes of small size. Alternatively, by adjusting the permeability of liposomes to entrapped drugs [21–23], slow release of the latter in the circulation may help to improve their chemotherapeutic capacity. A successful compromise in terms of liposomal size and charge and cholesterol content may enable drugs to reach tumours more efficiently, with the reticuloendothelial system serving as a sink for the excess. It is hoped that hepatic and splenic macrophages will be less vulnerable to cytotoxic drugs than normal rapidly dividing cells which are usually exposed to such drugs in conventional chemotherapy.

Immunopotentiation

In early work on the potential of liposomes as enzyme carriers it was found that immune response to liposomal enzymes in injected animals was much higher than when enzymes were given as such [68]. It thus appeared that liposomes were acting as immunological adjuvants to entrapped antigens, a property which could be of value in human and animal immunization where there is a real need for an effective and safe adjuvant. The adjuvant property of liposomes, initially established for diphtheria toxoid [68] and influenza virus subunits [14], has now been extended to the hepatitis B surface antigen (HB_sAg). Our recent work [77] has shown that HB_sAg can be incorporated into large multilamellar liposomes with some of the entrapped antigen available on the liposomal surface for interaction with anti-HB_s antibodies. In experiments with guinea pigs, antibody titres to subcutaneously injected liposomal HB_sAg were, at the end of 50 days, about 750 times greater than those obtained with similar amounts of the free antigen (Fig. 6). Furthermore, skin tests for delayed hypersensitivity in these animals showed that immune response was also cell-mediated [77]. Elevated antibody response to HB_sAg as a result of active or passive immunization has been shown to confer immunity to natural infection with hepatitis B virus. Therefore, a vaccine against the disease will be closer to its realization when injected materials are safe and

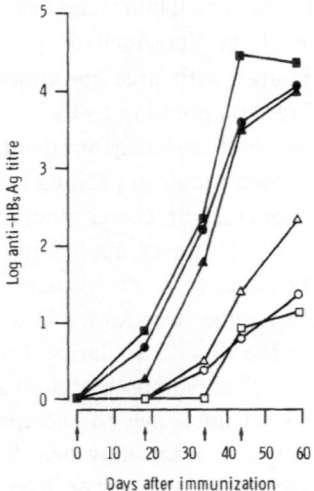

Fig. 6. Rise of anti-HB$_s$ titres in guinea pigs immunized with HB$_s$Ag. Animals were treated (arrows) with free HB$_s$Ag alone (O) or mixed with saponin (△) or *Bordetella pertussis* (□) and with liposomal HB$_s$Ag alone (●) or mixed with saponin (▲) or *B. pertussis* (■). They were bled by cardiac puncture on days 18, 34, 44 and 59. Each dose (0.6 ml) given subcutaneously in both hind limbs contained 1.4 μg free or liposomal (0.8 mg lipid) HB$_s$Ag and when appropriated, 1.2×10^{10} bacteria or 50 μg saponin. From Manesis et al. [77].

also more efficient towards the neutralization of the virus. The relatively low and aberrant immunogenicity of the HB$_s$Ag or its polypeptides will almost certainly require an adjuvant acceptable to man. The immunological adjuvant property of liposomes, together with the simplicity of their preparation, could render these suitable as components of a vaccine for mass trials.

CONCLUSIONS

The use of liposomes as membrane models has now been extended to that of a drug carrier. The popularity of liposomes in biological and medical research is based on two attractive features of the system, namely similarity to natural membranes and versatility. Because of their semi-synthetic nature, liposomes can vary widely in size, composition and surface characteristics and be made to accommodate an extraordinary range of pharmacologically active substances ranging from antitumour and antimicrobial drugs to enzymes, hormones, vaccines and informational molecules [14]. However, in spite of the multitude of potential or ongoing applications, knowledge on how liposomes interact with the biological milieu remains relatively poor. It is also not an exaggeration to say that, more often than not, the use of the liposomal carrier in terms of lipid composition, size etc. has been almost random. Indeed, it is only recently that serious attempts at rationalized approaches have been made. Undoubtedly, there are difficulties to face. Nonetheless, it should be remembered that with many diseases affecting very large numbers of individuals, drugs have not fulfilled original hopes that followed their discovery. Similarly, many problems encountered in biological research remain, for reasons discussed earlier, unsolved. It follows that, until there is considerable progress in achieving drug specificity, liposomes are likely to play important roles in optimizing drug action.

Acknowledgment. We thank Mrs Dorothy Seale for excellent secretarial work.

REFERENCES

1. Gregoriadis G: Targeting of drugs. Nature 265: 407, 1977.
2. Gregoriadis G: Liposomes. In: Gregoriadis G (ed) Drug carriers in biology and medicine. London, Academic Press, 1979, pp 287–341.
3. Gregoriadis G: The drug-carrier potential of liposomes in biology and medicine. N Engl J Med 295: 704, 1976.
4. Gregoriadis G: The drug-carrier potential of liposomes in biology and medicine. N Engl J Med 295: 765, 1976.
5. Bangham AD, Standish MM, Watkins JC: Diffusion of univalent ions across the lamellae of swollen phospholipids. J Mol Biol 13: 238, 1965.
6. Gregoriadis G, Leathwood PD, Ryman BE: Enzyme entrapment in liposomes. FEBS Lett 14: 95, 1971.
7. Gregoriadis G, Ryman BE: Fate of protein containing liposomes injected into rats. An approach to the treatment of storage diseases. Eur J Biochem 24: 485, 1972.
8. Gregoriadis G, Ryman BE: Lysosomal localization of β-fructofuranosidase-containing liposome injected into rats. Some implications in the treatment of genetic disorders. Biochem J 129: 123, 1972.
9. Black CDV, Gregoriadis G: Intracellular fate and effect of liposome-entrapped actinomycin D injected into rats. Biochem Soc Trans 2: 869, 1974.
10. Gregoriadis G, Buckland RA: Enzyme-containing liposomes alleviate a model for storage diseases. Nature 224: 170, 1973.
11. Gregoriadis G, Allison AC (eds): Liposomes in biological systems. Chichester, John Wiley and Sons, 1980.
12. Tyrrell DA, Heath TD, Colley CM, Ryman BE: New aspects of liposomes. Biochim Biophys Acta 457: 259, 1976.
13. Kimelberg HK, Mayhew E: Properties and biological effects of liposomes and their uses in pharmacology and toxicology. In: Goldberg L (ed) CRC critical reviews in toxicology. West Palm Beach FL, CRC Press, 1978, pp 25–79.
14. Gregoriadis G: The liposome drug-carrier concept: its development and future. In: Gregoriadis G, Allison AC (eds) Liposomes in biological systems. Chichester, John Wiley and Sons, 1980, pp 25–86.
15. Juliano RL, Stamp D: The effect of particle size and charge on the clearance rates of liposomes and liposome-encapsulated drugs. Biochem Biophys Res Commun 63: 651, 1975.
16. Gregoriadis G, Neerunjun ED, Hunt R: Fate of a liposome-associated agent injected into normal and tumour-bearing rodents. Attempts to improve localization in tumour tissues. Life Sci 21: 357, 1977.
17. Kimelberg HK: Differential distribution of liposome-entrapped [^{3}H]methotrexate and labelled lipids after intravenous injection in a primate. Biochim Biophys Acta 448: 531, 1976.

18. Zborowski J, Roerdink F, Scherphof G: Leakage of sucrose from phosphatidylcholine liposomes induced by interaction with serum albumin. Biochim Biophys Acta 497: 183, 1977.
19. Gregoriadis G: Drug entrapment in liposomes. FEBS Lett. 36: 292, 1973.
20. Kimelberg HK, Mayhew E, Papahadjopoulos D: Distribution of liposome-entrapped cations in tumour-bearing mice. Life Sci 17: 715, 1975.
21. Davis C, Gregoriadis G: The effect of lipid composition of liposomes on their stability in vivo. Biochem Soc Trans 7: 680, 1979.
22. Gregoriadis G, Davis C: Stability of liposomes in vivo and in vitro is promoted by their cholesterol content and the presence of blood cells. Biochem Biophys Res Commun 89: 1287, 1979.
23. Kirby C, Clarke J, Gregoriadis G: The effect of the cholesterol content of small unilamellar liposomes on their stability in vivo and in vitro. Biochem J 186: 591–598, 1980.
24. Ladbrooke BD, Williams RM, Chapman D: Studies on lecithin-cholesterol-water inter-actions by differential scanning calorimetry and X-ray diffraction. Biochim Biophys Acta 150: 333, 1968.
25. Scherphof G, Morselt H, Regts J, Wilschut JC: The involvement of the lipid phase transition in the plasma-induced dissolution of multilamellar phosphatidylcholine vesicles. Biochim Biophys Acta 556: 196, 1979.
26. Kirby C, Clarke J, Gregoriadis G: Cholesterol content of small unilamellar liposomes controls phospholipid loss to high density lipoproteins in the presence of serum. FEBS Lett 111: 324, 1980.
27. James AT, Lovelock JE, Webb PW: The lipids of whole blood. 1. Lipid biosynthesis in human blood in vitro. Biochem J 73: 106, 1959.
28. Juliano RL, Stamp D: Pharmacokinetics of liposome-encapsulated anti-tumour drugs. Biochem Pharmacol 27: 21, 1978.
29. Gregoriadis G, Davisson PJ, Scott S: Binding of drugs onto liposome-entrapped macro-molecules prevents diffusion of drugs from liposomes in vitro and in vivo. Biochem Soc Trans 5: 1323, 1977.
30. Gregoriadis G, Neerunjun ED: Control of the rate of hepatic uptake and catabolism of liposome-entrapped proteins injected into rats. Possible therapeutic applications. Eur J Biochem 47: 179, 1974.
31. Black CDV, Gregoriadis G: Interaction of liposomes with blood plasma proteins. Biochem Soc Trans 4: 256, 1976.
32. Segal AW, Wills EJ, Richmond JE, Slavin G, Black CDV, Gregoriadis G: Morphological observations on the cellular and subcellular destination of intravenously administered liposomes. Br J Exp Pathol 55: 320, 1974.
33. Wisse E, Gregoriadis G, Daems WTh: The uptake of liposomes by the rat liver. In: Reichard SM, Escobar MR, Friedman H (eds) The reticuloendothelial system in health and disease: functions and characteristics. New York, Plenum, 1976, pp 237–245.
34. Rahman Y-E, Wright BJ: Liposomes containing chelating agents. Cellular penetration and a possible mechanism of metal removal. J Cell Biol 65: 112, 1975.
35. Dapergolas G, Neerunjun ED, Gregoriadis G: Penetration of target areas in the rat by liposome-associated bleomycin, glucose oxidase and insulin. FEBS Lett 63: 235, 1976.
36. Segal AW, Gregoriadis G, Black CDV: Liposomes as vehicles for the local release of drugs. Clin Sci Mol Med 49: 99, 1975.
37. Richardson VJ, Jeyasingh K, Jewkes RF, Ryman BE, Tattersall MH: Properties of [^{99m}Tc] technetium-labelled liposomes in normal and tumour-bearing mice. Biochem Soc Trans 5: 290, 1977.
38. Gregoriadis G, Putman D, Louis L, Neerunjun ED: Comparative fate and effect of non-entrapped and liposome-entrapped neuraminidase injected into rats. Biochem J 140: 323, 1974.
39. Steger LD, Desnick RJ: Enzyme therapy. VI. Comparative in vivo fates and effects on lysosomal integrity of enzyme entrapped in negatively and positively charged liposomes. Biochim Biophys Acta 464: 530, 1977.

40. Gregoriadis G: Liposomes in therapeutic and preventive medicine. The development of the drug carrier concept. Ann NY Acad Sci 308: 343, 1978.
41. Caride VJ, Zaret BL: Liposome accumulation in regions of experimental myocardial infarction. Science 198: 735, 1977.
42. Dapergolas G, Gregoriadis G: Hypoglycaemic effect of liposome-entrapped insulin administered intragastrically into rats. Lancet 2: 824, 1976.
43. Grant CWM, McConnell HM: Fusion of phospholipid vesicles with viable Acholeplasma laidlawii. Proc Natl Acad Sci USA 70: 1238, 1973.
44. Papahadjopoulos D, Poste G, Mayhew E: Cellular uptake of cyclic AMP captured within phospholipid vesicles and effect on cell growth behaviour. Biochim Biophys Acta 363: 404, 1974.
45. Pagano RE, Huang L: Interaction of phospholipid vesicles with cultured mammalian cells. J Cell Biol 67: 49, 1975.
46. Gregoriadis G: Structural requirements for the specific uptake of macromolecules and liposomes by target tissues. In: Tager JM, Hooghwinkel GJM, Daems WTh (eds) Enzyme therapy in lysosomal storage diseases. Amsterdam, North-Holland, 1974, pp 131–148.
47. Gregoriadis G, Neerunjun ED: Homing of liposomes to target cells. Biochem Biophys Res Commun 65: 537, 1975.
48. Gregoriadis G: Catabolism of glycoproteins. In: Dingle JT, Dean RT (eds) Lysosomes in biology and pathology. Amsterdam, North-Holland, 1975, pp 265–294.
49. Magee WE, Gronenberger JH, Thor DE: Marked stimulation of lymphocyte-mediated attack on tumour cells by target-directed liposomes containing immune RNA. Cancer Res 38: 1173, 1979.
50. Weinstein JN, Blumenthal R, Sparrow SO, Henkart PA: Antibody-mediated targeting of liposomes. Binding to lymphocytes does not ensure incorporation of vesicle contents into the cells. Biochim Biophys Acta 509: 27, 1978.
51. Weismann G, Bloomgarden D, Kaplan R, Cohen C, Hoffstein S, Collins T, Gottlieb A, Nagle D: A general method for the introduction of enzymes, by means of immunoglobulin-coated liposomes, into lysosomes of deficient cells in vitro. Proc Natl Acad Sci USA 72: 88, 1975.
52. Cohen CM, Weismann G, Hoffstein S, Awasthi YC, Srivastava SK: Introduction of purified hexosaminidase A into Tay-Sachs leucocytes by means of immunoglobulin-coated liposomes. Biochemistry 15: 452, 1976.
53. Juliano RL, Stamp D: Lectin-mediated attachment of glycoprotein bearing liposomes to cells. Nature 261: 235, 1976.
54. Surolia A, Bachhawat BK: Monosialoganglioside liposome-entrapped enzyme uptake by hepatic cells. Biochim Biophys Acta 497: 760, 1977.
55. Inbar M, Shinitzky M: Increase of cholesterol level in the surface membrane of lymphoma cells and its inhibitory effect on ascites tumour development. Proc Natl Acad Sci USA 71: 2128, 1974.
56. Martin FJ, McDonald RC: Lipid vesicle-cell interaction. III. Introduction of a new antigenic determinant into erythrocyte membranes. J Cell Biol 70: 515, 1976.
57. Papahadjopoulos D, Poste G, Wail WJ, Biedler JL: Use of lipid vesicles as carriers to introduce actinomycin D into resistant tumour cells. Cancer Res 36: 2988, 1976.
58. Schiffman Fl, Klein I: Rapid induction of amphotericin B sensitivity in L1210 leukemia cells by liposomes containing ergosterol. Nature 269: 65, 1977.
59. Straub SX, Garry RF, Magee WE: Interferon induction by poly (I):poly(C) enclosed in phospholipid particles. Infect Immun 10: 783, 1974.
60. Magee WE, Talcott ML, Straub SX, Vriend CY: A comparison of negatively and positively charged liposomes containing entrapped polyinosinic polycytidylic acid for interferon induction in mice. Biochim Biophys Acta 451: 610, 1976.
61. Mayhew E, Papahadjopoulos D, O'Malley J, Carter WA, Vail WJ: Cellular uptake and protection against virus infection by polyinosinic-polycytidylic acid entrapped within phospholipid vesicles. Mol Pharmacol 13: 488, 1977.

62. Dimitriadis GJ: Translation of rabbit globin mRNA introduced by liposomes into mouse lymphocytes. Nature 274: 423, 1978.
63. Ostro MJ, Giacomoni D, Laveble D, Paxton W, Dray S: Evidence for translation of rabbit globin mRNA after liposome-mediated insertion into a human cell line. Nature 274: 921, 1978.
64. Mukherjee AB, Orloff S, Butler JD, Triche T, Lalley P, Schulman JD: Entrapment of metaphase chromosomes into phospholipid vesicles (lipochromosomes): carrier potential in gene transfer. Proc Natl Acad Sci USA 75: 1361, 1978.
65. Poste G, Papahadjopoulos D, Vail WJ: Lipid vesicles as carriers for introducing materials into cultured cells: influence of vesicle lipid composition on mechanism(s) of vesicle incorporation into cells. In: Prescott DM (ed) Methods of cell biology, vol 14. New York, Academic Press, 1976, pp 33–71.
66. Pagano RE, Weinstein JN: Interactions of liposomes with mammalian cells. Annu Rev Biophys Bioeng 7: 435, 1978.
67. Gregoriadis G: Liposomes in the treatment of lysosomal storage diseases. Nature (London) 275: 695, 1978.
68. Allison AC, Gregoriadis G: Liposomes as immunological adjuvants. Nature 252: 252, 1974.
69. Belchetz PE, Braidman IP, Crawley JCW, Gregoriadis G: Treatment of Gaucher's disease with liposome-entrapped glucocerebroside:β-glucosidase. Lancet 2: 116, 1977.
70. Beutler E, Dale GL, Kuhl W: Enzyme replacement with red cells. N Engl J Med 296: 942, 1977.
71. Gregoriadis G, Neerunjun ED, Meade TW, Goolamali SK, Weereratne H, Bull GM: Experiences after long-term treatment of a type I Gaucher's disease patient with liposome-entrapped glucocerbroside: β-glucosidase. In: Enzyme therapy in genetic diseases. Birth Defects Orig Artic Ser 1980, pp 383–392.
72. Bonventre P, Gregoriadis G: Killing of intraphagocytic Staph. aureus by dehydrostreptomycin entrapped in liposomes. Antimicrob Agents Chemother 13: 1049, 1978.
73. Black CDV, Watson GJ, Ward RJ: The use of Pentostam liposomes in the chemotherapy of experimental leishmaniasis. Trans Roy Soc Trop Med Hyg 71: 550, 1977.
74. New RRC, Chance ML, Thomas SC, Peters W: Antileishmanial activity of antimonials entrapped in liposomes. Nature 274: 55, 1978.
75. Vakirtzi-Lemonias C, Gregoriadis G: Uptake of liposome-entrapped agents by the trypanosome Crithidia fasciculata. Biochem Soc Trans 6: 1241, 1978.
76. Gregoriadis G: Targeting of drugs: possibilities in viral chemotherapy and prophylaxis. Pharmacol Ther 10: 103–118.
77. Manesis EK, Cameron C, Gregoriadis G: Hepatitis B surface antigen-containing liposomes enhance humoral and cell-mediated immunity to the antigen. FEBS Lett 102: 107, 1979.

22. FUNDAMENTAL STUDIES ON THE CELLULAR UPTAKE OF LIPOSOMES

G.L. SCHERPHOF, J. DAMEN, D. HOEKSTRA,
A.J.B.M. VAN RENSWOUDE, AND F.H. ROERDINK

STABILITY OF LIPOSOMES

When we first became involved in the field of biological applications of phospholipid vesicles (1972) we soon noticed that such vesicles, when prepared from the most commonly used lipid mixture in those days, i.e., lecithin, cholesterol, and phosphatidic acid or dicetylphosphate in a molar ratio of approximately 7:2:1, rapidly lost most of their contents when injected intravenously into rats or when incubated in vitro with (diluted) plasma. Under the same conditions, multilamellar vesicles containing sucrose, inulin, or albumin were shown to release a high proportion of the entrapped solutes [1, 2] (Fig. 1). We were able to mimic this effect of plasma by replacing it by albumin, and at the same time we found that, instead of albumin becoming bound to the liposomes as we had expected, some liposomal phospholipid became associated with the albumin [1].

In a later study, however, we found that when liposomes were incubated in whole plasma rather than in an albumin solution, almost no liposomal lipid

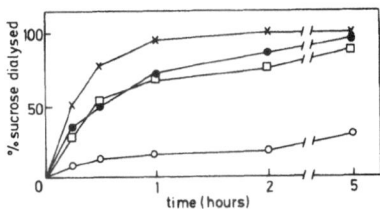

Fig. 1. Release of entrapped sucrose from liposomes during exposure to blood. Multilamellar liposomes (0.5 μmol lipid in 0.033 ml buffer) composed of rat-liver lecithin and phosphatidic acid (molar ratio 96:4) and containing [^{14}C]-sucrose were diluted to 1 ml with buffer or rat blood and dialyzed in a disk-shaped cell with a total volume of 2 ml against 1 ml buffer. Appearance of label in the buffer compartment was monitored over a 5-h period. X-X, free, nonentrapped sucrose; O——O, dilution with buffer; ●——●, dilution with blood + EDTA; □——□, dilution with heparinized blood. By permission *Biochim Biophys Acta* 497: 183–191, 1977.

Abbrevations: CF, carboxyfluorescein; chol, cholesterol; DML, dimyristoyl lecithin; FITC, fluorescein isothiocyanate; PC, phosphatidylcholine (= lecithin); PL, phospholipid; PVP, polyvinylpyrollidone; RNase, ribonuclease; sphingo, sphingomyelin; SUV, small (sonicated) unilamellar vesicle.

W.Th. Daems et al. (eds.), Cell Biological Aspects of Disease, 281–297. All rights reserved.
Copyright © 1981 by Martinus Nijhoff Publishers bv, The Hague/Boston/London.

282

became albumin-associated. Under these conditions we observed that sonicated multi- as well as unilamellar vesicles can release considerable quantities
of phospholipid, almost all of which was recovered in a lipoprotein fraction
which closely resembled the high-density lipoprotein fraction of plasma with
respect to both size and immunoelectrophoretic properties (Fig. 2). The small
fraction of albumin-associated phospholipid turned out to be mainly lysolecithin, whereas the lipoprotein-associated phospholipid was still intact lecithin [2].

After the discovery of the involvement of high-density lipoproteins in the
apparent disintegration of liposomes by plasma, we lost interest in the albumin phenomenon. In retrospect, we must admit that at that time we had not
taken any precautions to purify the commercial albumin preparations we
used and we therefore cannot exclude the possibility that our findings with
albumin were influenced by contamination with high-density lipoproteins.
Others have repeated our experiments or have done similar work with very
pure albumin preparations and found very little or no effect on liposomal
integrity (J.N. Weinstein and J. Goerke, personal communication) [3].

Initially, our feeling was that the observed release of entrapped solutes
from liposomes and the transfer of liposomal phospholipid to a lipoprotein
particle were so closely related that the former was supposed to be caused by
the latter. The phospholipid transfer we found was shown to represent net
release from the vesicles which, by necessity, must involve disintegration of

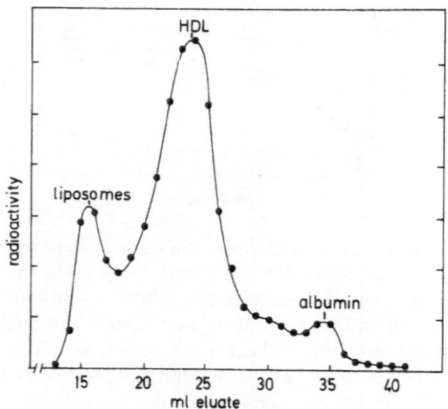

Fig. 2. Transfer in plasma of liposomal lecithin from vesicles to (high-density) lipoprotein after
intravenous injection of liposomes into rats. Small unilamellar vesicles consisting of 1 μmol [14]C-
labeled egg lecithin were injected intravenously into a rat. After 5 min the rat was anesthesized
and 5 ml blood was withdrawn from the caval vein. Cells were spun down and 2 ml plasma was
chromatographed on an Ultrogel AcA34 column. Remaining liposomes elute in the void volume.
The bulk of the radioactivity is associated with a fraction which was identified as high-density
lipoprotein or a very similar particle. By permission *Biochim Biophys Acta* 556: 196–207, 1979.

vesicles. Yet, we later found that the extent of phospholipid release from multilamellar vesicles was limited compared with that from unilamellar vesicles, whereas release of contents from such multilamellar vesicles as a result of plasma interaction was still considerable. We now believe that release of contents and release of phospholipid are not necessarily linked.

It is conceivable that plasma constituents other than high-density lipoproteins interact with the liposomes such that their permeability for entrapped solutes is increased but without disrupting the vesicles, i.e., by transforming them into newly formed lipoprotein particles. We have shown that numerous plasma proteins become liposome-associated during incubation of liposomes in plasma [4]. Conversely, we demonstrated that under conditions that strongly limit solute release from plasma-incubated liposomes (see below), significant phospholipid transfer can still take place. Presumably, transfer in this case represents exchange of phospholipid molecules between liposome and lipoprotein rather than net release. Although it does not lead to liposomal disintegration, such phospholipid exchange may nevertheless have an undesired effect in studies on the fate of intravenously injected liposomes. Radioactive phospholipid used as a liposomal marker will thus circulate as part of a lipoprotein particle rather than of a liposome. This problem can be largely overcome by the use of sphingomyelin rather than lecithin as the phospholipid backbone of the liposome (Table 1).

Table 1 also shows the conditions which lead to greatly enhanced stability of liposomes in plasma, both in terms of solute release and of phospholipid

Table 1. Effect of cholesterol on liposomal stability in plasma.

Lipid composition	% PL transfer in 30 min	% Inulin release in 30 min
Egg PC	61	29
Egg PC:chol (2:1)	42	—
Egg PC:chol (3:2)	—	9
Egg PC:chol (1:1)	24	6
sphingo	29	87
sphingo:chol (3:2)	19	4
sphingo:chol (1:1)	6	—

PL, phospholipid; PC, phosphatidylcholine (lecithin); chol, cholesterol; sphingo, sphingomyelin.

Aliquots of 0.5 μmol [^{14}C]-egg lecithin or sphingomyelin with or without cholesterol, in the indicated molar ratios, were sonicated into small unilamellar vesicles. The vesicles were incubated for 30 min at 37° C in 2 ml 50% rat plasma and the mixtures were then chromatographed on Sepharose 6B columns to separate the radioactive lipoprotein formed from the remaining vesicles. Phospholipid transfer was calculated as the proportion of total radioactivity associated with the lipoprotein fractions. For inulin release, [^{3}H]-inulin was entrapped in (sonicated) multilamellar vesicles of the same composition. After 30 min of incubation at 37°C in 50% plasma, samples were passed through Sephadex G-50 columns to separate released inulin from that which was still entrapped. The percent release was then calculated.

transfer. Incorporation of sizable quantities of cholesterol into the liposomal membrane greatly reduces plasma-induced release of inulin. However, when inulin release is down to very low levels, lecithin transfer (presumably exchange) is still considerable. When sphingomyelin is substituted for lecithin, also phospholipid transfer is reduced to minimal values. It should be kept in mind that the percent transfer is a maximal value because the method used to determine the lipid transfer involves gelfiltration on Sepharose. This means that, because of imperfect separation of liposomes and lipoprotein, some radioactivity will always be found at the position where the lipoprotein elutes, even in the absence of transfer.

The beneficial effect of cholesterol was also found when the solubilization of large, nonsonicated multilamellar vesicles consisting of dimyristoyl lecithin was studied. This synthetic lecithin contains two identical saturated fatty acyl residues with a chain length of 14 carbon atoms and, like other pure phospholipids, undergoes a transition from gel to liquid-crystalline phase in aqueous dispersions at a well-defined temperature characteristic of the particular phospholipid (see ref. 5 for a review). For dimyristoyl lecithin (DML) this temperature is close to 24° C. Below this temperature the fatty acyl chains of DML are in a strongly ordered gel-like state. At 24° C there is a highly cooperative transition to a state in which the hydrocarbon chains are much less ordered and which is called the liquid-crystalline state. Precisely at the temperature of transition the two phases coexist, and it has been shown that solutes then very rapidly penetrate the phospholipid bilayer [6–8]. Also, it has been demonstrated that phospholipids at the transition temperature are extremely susceptible to hydrolysis by phospholipases [9, 10]. It is believed that when patches of gel- and liquid-crystalline phases coexist, there are structural irregularities at the boundaries of such lipid domains. Solutes as well as protein would have relatively easy access through or to the lipid bilayer at such phase boundaries. Accordingly, we found that at, and not below or bove, the phase transition temperature such liposomes are readily solubilized in plasma, even when they are present as very large unsonicated aggregates (Fig. 3). When present as nonsonicated liposomes, egg lecithin — which because of its heterogeneous fatty acid composition, including unsaturated fatty acids has a broad transition range below 0° C — is not susceptible at all to solubilization at 37° C, at which temperature all of the lipid is in the liquid-crystalline state. Only when the radius of curvature of such liposomes is reduced by using sonication to break the liposomes into smaller vesicles, will the strain thus introduced into the lipid bilayers allow significant lipoprotein attack and subsequent solubilization [11].

Incorporation of increasing amounts of cholesterol into the phospholipid bilayers gradually abolishes the phase transition as a result of complex formation between lecithin and cholesterol, until at a molar ratio of one choles-

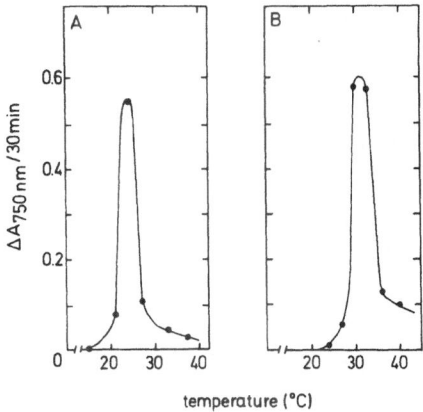

Fig. 3. Solubilization of nonsonicated liposomes in plasma at the phase-transition temperature. 2.2 μmol dimyristoyl lecithin (A) or of an equimolar mixture of dimyristoyl and dipalmitoyl lecithin (B) was dispersed without sonication in NaCl/Tris buffer and incubated at various temperatures in a total volume of 3 ml 50% rat plasma. The turbidity, measured as absorbance at 750 nm, was monitored for several hours and taken as a measure of solubilization. Absorbance decrease during the first 30 min of incubation served as a parameter of the initial rate of solubilization. Pure dimyristoyl lecithin has a gel to liquid-crystalline phase-transition temperature of 24°C, whereas the transition takes place at about 33°C in an equimolar mixture of dimyristoyl and dipalmitoyl lecithin. By permission *Biochim Biophys Acta* 556: 196–207, 1979.

terol to two lecithins the phase transition has completely vanished [12]. At that ratio, DML/cholesterol liposomes proved to be completely resistant to lipoprotein attack (Fig. 4).

Recently, a very elegant application of the preferential attack by lipoproteins on liposomes at the phase-transition temperature was reported. Complete release of a liposome-entrapped cytostatic drug in a tumor heated to that temperature by short-wave irradiation led to preferential uptake of the drug by the tumor [13, 14].

IN VIVO FATE OF LIPOSOMAL CONSTITUENTS

It has been known for several years now that the liver and spleen play a major role in the clearance of liposome-associated material from the blood after intravenous injection [15–18], but the participation of the hepatocytes in the clearing process has been controversial for some time [19–21]. Depending on the type of liposomal marker used, different results were obtained. In a study using radiolabeled lecithin as a marker of the liposomal envelope and either horseradish peroxidase as a cytochemically detectable marker or ^{125}I-albumin as a radioactive marker of the aqueous contents, we found a clear discrepancy between the markers of the liposomal envelope and

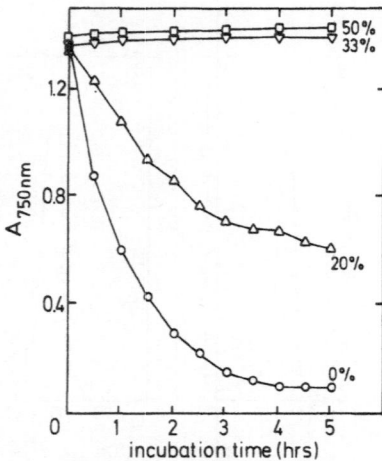

Fig. 4. Cholesterol effect on solubilization of dimyristoyl lecithin liposomes by plasma. Nonsonicated liposomes were prepared from pure dimyristoyl lecithin (○) or from mixtures of this lecithin with cholesterol in molar ratios of lecithin to cholesterol of 4:1 (△), 2:1 (▽), or 1:1 (□); 1.9 μmol of total lipid was incubated at 24°C in 2.6 ml 50% rat plasma. Solubilization was monitored as absorbance change at 750 nm. By permission *Biochim Biophys Acta* 556: 196–207, 1979.

aqueous space with respect to both the plasma clearance and the intrahepatic localization [22]. The radioactive phospholipid was mainly recovered in the hepatocytes, whereas little or none of the entrapped proteins was found in those cells. As to the labeled albumin, we were unable to establish in which of the nonparenchymal cells it was located, because at that time we had no means to separate endothelial cells from Kupffer cells. Electron microscopy revealed that the peroxidase, after intravenous administration in liposomes, was situated in endocytic vacuoles of both Kupffer and endothelial cells [22]. Since free peroxidase showed a distribution pattern similar to that of the entrapped enzyme, we could not exclude the possibility that any peroxidase that had entered the endothelial cells had first been released from the liposomes and subsequently been taken up in free form. As outlined in the preceding section, liposomes without high proportions of cholesterol are subject to attack by lipoproteins and possibly by other plasma proteins, which causes rapid release of entrapped solutes. (Depending on the cholesterol content and on the size of the liposomes, the lipoprotein attack may lead to total disintegration of the vesicles, but apparently this is not a prerequisite for the occurrence of considerable leakage.) Preliminary experiments with stabilized liposomes (33 mol% cholesterol) containing ^{125}I-labeled polyvinyl pyrrolidone (PVP) showed that the contribution of the endothelial cells to the total hepatic uptake of radioactivity was indeed negligible (J. Dijkstra, G. Hartman, F.H. Roerdink, and G.L. Scherphof, unpublished results). Recently developed methods to separate Kupffer cells and endothelial cells by elutriation centrifugation [23, 24] enabled us to perform this kind of experiment. These results confirm our view that our earlier results were influenced by a partial release of entrapped solutes. Depending on the nature of the solute, it may enter various types of cell and the result may be mistaken for uptake of liposomes.

Similar erroneous conclusions may be drawn from experiments in which the phospholipid label of the liposomes is monitored. As described in the first section of this chapter, liposomal lecithin can become part of a lipoprotein particle which shares several properties with high-density lipoprotein. We have isolated this particle containing radioactive lecithin derived from liposomes and injected it intravenously into rats. It was cleared from the circulation with a half-life of slightly over 1 h, i.e., similar to that of unilamellar vesicles made up of radioactive lecithin, and almost all of the radioactivity was recovered as lecithin from the parenchymal cells of the liver (Table 2). In our opinion, this explains how lecithin injected as unilamellar vesicles ends up in the hepatocytes: the vesicles are very rapidly solubilized to form the lipoprotein particle which donates its phospholipid to the liver parenchymal cells in an as yet unknown way.

For the larger, briefly sonicated, multilamellar vesicles, this cannot be the whole story; they are not solubilized rapidly enough to explain the rapid appearance of phospholipid label in the hepatocytes via the lipoprotein-mediated mechanism. Most of the multilamellar liposomes used in our studies are larger than the $0.1\text{-}\mu$ fenestrations [25] in the liver endothelial cells lining the sinusoids. This would preclude a major contribution by the underlying hepatocytes to the process of direct vesicle uptake. In addition, in vitro experiments with isolated hepatocytes (the third section) give the impression that these cells are not very active at all in liposome uptake. Possibly, phos-

Table 2. Fate of [^{14}C]-lecithin injected intravenously either as unilamellar vesicles or as lipoprotein particles.

^{14}C-lecithin injected as:	SUV	Lipoprotein
Half-life in blood (min)	73	65
^{14}C in liver after 1 h (% of injected dose)	26.5	24.5
^{14}C in parenchymal cells after 1 h (% of injected dose)	24.4	21.6
^{14}C recovered as lecithin (% of total amount in homogenate)	96	94

Small unilamellar vesicles (SUV) composed of [^{14}C]-egg lecithin were either directly injected i.v. (1 μmol) into rats or incubated for 1 h at 37° C in 50% rat plasma. The incubation mixture was chromatographed on Ultrogel AcA34, and the ^{14}C-containing lipoprotein fractions were pooled and concentrated. The equivalent of 1 μmol ^{14}C-lecithin was then injected i.v. into rats. Blood radioactivity levels were monitored for 1 h. After that, the animals were killed, the livers were perfused with collagenase, and parenchymal and nonparenchymal cells were isolated. Homogenates of whole liver pieces and of cell fractions were extracted with chloroform/methanol. The lipid extract containing virtually all of the radioactivity in the homogenates was chromatographed on thin-layer silica plates to separate the phospholipids.

pholipid which initially is endocytosed by Kupffer cells in the form of liposomes is transferred to the hepatocytes after being processed inside the lysosomal system of the Kupffer cells to an unknown extent. Experiments in our
laboratory with doubly labeled lecithin showed that the lecithin recovered
from the hepatocytes after injection of liposomes does not have the same
isotopic ratio as the starting material (Table 3), which indicates at least partial
metabolization of the phospholipid.

To summarize our points of view we would say that intravenously injected
liposomes that are not stabilized by incorporation of high cholesterol concentrations are subject to attack by plasma (lipo) proteins. Small unilamellar
vesicles are almost instantaneously solubilized, their lipid becomes part of a
lipoprotein particle and their contents are set free in the circulation. The
lipoprotein-bound lipid is mainly donated to the parenchymal cells of the
liver. The plasma clearance and tissue distribution of the contents will be
virtually identical to what is found for the substance when injected non-
entrapped. Multilamellar vesicles and their contents will partly share this fate.
However, lipoprotein formation will be limited and release of entrapped
solute will be mainly caused by other plasma components, e.g., complement
[3]. The released solute will of course be cleared from the circulation in the
same way as the nonentrapped compound. Nondegraded liposomes, plus any
remaining entrapped solute, are endocytosed by tissue macrophages such as
the Kupffer cells. In the liver, phospholipid is then somehow transferred to
the hepatocytes. It is obvious that some of these postulations need further
substantiation by additional experiments.

The apparent avidity with which macrophages in the body take up injected
liposomes presents a problem to those who wish to direct drug-loaded lipo-

Table 3. Hepatic uptake and metabolism of $[^3H/^{14}C]$-labeled lecithin after intravenous injection
as unilamellar vesicles.

Exp.	Time after injection	$^3H/^{14}C$ ratio in		
		Vesicles (before injection)	Whole liver	Hepatocytes
1	1 h	12.6	7.5	9.2
2	1 h	12.3	7.7	8.2
3	2 h	12.3	6.6.	7.6
4	3 h	12.6	6.3	7.1

Rat-liver lecithin labeled at the 1-position with $[^3H]$-oleate was mixed with egg lecithin labeled in
the polar head group with $[^{14}C]$-choline so as to give a lecithin preparation with an isotopic ratio
of ca. 12.5. This doubly labeled lecithin was transformed into sonicated unilamellar vesicles and 3
μmol was injected intravenously into rats. After 1, 2, or 3 h, the animals were killed and
hepatocytes were isolated. Homogenates from whole liver pieces as well as hepatocytes were
extracted with chloroform/methanol and lecithin was isolated from the lipid extract by thin-layer
chromatography. The $^3H/^{14}C$ ratio in the isolated lecithin was estimated.

somes to other cell types such as those in tumor tissues. To circumvent this problem one might try to temporarily block the macrophage activity, thus allowing more time for other tissues to interact with the vesicles. We are currently investigating the possibility of blocking Kupffer cell activity reversibly by injection of lanthanium or gadolinium salts [26]. Clearance of liposomes can be considerably delayed and liver uptake suppressed by giving the animals a few μmol of these salts 24 h before the injection of liposomes. A week after lanthanium administration, clearance and liver uptake are back to normal. Another possibility might be to coat the liposomes with substances that would prevent opsonization and thus phagocytosis.

If attempts to suppress macrophage activity succeed, it will remain to be seen whether prolonged survival time in the circulation will lead to increased uptake by the tissue or cell type of interest. As will be shown in the following section, the potential of cells other than macrophages to take up liposomes and their contents appears to be limited. Furthermore, morphological barriers such as basement membranes or nonfenestrated endothelium may prevent massive access of liposomes to the target cells. Even so, however, liposomes could still be put into use as drug carriers, since they might provide a suitable depot from which a drug could be released at optimal rates, regulated by the lipid composition, e.g., the cholesterol content. If such release could be caused to take place in selected areas of the body, toxic side effects of the drug could thus be minimized. Specific targetting by means of antibody-antigen interaction between cells and antibody-coated liposomes could fulfill this requirement [27, 28]. Alternatively, liposomes of a composition making them susceptible to phase-transition-induced release of contents at a temperature slightly above that of the body could be used to release a drug in an area treated by hyperthermia [14]. As pointed out above, the feasibility of such an approach was recently demonstrated for methotrexate-containing vesicles injected in tumor-bearing mice [15].

INTERACTIONS WITH CELLS IN VITRO

Suppose we succeed in creating conditions allowing injected liposomes to remain in circulation for prolonged periods without being phagocytosed by macrophages, and to aim more or less specifically at a certain target tissue. The question then to be answered is, do the target cells take up the liposomes which gain access to them and, if so, by what mechanism? Obviously, the latter question is important with respect to the intracellular site(s) to be reached by the entrapped drug.

Endocytosis would bring the liposomes into the lysosomal system, where they would have to be degraded or at least labilized to release the entrapped drug. Fusion of unilamellar vesicles with the plasma membrane would release vesicle contents directly into the cytoplasm. Fusion of the outer lamella of a multilamellar vesicle with the plasma membrane would release the contents of the outermost compartment as well as the remainder of the liposome with its contents directly into the cytoplasm. Formation of an autophagocytic vacuole could render the liposomal 'remnant' lysosome-bound once again. Alternatively, contents could slowly leak out of this remnant. The properties and mechanism of action of the drug to be delivered would determine which of the uptake mechanisms, if any, would be preferred.

To investigate the capacity of individual cell types to internalize phospholipid vesicles, we followed a number of different approaches with various types of cells. With cultured skin fibroblasts from a patient with Pompe's disease (glycogenosis type II), we established that the decrease in glycogen content, which is measured after incubating such cells with glucosidase-containing liposomes, is due to depletion of the cytoplasmic glycogen stores and not of those present in the lysosomes [29]. This would favor an uptake mechanism in which the outer bilayer of the multilamellar vesicles fuses with the plasma membrane.

Rat hepatocytes were found to degrade radiolabeled albumin entrapped in multilamellar vesicles (Fig. 5). In the same study, however, we obtained

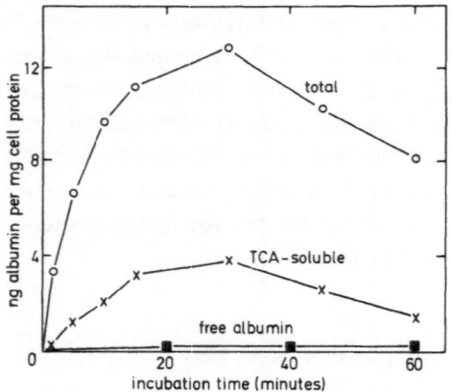

Fig. 5. Uptake and intracellular degradation of [125I]-labeled albumin entrapped in multilamellar vesicles by hepatocytes in monolayer culture. 3 μmol multilamellar vesicles consisting of lecithin, cholesterol, and dicetylphosphate (molar ratio 7:2:1) and containing ca. 20 μg [125I]-albumin per μmol lipid were added to 6.10^6 hepatocytes in primary monolayer culture. At various intervals, medium containing the vesicles was removed and the cells were thoroughly washed. Total cell-associated as well as TCA-soluble radioactivity were measured in cell homogenates. For each time point the average results from two separate culture dishes were used. In control experiments cells were incubated with the same amount of nonentrapped albumin. Results were calculated as ng albumin per mg total cell protein. (O), total cell-associated radioactivity; (×), TCA-soluble radioactivity; (■), total cell-associated radioactivity following incubation with nonentrapped albumin.

evidence that a nondegrading mechanism also plays a role in the uptake of liposome-entrapped albumin by hepatocytes [30].

The use of fluorescent dyes as markers of the entrapped volume of phospholipid vesicles has recently begun to contribute substantially to an understanding of the mechanisms of vesicle-cell interaction [31]. In high concentrations, fluorescence of these dyes is almost completely quenched. When such high concentrations of dye are entrapped in lysosomes, the introduction of the dye into the cytoplasm of the cells after liposome-cell interaction will show up as a fluorescent signal due to intracellular dilution of the dye. Liposomes which merely adhere to the cell surface without being internalized will not give rise to a fluorescent signal unless a detergent is added, as a result of which the dye is diluted, self-quenching is relieved, and a fluorescent signal is developed. Thus, uptake and adsorption of vesicles can, in principle, be readily discriminated.

With Zajdela ascites hepatoma cells we found that carboxyfluorescein or fluorescein isothiocyanate-labeled dextran (FITC-dextran, average molecular weight ca. 3000), when offered to the cells entrapped in unilamellar phospholipid vesicles, is internalized by the cells by a mechanism not involving endocytosis [32]. Similar observations were made with lymphosarcoma cells, which, however, were more active in total vesicle uptake. This quantitative difference between these two tumor cell lines was also expressed in the sensitivity to liposome-entrapped RNase of their protein-synthesizing capacity. The dramatic inhibition of leucine incorporation by the cells of both types as a result of incubation with RNase-containing unilamellar phosphatidylserine vesicles is shown in Fig. 6. These results also suggest that the RNase enters the cell by a mechanism which does not involve endocytosis or only endocytosis. Uptake via the lysosomal pathway would almost certainly destroy RNase activity by acid proteases, so the protein-synthesizing machinery of the cell would go unharmed.

The approach with self-quenched fluorescent dyes was also applied to hepatocytes, and showed that these cells internalize 2–3 times more liposome-entrapped carboxyfluorescein per cell than do the Zajdela hepatoma cells [33]. Another difference between these two related cell types (the tumor cell line is a chemically induced rat hepatoma) is the fraction of vesicles found sticking to the cell surface without being internalized. In the absence of fetal calf serum, the hepatocytes adsorb a much larger proportion of vesicles to their cell surface than do the hepatoma cells. This adsorption phenomenon is greatly reduced when cells and vesicles are incubated in the presence of 15% fetal calf serum. However, the actual internalization of carboxyfluorescein does not appear to be influenced by the calf serum. Experiments with liposomes labeled with radioactive lecithin or cholesteryl oleate essentially confirmed these observations. In addition, we found that there is a specific

292

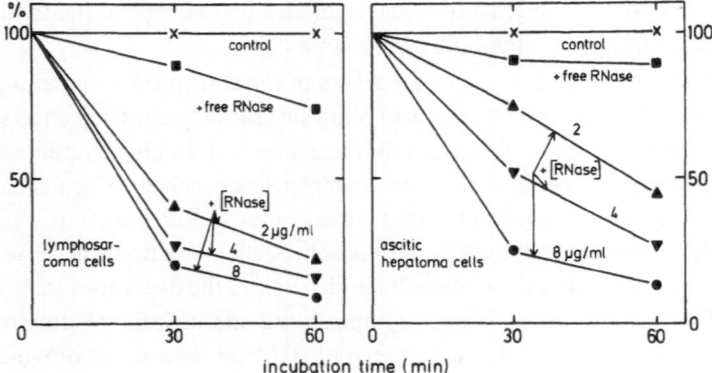

incubation time (min)

Fig. 6. Inhibition of [^{14}C]-leucine incorporation by lymphosarcoma cells and Zajdela ascites hepatoma cells as a result of incubation with RNase-containing phospholipid vesicles. Variable amounts of RNase A were entrapped in small unilamellar vesicles made from phosphatidyl-serine. 5.10^6 cells per ml were incubated with 0.4 mM vesicle lipid containing the indicated amounts of RNase, in the presence of [1-^{14}C]leucine. Ca^{2+} was added (4.3 mM) to promote fusion. Trichloroacetic acid-precipitable material was assayed for radioactivity after 30 and 60 min of incubation. Values were corrected for anisomycin/puromycin backgrounds, and therefore represent de novo protein synthesis. Control incubations were done with empty vesicles ($\times$), which did not at all inhibit leucine incorporation, and with empty vesicles plus 16 μg free RNase (■); ▲, vesicles containing 2 μg RNase; ▼, vesicles containing 4 μg RNase; ●, vesicles containing 8 μg RNase. Incorporation is plotted as % of control values: ca. 3 nmol/h per 10^6 cells for lymphosarcoma cells (A) and ca. 0.8 nmol/h per 10^6 cells for Zajdela cells (B).

molecular exchange of lecithin between vesicles and cells, which is also dras-tically diminished in presence of serum (Fig. 7). This shows that the inter-action between cells and vesicles not only can lead to internalization of vesicle contents but may result in transfer of specific lipid components to the cell as well. This confirms recent work by Pagano and co-workers, and adds an important element to the biological use of liposomes as potential modifiers of cell membranes [34].

Our experiments with isolated hepatocytes were based on considerations of the in vivo situation outlined in the preceding section: if injected liposomes are able to come close to the parenchymal cells of the liver, will they be taken up and, if so, by what mechanism? Continuing along this line, we tried to design liposomes with increased affinity for hepatocytes. To that end we incorpo-rated glycolipids with a terminal galactoside in the liposomal bilayers. The presence of a specific galactose receptor on the hepatocyte surface, reported some years ago [35], was expected to bind relatively large quantities of these vesicles, possibly leading to enhanced uptake of entrapped material. We found that the presence of GM$_1$ ganglioside or lactosylceramide in the lipo-somal bilayer indeed increased the association of labeled liposomal lecithin several-fold. However, with entrapped carboxyfluorescein the transfer of lipo-

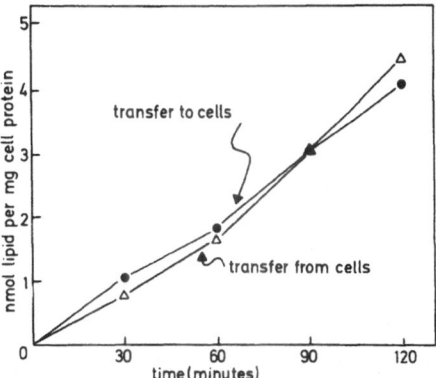

Fig. 7. Phosphatidylcholine exchange between phospholipid vesicles and isolated hepatocytes. Hepatocytes were incubated with [^{14}C-Me]choline to label cellular lecithin. The labeled cells were incubated with unlabeled small unilamellar vesicles consisting of lecithin, cholesterol, and dicetylphosphate in a molar ratio of 4:3:0.45. Alternatively, unlabeled cells were incubated with similar liposomes which contained a trace of [^{14}C]cholesteryl oleate and whose lecithin was also radiolabeled. At various times of incubation (1 μmol vesicles, 3.10^6 cells), cells and vesicles were separated by centrifugation and washing. The amount of lecithin transfer was calculated on the basis of ^{14}C-lecithin transfer (from cells to vesicles or vice versa) or of ^{14}C-cholesteryl oleate transfer (from vesicles to cells). Plotted against time are the amount of lecithin transferred from cells to vesicles (triangles) and the *difference* between ^{14}C-lecithin and ^{14}C-cholesteryl oleate transfer from vesicles to cells (circles). The latter values are taken to represent that amount of lecithin transfer which is not representative of whole vesicles but rather of molecular exchange of lecithin between cells and vesicles.

somal contents was barely above the control level, and the fraction of liposomes adsorbed to the cell surface was also only marginally increased (Table 4). This was confirmed by experiments in which radiolabeled cholesteryl oleate was used as a liposomal marker, and our conclusion was that the incorporation of galactose residues into the liposomal surface served mainly to stimulate the phospholipid exchange between cells and vesicles.

CONCLUDING REMARKS

When liposomes are thought of as in vivo carriers of entrapped drugs it should be kept in mind that such particles have only limited stability in the blood circulation. As described in the foregoing, this is due to interactions with plasma (lipo)proteins, but we recently found that the very contact of liposomes with cell surfaces may also have a labilizing effect on the vesicles with respect to solute retention [36]. For the purpose of drug delivery via cellular uptake of liposomes, this may be unfortunate; but from the point of view of depot action, limited instability may be even advantageous for the achievement of optimal release rates. The avidity of macrophages for injected

Table 4. Effect of galactolipid incorporation into liposomes on their uptake by isolated hepatocytes.

	Vesicles without GM_1	Vesicles with GM_1
CF inside cells (pmol/10^6 cells)	7.5	8.3
CF adsorbed to cells (pmol/10^6 cells)	25.2	34.4
Total cell-associated lipid (nmol/10^6 cells) based on:		
CF	0.53	0.75
Chol. oleate	0.59	0.78
Lecithin	0.74	4.1

Unilamellar vesicles were prepared from [^{14}C]-egg lecithin, cholesterol, dicetylphosphate (with or without GM_1 ganglioside) in a molar ratio of 4:3:0.45 (:0.6) and a trace of cholesteryl-[1-^{14}C]-oleate. The vesicles contained 100 mM carboxyfluorescein (CF) which, at this concentration, is nonfluorescent because of self-quenching but becomes fluorescent when it is diluted by transfer into the cells after vesicle-cell interaction or by addition of Triton X-100. Fluorescence measurement before and after Triton addition allows discrimination between CF transferred into the cells and CF in vesicles adsorbed to the cells (upper part of table); 2×10^6 hepatocytes were incubated for 5 min with 1.25 μmol total vesicle lipid in a volume of 10 ml. Association of total vesicle lipid with the cells was assayed on the basis of [^{14}C]phosphatidyl-choline, [^{14}C]-cholesteryl oleate, and CF (lower part of table).

liposomes can, obviously, present serious difficulties. On the other hand, this problem too has a sunny side, as has been elegantly shown by Alving and co-workers [37, 38] and New et al. [39] in studies on the use of liposomes as carriers of anti-leishmaniasis drugs. The Leishmania parasites reside in the Kupffer cells of the host, and the encapsulation in liposomes of the usual antimonial drugs to combat this disease resulted in a several hundred-fold increase in drug efficiency. For applications other than those requiring uptake by macrophages, ways have to be found to prevent such uptake. Studies to find a means to block the activity of macrophages or prevent them in some other way from taking up injected liposomes are in progress.

To be able to take optimal advantage of interactions between drug-containing liposomes and nonphagocytic cells it is important to understand the precise nature of these interactions. For this purpose, studies on isolated cells in vitro are of essential importance. In addition to the use of fluorescent dyes, the application of fluorogenic substrates which become fluorescent only after enzymatic cleavage [40] may be very helpful in elucidating the mechanisms by which liposomes interact with cells and the factors which determine the nature and extent of this interaction. We recently showed that such substrates can be put to use in monitoring the fusion of phospholipid vesicles [41]. Application of the same approach to vesicle-cell interaction would seem a matter of designing proper fluorogenic substrates for specific intracellular enzymes.

295

Acknowledgments. The work described in this chapter was financially supported by The Netherlands Organization for the Advancement of Pure Research, the Koningin Wilhelmina Fonds, and NATO. The technical assistance of Joke Regts, Henriëtte Morselt, Ron Tomasini, Henk Westenberg, Bert Dontje, and Jan Wybenga is gratefully acknowledged. We thank Mrs. Rinske Kuperus for preparing the manuscript and Theo Deddens and Bert Tebbes for the artwork.

REFERENCES

1. Zborowski J, Roerdink F, Scherphof G: Leakage of sucrose from phosphatidylcholine liposomes induced by interaction with serum albumin. Biochim Biophys Acta 497: 183–191, 1977.
2. Scherphof G, Roerdink F, Waite M, Parks J: Disintegration of phosphatidylcholine liposomes in plasma as a result of interaction with high-density lipoproteins. Biochim Biophys Acta 542: 296–307, 1978.
3. Finkelstein MC, Weissmann G: Enzyme replacement via liposomes. Variations in lipid composition determine liposomal integrity in biological fluids. Biochim Biophys Acta 587: 202–216, 1979.
4. Hoekstra D, Scherphof G: Effect of fetal calf serum and serum protein fractions on the uptake of liposomal phosphatidylcholine by rat hepatocytes in primary monolayer culture. Biochim Biophys Acta 551: 109-121, 1979.
5. Lee AG: Lipid phase transitions and phase diagrams. Biochim Biophys Acta 472: 237–344, 1977.
6. Papahadjopoulos D, Jacobson K, Nir S, Isac T: Phase transitions in phospholipid vesicles. Fluorescence polarization and permeability measurements concerning the effect of temperature and cholesterol. Biochim Biophys Acta 311: 330–348, 1973.
7. Blok MC, Van der Neut-Kok ECM, Van Deenen LLM, De Gier J: The effect of chain length and lipid phase transitions on the selective permeability properties of liposomes. Biochim Biophys Acta 406: 187–196, 1975.
8. Fukuzawa K, Ikeno H, Tokumura A, Tsukatani H: Effect of α-tocopherol incorporation on glucose permeability and phase transition of lecithin liposomes. Chem Phys Lipids 23: 13–22, 1979.
9. Op den Kamp JAF, Kauerz MT, Van Deenen LLM: Action of pancreatic phospholipase A$_2$ on phosphatidylcholine bilayers in different physical states. Biochim Biophys Acta 406: 169–177, 1975.
10. Wilschut JC, Regts J, Westenberg H, Scherphof G: Hydrolysis of phosphatidylcholine liposomes by phospholipases A$_2$. Effects of the local anesthetic dibucaine. Biochim Biophys Acta 433: 20–31, 1976.
11. Wilschut JC, Regts J, Westenberg H, Scherphof G: Action of phospholipases A$_2$ on phosphatidylcholine bilayers. Effects of the phase transition, bilayer curvature and structural defects. Biochim Biophys Acta 508: 185–196, 1978.
12. Mabrey S, Mateo PL, Sturtevant JM: High-sensitivity scanning calorimetric study of mixtures of cholesterol with dimyristoyl and dipalmitoyl phosphatidylcholines. Biochemistry 17: 2464–2468, 1978.
13. Yatvin MB, Weinstein JN, Dennis WH, Blumenthal R: Design of liposomes for enhanced release of drugs by hyperthermia. Science 202: 1290–1294, 1978.
14. Weinstein JN, Magin RL, Yatvin MB, Zaharko DS: Liposomes and local hyperthermia: selective delivery of methotrexate to heated tumors. Science 204: 188–191, 1979.
15. Rahman Y-E, Wright BJ: Liposomes containing chelating agents. Cellular penetration and a possible mechanism of metal removal. J Cell Biol 65: 112–122, 1975.
16. Gregoriadis G, Putman D, Louis L, Neerunjun DE: Comparative effect and fate of non-entrapped and liposome-entrapped neuraminidase injected into rats. Biochem J 140: 323–330, 1974.

17. McDougall IR, Dunnick J, McNamee MG, Kriss JP: Distribution and fate of synthetic lipid vesicles in the mouse: a combined radionuclide and spin label study. Proc Natl Acad Sci USA 71: 3487–3491, 1974.
18. Hinkle GH, Born GS, Kessler WV, Shaw SM: Preferential localization of radiolabeled liposomes in liver. J Pharm Sci 67: 795–798, 1978.
19. Gregoriadis G, Neerunjun DE: Control of the rate of hepatic uptake and catabolism of liposome-entrapped proteins injected into rats. Eur J Biochem 47: 179–185, 1974.
20. Wisse E, Gregoriadis G, Daems WTh: Electronmicroscopic cytochemical localization of intravenously injected liposome-encapsulated horse radish peroxidase in rat liver cells. In: Reichard SM, Escobar MR, Friedman H (eds) The reticuloendothelial system in health and disease: functions and characteristics. New York, Plenum, 1976, pp 237–245.
21. Scherphof G, Roerdink F, Hoekstra D, Zborowski J, Wisse E: Stability of liposomes in presence of blood constituents: consequences for uptake of liposomal lipid and entrapped compounds by rat liver cells. In: Gregoriadis G and Allison AC (eds) Liposomes in biological systems. London, John Wiley and Sons, 1980, pp 179–209.
22. Roerdink FH, Wisse E, Morselt HWM, Van der Meulen J, Scherphof GL: Cellular distribution of intravenously injected protein-containing liposomes in the rat liver. In: Wisse E, Knook DL (eds) Kupffer cells and other liver sinusoidal cells. Amsterdam, Elsevier/North-Holland, 1977, pp 263–272.
23. Munthe-Kaas AC, Berg T, Seljelid R: Distribution of lysosomal enzymes in different types of rat liver cells. Exp Cell Res 99: 146–154, 1976.
24. Knook DL, Sleyster EC: Separation of Kupffer and endothelial cells of the rat liver by centrifugal elutriation. Exp Cell Res 99: 444–449, 1976.
25. Wisse E: In: Wisse E, Knook DL (eds) Kupffer cells and other liver sinusoidal cells. Amsterdam, Elsevier/North-Holland, 1977, pp 33–60.
26. Lazar G: The reticuloendothelial-blocking effect of rare earth metals in rats. J Reticuloendothel Soc 13: 231–237, 1973.
27. Weismann G, Bloomgarden D, Kaplan R, Cohen C, Hoffstein S, Collins T, Gotlieb A, Nagle D: A general method for the introduction of enzymes by means of immunoglobulin-coated liposomes, into lysosomes of deficient cells. Proc Natl Acad Sci USA 72: 88–92, 1975.
28. Gregoriadis G, Neerunjun DE: Homing of liposomes to target cells. Biochem Biophys Res Commun 65: 537–544, 1975.
29. Roerdink FH, Hulstaert CE, Nienhaus AJ, Scherphof GL: Effect of liposome-entrapped glucosidase on glycogen stores in cultured fibroblasts from a patient with Pompe's disease (glycogenosis type II). In: Hommes FA (ed) Models for the study of inborn errors of metabolism. Amsterdam, Elsevier/North Holland Biomedical Press, 1979, pp 333–340.
30. Hoekstra D, Tomasini R, Scherphof G: Interaction of phospholipid vesicles with rat hepatocytes in monolayer culture. Biochim Biophys Acta 542: 456–469, 1978.
31. Weinstein JN, Yoshikami S, Henkart P, Blumenthal R, Hagins WA: Liposome-cell interaction: transfer and intracellular release of a trapped fluorescent marker. Science 195: 489–492, 1977.
32. Van Renswoude AJBM, Westenberg P, Scherphof GL: In vitro interaction of Zajdela ascites hepatoma cells with lipid vesicles. Biochim Biophys Acta 558: 22–40, 1979.
33. Hoekstra D, Van Renswoude AJBM, Tomasini R, Scherphof GL: Interaction of phospholipid vesicles with rat hepatocytes. Further characterization of vesicle-cell surface interaction; use of serum as a physiological modulator. Membr Biochem (submitted for publication).
34. Sandra A, Pagano RE: Liposome-cell interactions. Studies of lipid transfer using isotopically asymmetric vesicles. J Biol Chem 254: 2244–2249, 1979.
35. Ashwell G, Morell AG: The role of surface carbohydrates in the hepatic recognition and transport of circulating glycoproteins. Adv Enzymol 41: 99–128, 1974.
36. Van Renswoude AJBM, Hoekstra D: Cell-induced leakage of liposome contents. Biochemistry (in press).
37. Alving CR, Steck EA, Hanson WL, Loizeaux PS, Chapman WL, Waits VB: Improved therapy of experimental Leishmaniasis by use of a liposome-encapsulated antimonial drug. Life Sci 22: 1021–1026, 1978.

38. Alving CR, Steck EA, Chapman WL, Waits VB, Hendricks LD, Swartz GM, Hanson WL: Therapy of Leishmaniasis: superior efficacies of liposome-encapsulated drugs. Proc Natl Acad Sci USA 75: 2959-2963, 1978.
39. New RRC, Chance ML, Thomas SC, Peters W: Anti Leishmanial activity of antimonials entrapped in liposomes. Nature 272: 55–56, 1978.
40. Yaron A, Carmel A, Katchalski-Katzir E: Intramolecularly quenched fluorogenic substrates for hydrolytic enzymes. Anal Biochem 95: 228–235, 1979.
41. Hoekstra D, Yaron A, Carmel A, Scherphof GL: Fusion of phospholipid vesicles containing a trypsin-sensitive fluorogenic substrate and trypsin: a new method to study membrane fusion in a model system. FEBS Lett 106: 176–180, 1979.

23. THE USE OF DRUG-CARRIER CONJUGATES IN THERAPY

A. TROUET

The chemotherapeutic selectivity of antitumoral and antiinfectious drugs can be enhanced very significantly by linking to carriers [1]. To achieve such improvement, several conditions must be fulfilled: (a) the drug-carrier link should remain stable in the bloodstream and be cleaved inside the target cells so as to induce the release of the drug in an active form; (b) the drugs to be carried must act only intracellularly and not require a metabolic transformation step in nontarget cells; and (c) the carrier should be unable to permeate across the cell membrane, be degradable, possess to some extent the ability to interact with a given cell type, and be endocytosable. If all these conditions are fulfilled, the carried drug will remain inactive until it is endocytosed with its carrier and released inside the lysosomal system after digestion of the carrier or of the carrier-drug bond. Unlike that of classic drugs, whose selectivity is rarely determined by the mode of cellular uptake, the drug-carrier activity will rely on the differential uptake by various types of cell. Since the endocytic properties of cells are known to vary greatly with respect to different macro-molecules, the type of carrier will influence the type of cell that will activate the drug. Another important factor will be the necessity for the drug-carrier conjugate to cross barriers such as the capillary walls, whose permeability may be very high in tissues such as bone marrow and spleen or at an extremely low level in the case of the blood-brain barrier. The nature of the carrier will thus influence the availability of the drug to several tissues and organs.

We distinguish three levels of increased selectivity that can be imparted to drugs by binding to carriers. The first level results from the absence of uptake of the drug carrier by those nontarget cells which, although sensitive to the toxic action of the free drug, do not endocytose the carrier or are separated from the bloodstream by anatomical barriers impermeable to the carrier. A second level will be reached when the target cells are very active in binding and endocytosing the carrier; as a result, the concentration of the carrier drug

---

Abbreviations: DNA, deoxyribonucleic acid; DNR, daunorubicin; DOX, doxorubicin; EB, ethidium bromide; MST, median survival time; ILS, increase in life span; VCR, vincristine; PQ, primaquine; W.ch., weight change; Lip, liposome; MLV, multilamellar large liposomes; SUV, small unilamellar liposomes; PC:CHOL:PS, liposomes composed of phosphatidylcholine, chol-esterol, phosphatidylserine; LTS, long-term survivors; PC:CHOL:SA, liposomes composed of phosphatidylcholine, cholesterol, stearylamine; SA, serum albumin; AA, amino acid.

W.Th. Daems et al. (eds.), Cell Biological Aspects of Disease, 299–307. All rights reserved.
Copyright © 1981 by Martinus Nijhoff Publishers bv, The Hague/Boston/London.

will be selectively increased in those cells. A third and optimal level will be achieved when only target cells bind and activate the drug carrier conjugate; this could theoretically be the case for carriers, such as some glycoproteins which react with and are endocytosed by one given cell type, for instance hepatocytes [2] or macrophages [3].

To test this hypothesis in the field of chemotherapy for cancer and protozoal diseases, we have studied DNA and liposomes as carriers and are developing methods for linking drugs to proteins. We shall briefly summarize our results and draw some conclusions about the suitability of DNA and liposomes as carriers for antitumoral and antiprotozoal drugs.

DRUG-DNA COMPLEXES

Antitumoral anthracyclines-DNA

Since antitumoral anthracyclines, e.g., daunorubicin (DNR) and doxorubicin (DOX), have a high affinity for DNA, we have compared in mice the toxic and chemotherapeutic properties of the free drugs and of the complexes formed in vitro between these drugs and high molecular weight DNA extracted from calf thymus or herring sperm [4, 5]. The most encouraging results were obtained with DOX-DNA, the toxicity of which was decreased while its activity against the L1210 leukemia was very significantly enhanced. Similar but less impressive results were obtained with DNR-DNA [6]. Pharmacokinetic studies have shown that DOX-DNA is a much more stable complex than DNR-DNA after intravenous administration, the latter behaving more like a slow-release form of DNR [7]. Clinical trials performed on almost 600 patients indicate that for an activity at least equal to that of the free drug on several types of malignant diseases, DNR-DNA and DOX-DNA are less cardiotoxic than their free counterparts [8]. This decrease in cardiotoxicity was one of our claims, since we postulated, on the assumption of a limited endocytosis of DNA by myocardial cells, that the uptake of anthracyclines by heart-muscle cells would be decreased after administration of DNA complexes. Experiments in mice have indeed shown that the uptake of anthracyclines by the heart is reduced about three times by the use of DNA complexes [7].

Antiprotozoal ethidium bromide-DNA

The chemotherapeutic activity of an antiprotozoal drug-carrier conjugate would be increased if extracellular protozoa endocytose the carrier very actively or if the intracellular protozoa infect cells possessing a high endocytic

Table 1. Chemotherapeutic effect of EB and EB-DNA in experimental Chaga's disease.

Drug	Days of injection	MST	ILS
0	0	13.8	0
EB	1, 2, 3	14	1
EB-DNA	1, 2, 3	>168	>1114
EB	3, 4, 5	31	124
EB-DNA	3, 4, 5	>168	>1114
EB	5, 6, 7	30	117
EB-DNA	5, 6, 7	>168	>1114
EB	7, 8, 9	13.8	0
EB-DNA	7, 8, 9	13.7	—1

NMRI mice were inoculated i.p. with 10^5 *Trypanosoma cruzi* on day 0 and received 3 i.p. injections of EB or EB-DNA at a dose of 20 mg EB/kg/injection. MST, median survival time (in days); ILS, increase in life span over controls (in percent).

activity. To test these possibilities, we compared the toxicity and the activity of free ethidium bromide (EB) and EB-DNA complexes in mice infected intraperitoneally with *Trypanosoma cruzi* [9]. Whereas the toxicity of EB is significantly reduced after intraperitoneal administration of a DNA complex, its chemotherapeutic activity against experimental Chaga's disease is, as shown in Table 1, greatly increased when the injections of the drugs are given within the seven days after the parasite inoculation. Pharmacokinetic studies have shown that the stability of EB-DNA is weak in the bloodstream and that at least part of the enhanced chemotherapeutic effect could be the result of increased levels of EB maintained for a longer period in the peritoneal cavity.

DNA as carrier

The main advantage of DNA as a carrier is the ease with which the drug can be bound without chemical manipulation. Its usefulness is, however, restricted to those drugs which, like anthracyclines and to a lesser extent like ethidium bromide, have a high affinity for DNA. Due to the noncovalent type of linkage the stability of the complex may be poor in the bloodstream, and we have calculated that for a DNA-drug complex to be sufficiently stable, the drug should have an affinity constant of at least 10^6 as determined at 37°C and in the presence of serum proteins [10].

LIPOSOME-ENTRAPPED DRUGS

Daunorubicin and vincristine

In collaboration with D. Deprez-De Campeneere, D. Layton, and E. Mayhew, we have entrapped DNR and vincristine (VCR) and in liposomes of different types: multilamellar, unilamellar, and positively and negatively charged. As illustrated in Tables 2 and 3, the entrapment of DNR or VCR in liposomes does not result in an increase of the chemotherapeutic activity when given intraperitoneally against the intraperitoneal form of L1210 leukemia or when given intravenously against the intravenously inoculated P388 leukemia. Contrary to our expectations, multilamellar liposomes composed of phosphatidylcholine, cholesterol, and stearylamine and containing VCR were much more toxic than VCR alone.

We think that liposomes are poorly suited to carry antitumoral drugs because they are mainly taken up by the liver, spleen, and lung [11], which makes it very difficult to direct them toward tumoral cells localized in other tissues. As a consequence of this, however, liposomes may be more useful when drugs are needed at sites of intracellular infection localized in liver or spleen.

Table 2. Chemotherapeutic activity against L1210 leukemia of daunorubicin entrapped in liposomes.

Drug	Dose (mkg/kg/day)	ILS	LTS	W.ch.
DNR	1	43	0/9	+ 0.3
	2	47	0/9	+ 0.1
	4	45	0/9	− 2.2
DNR-Lip	1	41	0/9	+ 0.1
MLV	2	47	0/9	+ 0.2
(PC:CHOL:PS)	4	41	1/9	− 0.4
DNR-Lip	1	45	1/9	+ 0.4
SUV	2	44	1/17	+ 0.4
(PC:CHOL:PS)	4	51	0/8	− 1.7

DBA$_2$ mice were inoculated i.p. on day 0 with 10^4 L1210 cells and treated i.p. with free DNR or DNR entrapped in liposomes (DNR-Lip) on days 1 and 2. MLV, multilamellar large liposomes; SUV, small unilamellar liposomes; PC:CHOL:PS, liposomes composed of phosphatidylcholine, cholesterol, and phosphatidylserine in a molar ratio of 4:5:1; ILS, increase in life span in percent over controls; LTS, long-term survivors on day 30; W.ch., weight change (in grams) observed on day 8.

Table 3. Chemotherapeutic activity against P388 leukemia of vincristine entrapped in liposomes.

Drug	Dose (mg/kg/day)	Day of injection	ILS	LTS
VCR	1.4	1, 2	16	0/8
VCR-Lip (PC:CHOL:SA)	1.4	1, 2	−73	0/10
VCR	0.8	1, 5	25	0/10
VCR-Lip (PC:CHOL:SA)	0.8	1, 5	−45	0/10
VCR	0.6	1, 5, 9	22	0/7
VCR-Lip (PC:CHOL:PS)	0.6	1, 5, 9	15	0/8
VCR	0.3	1, 5, 9	13	0/9
VCR-Lip (PC:CHOL:PS)	0.3	1, 5, 9	19	0/10

C_{57} black mice were inoculated i.v. on day 0 with 2.10^4 P388 cells and treated i.v. with free VCR or VCR entrapped in multilamellar large liposomes (VCR-Lip). PC:CHOL:SA, liposomes composed of phosphatidylcholine, cholesterol, and stearylamine in a molar ratio of 7:2:1; PC:CHOL:PS, liposomes composed of phosphatidylcholine, cholesterol, and phosphatidylserine in a molar ratio of 7:2:1; ILS, increase in life span (in percent of control value); LTS, long-term survivors on day 30.

Table 4. Chemotherapeutic activity of primaquine entrapped in liposomes in murine *Plasmodium berghei* infection.

Drug	Dose (mg/kg)	MST	ILS	LTS
PQ	0	11	0	0
	20	21	91	0
	25	> 50	> 355	53
	30	0	− 91	22
PQ-Lip	0	11	0	0
	20	23	109	29
	25	39	255	50
	30	41	273	50
	40	> 50	> 355	88
	50	> 50	> 355	79
	60	> 50	> 355	100

Primaquine (PQ) and primaquine entrapped in liposomes (PQ-Lip) were injected intravenously into TB_{ESP} mice 3 h after ± 10,000 *Plasmodium berghei* sporopzoite inoculation. MST, median survival time (in days); increase in life span (in percent of control value); LTS, long-term survivors on day 50 (in percent).

Primaquine

When primaquine (PQ) is entrapped in small multilamellar liposomes (PQ-Lip) (phosphatidylcholine: cholesterol: phosphatidylserine in molar ratios of 4:5:1), its toxicity is very significantly decreased after intravenous administration, since the LD_{50} of PQ-Lip is 139 mg/kg as compared with 38 mg/kg for free PQ. This 3.5-fold decrease in toxicity makes it possible, as shown in Table 4, to administer a 100% curative dose of PQ in a single intravenous injection to treat the exoerythrocytic stage of *Plasmodium berghei* infection (sporozoite-induced) of mice [12].

Liposomes as carriers

The use of liposomes as drug carriers faces two major problems, namely, the difficulty of obtaining a liposome preparation which remains stable in the bloodstream and the tropism of liposomes for liver and spleen. The major indications for liposome-drug conjugates seem to be the treatment of protozoal diseases such as leishmania [13] and the exoerythrocytic stage of malaria.

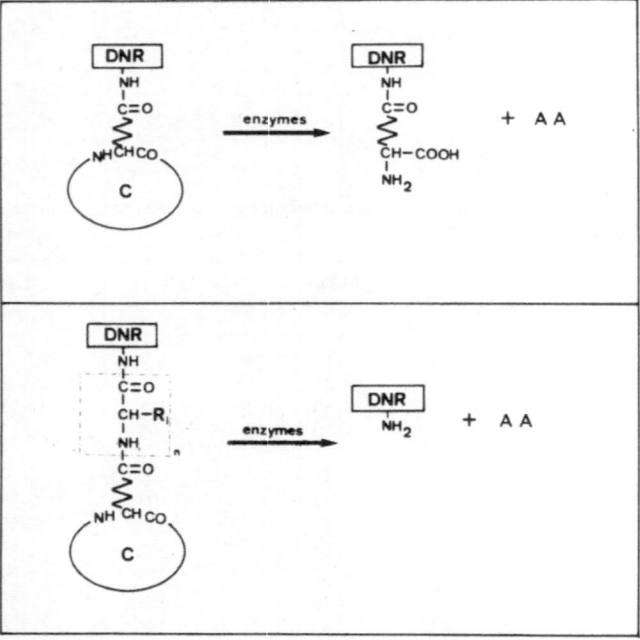

Fig. 1. Schematic representation of the effect of an amino acid or a peptidic spacer on the enzymatic release of intact daunorubicin from a daunorubicin-protein conjugate. Above: direct linking of DNR to a protein (c); below: linking of DNR via one amino acid (AA) or an oligopeptide of *n* amino acids.

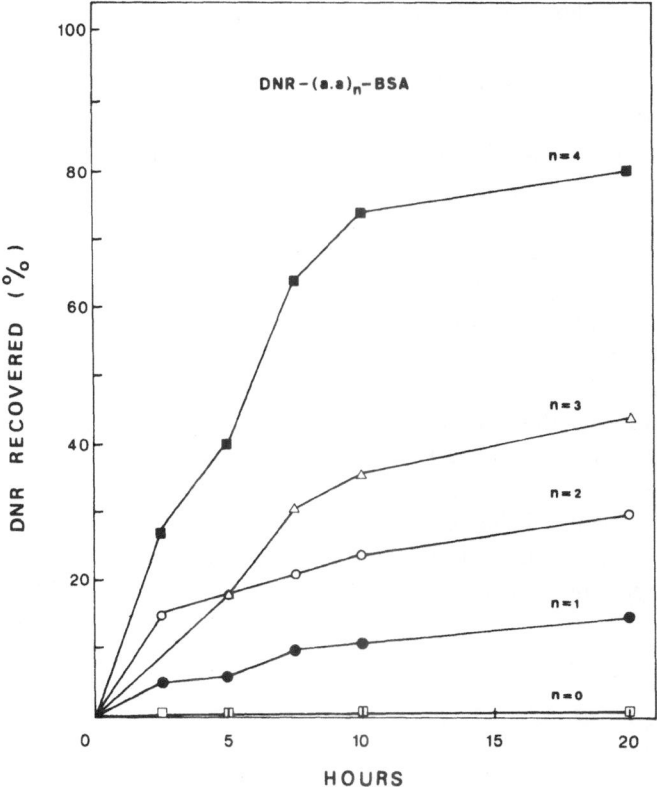

Fig. 2. Influence of the length of the peptidic spacer arm on the release, by lysosomal enzymes, of daunorubicin linked to serum albumin. Daunorubicin linked to serum albumin (DNR-(a.a)$_n$-SA) directly ($n = 0$), via one amino acid ($n = 1$), or via a di-, tri-, or tetrapeptidic spacer ($n = 2, 3$, and 4) was incubated for up to 20 h at 37° C and at pH 4.5 in the presence of lysosomal enzymes purified from rat liver. The release of DNR was measured by high-pressure liquid chromatography.

DRUG-PROTEIN CONJUGATES

The major problem in the development of effective drug-protein conjugates is to achieve a stable covalent linkage between the drug and the protein. This linkage must furthermore be sensitive to lysosomal hydrolases or to an acid pH and allow the release of the drug in an active form. To our knowledge, no such method has yet been described. To investigate this problem, R. Baurain and M. Masquelier have in our laboratory linked DNR to serum albumin (SA) in such a covalent and reversible manner. As illustrated in Fig. 1, it is easy to link the sugar amino group of DNR to a carboxylic side-chain of SA via an amide bond. However, such a bond cannot be a split by peptidases.

because the carboxyl moiety involved in the bond is not in an α position with respect to an asymmetric carbon. Theoretically, however, this problem can be solved (Fig. 1) by intercalating an amino acid or an oligopeptidic spacer arm between the drug and the protein. Under these conditions the peptidic bond adjacent to DNR can be split enzymatically, since the carboxyl group is not in an α position with respect to an asymmetric carbon.

We studied these possibilities by preparing conjugates of DNR and SA and while intercalating up to four amino acids between the drug and the protein. As a test for the suitability of the linkage we incubated these conjugates with purified lysosomal preparations in vitro and followed the release of intact DNR. As illustrated in Fig. 2, no DNR is released if no amino acid is intercalated, and the degree of release increases with the number of amino acids involved in the peptidic spacer arm. This release amounts to more than 80% of the linked DNR if a tetrapeptidic spacer arm is used.

The development of such a linkage technique will allow us to analyze how the physicochemical characteristics of a protein carrier — such as molecular weight, net electrostatic charge, or biological and immunological properties — influence the toxicity and chemotherapeutic properties of the drug it carries.

REFERENCES

1. Trouet A: Increased selectivity of drugs by linking to carriers. Eur J Cancer 14: 105–111, 1978.
2. Ashwell G, Morell AG: The role of surface carbohydrates in the hepatic recognition and transport of circulating glycoproteins. Adv Enzymol 41: 99–128, 1974.
3. Sly WS, Stahl P: Receptor-mediated uptake of lysosomal enzymes. In: Silverstein SC (ed) Transport of macromolecules in cellular systems. Berlin, Dahlem Konferenzen, 1978, pp 229–244.
4. Trouet A, Deprez-De Campeneere D, De Duve C: Chemotherapy through lysosomes with a DNA-daunorubicin complex. Nature [New Biol] 239: 110–112, 1972.
5. Trouet A, Deprez-De Campeneere D, De Smedt-Malengreaux M, Atassi G: Experimental leukemia chemotherapy with a 'lysosomotropic' adriamycin-DNA complex. Eur J Cancer 10: 405–411, 1974.
6. Trouet A, Deprez-De Campeneere D: Daunorubicin-DNA and doxorubicin-DNA: a review of experimental and clinical data. Cancer Chemother Pharmacol 2: 77–79, 1979.
7. Deprez-De Campeneere D, Baurain R, Huybrechts M, Trouet A: Comparative study in mice of the toxicity, pharmacology and therapeutic activity of daunorubicin-DNA and doxorubicin-DNA complexes. Cancer Chemother Pharmacol 2: 25–30, 1979.
8. Trouet A, Sokal G: Clinical studies with daunorubicin-DNA and adriamycin-DNA complexes: a review. Cancer Treat Rep 63 (5): 895–898, 1979.
9. Trouet A, Deprez-De Campeneere D, Maldague P, Jadin JM, Van Hoof F: The concept of lysosomotropic chemotherapy: applications to neoplastic and parasitic diseases. Drug design and adverse reactions. Alfred Benzon Symposium X. Copenhagen, Munksgaard, 1977, pp 77–88.

10. Schneider YJ, Baurain R, Zenebergh A, Trouet A: DNA-binding parameters of dauno-rubicin and doxorubicin in the conditions used for studying the interaction of anthracycline-DNA complexes with cells in vitro. Cancer Chemother Pharmacol 2: 7–10, 1979.
11. Juliano RL, Stamp D: Pharmacokinetics of liposome encapsulated anti-tumor drugs. Biochem Pharmacol 27: 21–27, 1978.
12. Pirson P, Steiger RF, Trouet A: Primaquine liposomes in the chemotherapy of experimental murine malaria. Ann Trop Med Parasitol (in press) 1980.
13. Alving Cr, Steck E, Chapman WL. Waits VB, Hendrickx LD, Swartz GM, Hanson WC: Therapy of leishmaniasis superior efficacies of liposome encapsulated drugs. Proc Natl Acad Sci USA 75: 2959–2963. 1978.

24. CELL BIOLOGY AND HEALTH CARE

INTRODUCTION

Although the subject assigned to me cannot be covered completely in the available space, I shall present some general data on causes of mortality and morbidity and then limit myself to the diagnosis and prevention of congenital disorders as an example to analyze the contribution of cell biological techniques. I shall end by discussing some problems which, in my opinion, limit the optimal development of research and the application of new technology in the field of health care.

It may seem at first sight ridiculous to devote attention to the role of cell biology in health care if one tries to imagine the enormous suffering that must be associated with the high rate of morbidity and mortality in the developing countries (Table 1). Since most of the millions of infant deaths are caused by starvation and infectious diseases, the highest priority must of course be given to improvement of the economic, social, hygienic, and nutritional conditions together with the treatment and prevention of infectious diseases. Cell biology does not play a role in the solution of these immense problems, but it might contribute to the development of new methods of contraception and thus help to decrease the high birth rate, which in time would indirectly influence the prevailing living conditions. So far, acceptance of the available contraceptives has been limited in most of the societies in developing countries, and in addition to religious, economic, and social factors, objections to

Table 1. Birth rate and infant mortality in various parts of the world*.

	Crude birth rate (per 1000)	Infant mortality (per 1000)
Industrialized countries	17	20
Africa	46	120
Latin America	37	60
Asia	38	121

In the developing countries, 37% of the overall mortality occurs during the first year of life and 15%–20% in the period between the age of 1–4 years. In the industrialized countries 2%–5% of the overall mortality occurs between 0 and 5 years of age.
* Data taken mainly from NcNamara's address on the Population Problem delivered at the Massachusetts Institute of Technology on 26 April 1977.

W.Th. Daems et al. (eds.), Cell Biological Aspects of Disease, 309–318. All rights reserved.
Copyright © 1981 by Martinus Nijhoff Publishers bv, The Hague/Boston/London.

the types of contraceptives now made available also play a role. It might be advantageous to have contraceptives that specifically affect male spermatogenesis in a reversible way and without systemic effects. A better understanding of the cell biological processes involved in the division and differentiation of male germ cells might be of great help in developing such contraceptives.

In the wealthy industrialized countries only 2%–5% of the overall mortality is due to death in early infancy. An illustration of the main causes of mortality in four age groups (see Table 2) shows that congenital disorders predominate in childhood, and cardiovascular diseases and malignant tumors in later life. Cell biology does not yet play an important role in the care of patients with these diseases, but cytochemical staining techniques and (automated?) microscopic evaluation of cell morphology and biochemistry will play an increasingly important role in the early diagnosis of several forms of malignancies [3]. Also, it is to be expected that basic research in cell biology and molecular biology will be essential for the elucidation of the etiology of both cardiovascular disease and cancer.

During the last 50 years, infant mortality in the Western countries has decreased by a factor of 10, to about 20/1000. Such countries might then decide to pay little attention to the remaining causes of death in childhood and use their limited funds for other purposes. From a political point of view it could indeed be defensible for a government to give a higher priority to helping many children in a developing country instead of spending the same amount of money for the treatment of a few children with a relatively rare disease in its own country. In practice, however, it appears that a wealthy society with a low infant mortality rate still wants to invest in the treatment and prevention of the diseases that are the remaining causes of death in childhood. Because of the increasing costs of health care, governments of industrialized countries pay more and more attention to the prevention of long-lasting crippling diseases rather than to the treatment of rapidly fatal

Table 2. Three main causes of mortality in difference age groups in an industrialized country.*

Age groups (y)	0–14	15–44	45–64	> 65
Total number of deaths per year	2811 (2.5%)	5686 (5.2%)	20,782 (19%)	80,814 (73.3%)
Congenital disorders and perinatal complications	47%	—	—	—
Accidents	20%	41%	6%	—
Malignant tumors	6.5%	22%	39%	24%
Respiratory diseases	—	15%	—	8%
Cardiac and vascular diseases	—	—	38%	51%

* Data for the Netherlands, 1977, from the *Centraal Bureau voor de Statistiek*, The Hague.

diseases. Also, in medical research and health care more and more emphasis is being put on the prevention of diseases and handicaps. Congenital disorders, which occur in 4%–6% of all liveborns [4–6] and are responsible for a considerable proportion of admissions to hospitals and institutes for the mentally and/or physically handicapped, are a good example of an important field of health care to which basic research in cell biology was contributed. In the following sections some of the contributions to early diagnosis and prevention will be briefly summarized.

CELL BIOLOGY AND CHROMOSOMAL ANOMALIES

Since the discovery by Lejeune et al. [7] that mongoloid idiocy or Down's syndrome is caused by a trisomy of chromosome no. 21, several dozens of syndromes with multiple congenital malformations have been attributed to numerical or structural aberrations of chromosomes [8]. From several newborn screening programs it has become clear that 1 in 200 newborns have a chromosomal anomaly, most of them leading to severe mental retardation and multiple physical handicaps. Some major aberrations of sex chromosomes are associated with growth disturbance and infertility. Chromosomal aberrations have also been found to be responsible for 40%–60% of all spontaneous abortions, and it is now generally assumed that one out of every two conceptions fails because of a chromosomal anomaly [9, 10].

The diagnosis of chromosomal aberrations must be based on karyotyping of short-term cultures of blood lymphocytes and, if mosaicism is found, chromosome analysis of cultured skin fibroblasts will give additional information. In cases of familial chromosome translocations, chromosome studies of healthy relatives of a patient may reveal balanced carriers of a chromosomal anomaly who in most instances have a relatively high risk of affected offspring. Population studies have also shown that the risk of having a child with Down's syndrome increases with maternal age (from 1:1600 at 20 years of age to 1:100 at 40 years and 1:20 at 45 years) and the same holds to a lesser extent for several other chromosomal aberrations. Recently, it became clear that a higher paternal age than 55 years also carries an increased risk (for reviews, see ref. 11).

During the last decade, couples at risk could be offered the option of prenatal chromosome analysis and abortion if an affected fetus was found. Several surveys indicate that up to 1978, at least 15,000 pregnancies had been monitored for a chromosomal anomaly and about 500 affected fetuses were detected [11–14]. At present, prenatal diagnosis and selective abortion have become routine in nearly all industrialized countries, and in the major centers 20–25 pregnant women are monitored every week. Early diagnosis of patients with a chromosomal aberration, family studies in translocation cases, followed by genetic counseling and prenatal karyotyping, now make an important contribution to the prevention of the birth of severely handicapped children.

Cell biological research has played an important role at various stages in the development of early diagnosis and prevention of this category of congenital disorders. First of all, many years of research on mitotic and meiotic cell division and the development of preparation techniques made it possible for Tjio and Levan to establish in 1956 the normal number of chromosomes in man [15]. The discovery by Caspersson and co-workers [16] that fluorescent alkylating agents enable the identification of each individual human chromosome, and even of specific parts within one chromosome, was a great stimulus for the development of a series of new staining techniques (for a review, see ref. 17). This advance not only meant an improvement in the diagnosis of chromosomal anomalies but also contributed significantly to the study of human gene mapping based on human × rodent cell hybrids [18]. The latter studies in turn helped in the elucidation of the nature of some genetic enzyme deficiencies (see next section).

The pioneering work on tissue culture done by Carrell, Fell, Gaillard, and others is another example of an important contribution made by cell biology. This work formed the basis for the first successful cultivation of fetal cells present in amniotic fluid. Advances in the obstetric techniques of early transabdominal amniocentesis and ultrasonography made it possible to obtain samples of amniotic fluid safely in the 16th week of pregnancy, and hence all requirements were fulfilled for the initiation of prenatal diagnosis of chromosomal anomalies in the late 1960s. Further improvement of preparative and staining methods and technical developments in automated evaluation of light-microscopic images may enable us to perform chromosome analysis on a larger scale and at lower cost in the future [3].

CELL BIOLOGY AND GENETIC METABOLIC DISEASES

A total of 3000 conditions are now known to be due to a single gene mutation [19], and in about 200 genetic diseases the responsible molecular defect has been identified [19, 20]. The overall incidence of genetic diseases with Mendelian inheritance is probably of the order of 0.5%–1.0% of all liveborns. The incidence of individual diseases varies between 1 in 10,000 to less than 1 in 100,000 newborns. Most genetic metabolic diseases are associated with severe physical and/or mental handicaps and a shortened life expectancy. In a few diseases the development of psychomotor deterioration can be prevented by early treatment either with a specific diet or by the administration of coenzymes, vitamins, hormones, or drugs. For some of these diseases, for instance phenylketonuria, early diagnosis and treatment is being accomplished by mass screening of newborns [21].

Once a child with a genetic disease has been born, the parents have a recurrence risk of 25% or 50%, depending on whether the disease is inherited as a recessive or a dominant trait. As a result of this high risk, many parents will be deterred from another pregnancy despite the fact that they would have liked to have a normal child. If both are carriers of the same recessive gene mutation or the male carries a dominant mutation, artifical insemination with donor sperm could be considered for couples at risk who want another child. In practice, this approach is not chosen very often. Fortunately, during the last decade another alternative for couples at risk has emerged in the form of prenatal monitoring followed by selective abortion. At present, more than 60 genetic metabolic diseases have been shown to be expressed in cultured amniotic fluid cells, and practical experience with prenatal diagnosis in the 16th–20th week of pregnancy has already been gained for 40 different recessive diseases. Worldwide experience probably amounts to 1500–2000 cases, in about 25% of which the fetus was found to be affected [11–14].

In autosomal-recessive diseases the diagnosis of a patient usually is the first indication that both parents are carriers of the same gene mutation. Genetic counseling and prenatal monitoring in subsequent pregnancies can only prevent the birth of a second affected child in the same family. It would of course be advantageous to know that two partners are carriers of the same mutation before the first pregnancy. Unfortunately, this is only possible in a few cases. In some X-linked disorders, such as Duchenne muscular dystrophy, classic hemophilia, the Lesch-Nyhan syndrome, Fabry's disease, mucopolysaccharidosis type II, and a few others, the presence of an affected brother, uncle, nephew, or other male relative may warn a woman that she might be a carrier. If this can be demonstrated by laboratory tests, she can be informed before reproduction that she runs a 1 in 4 risk of having an affected son, and preventive measures can be taken. In exceptional cases of autosomal-recessive diseases with a high incidence among certain ethnic groups, mass screening for carriership has been performed [22], but in most instances the incidence of such diseases is too low and the methodology of carrier detection is too uncertain to warrant such carrier screening programs [23]. In other genetic diseases that do have a high incidence, such as cystic fibrosis (1 in 2500 newborns), the responsible molecular defect is not yet known and therefore screening of neither patients nor carriers is possible.

Cell biology and biochemistry have so far been of great importance for the early diagnosis and prevention of genetic metabolic diseases, and these disciplines are likely to contribute in the future as well. In the past, the diagnosis of genetic diseases was mainly based on clinical examination and pedigree studies. Later, pathological investigation of organs and tissues provided additional help in delineating a certain syndrome. The application of more specific histochemical staining techniques and the performance of electron-microscopic studies on the subcellular morphology have been of great value in the identification of specific storage products present in many genetic diseases. The most illustrative example of this is the work of the Louvain group on lysosomal storage diseases (for reviews, see refs. 14, 20, and 24). Chemical analysis of metabolites in urine, blood, and other body fluids and biochemical assays of autopsy material and organ biopsies subsequently formed the main basis for the elucidation of the responsible molecular defects. New analytic techniques such as chromatography, and bacterial inhibition assays were often needed before significant advances in chemical diagnosis could be made. The knowledge about accumulation of certain chemical constituents or the lack of specific metabolites led to the discovery of particular genetically determined enzyme deficiences, and this in turn has greatly facilitated the biochemical diagnosis of genetic disease [14, 20]. In many instances the exact diagnosis can now be made by enzyme assays of white blood cells, tissue biopsies, or cultured skin fibroblasts.

Cell biological techniques have been particularly important in the investigation of cultured cells from patients with a genetic metabolic disease, in carrier detection in X-linked disorders, and in prenatal diagnosis. Autoradiography after incubation of cultured cells with [3]H- or ^{14}C-labeled compounds permitted the first (prenatal) analysis of human mutant fibroblasts or cultured amniotic fluid cells [25, 26], and at present an appreciable number of genetic diseases can be detected in utero with this method. Autoradiography also makes it possible to demonstrate metabolic defects in single cultured cells, and hence this technique is useful for the detection of carriers of some X-linked diseases by demonstrating two clonal cell populations in a skin biopsy (for a review, see ref. 14). Conventional biochemical techniques for enzyme assays usually require several milligrams of cell material. This means that many millions of cells must be cultivated, and cultivation periods of 4–6 weeks were no exception in the earlier days of prenatal diagnosis of genetic diseases [27]. The amount of cell material needed for enzyme assays could be significantly reduced by the application of ultramicrotechniques originally developed for the microchemical analysis of dissected tissue structures from freeze-dried sections [28–32]. Our own group in Rotterdam has adapted microspectrophotometric and microfluorometric methods for the (prenatal) analysis in small numbers of cells, and sometimes even in single cultured cells, of about 20 different genetic enzyme defects mainly involved in lysosomal storage diseases [14, 32]. During the last few years other centers have successfully scaled down chromatographic radiometric methods [14], and it is to be expected that in the future quantitative cytochemical techniques will find further application in the early diagnosis of genetic disease and in carrier detection.

An alternative approach to the (prenatal) detection of genetic metabolic defects is the demonstration of gene mutations directly at the level of DNA itself. Quite recently, the use of restriction enzymes and molecular hybridization with radioactive complementary DNA made it possible to demonstrate in relatively few cultured (amniotic fluid) cells the gene mutations responsible for β-thalassemia [33] and for sickle-cell anemia [34]. The potential of this approach is quite impressive, since it is no longer necessary for a particular genetic metabolic defect to be expressed in cultured cells, because the complete genetic information, including gene mutations, is present in all nucleated cells. By using linkage between a gene mutation and a specific polymorphism it will even be possible to demonstrate in cultured amniotic-fluid cells genetic diseases for which the responsible protein defect is still unknown [34].

SOME GENERAL REMARKS ABOUT THE RELATION BETWEEN BASIC RESEARCH AND HEALTH CARE

The examples given in the two preceding sections have illustrated that cell biology has made important contributions to the early diagnosis and prevention of certain categories of congenital disorders. Experts in other fields could no doubt give similar examples for other groups of diseases. Even a brief list of the advances made in molecular genetics, cell biopsy, biochemistry, and medical technology would be impressive and might lead one to wonder where the limitations of future research will be. The ethicists have not had time yet for proper studies to answer the successive questions that have arisen as a result of new applications in health care. To mention a few of these questions: Is abortion of an affected fetus justified, and if so, up to which gestational period?

How should 'affected' be defined, and what should the decision be, for instance, when a chromosomal or molecular defect is detected that cannot be related to specific handicaps with absolute certainty? What criteria do we use when we decide to put a premature baby in an intensive care unit and how do we act if such a baby has severe malformations? Should we screen all newborns for all kinds of genetic diseases, irrespective of whether treatment is available, just for the sake of early genetic counseling to prevent the birth of a second affected child? Do we want to know that our babies are suffering from a certain abnormality even if this will only be expressed clinically many years later or perhaps not until adulthood? What are the criteria to start with sophisticated treatment and when do we stop? And these are only a few of the questions that must be answered.

One often has the impression that expert committees are still working on 'old' ethical questions at a time when the practice of health care already requires daily action and basic research has already created 'new' problems. It is not surprising that some people and organizations have reacted to this situation by trying to retard, and sometimes even stop, new developments. One example of this is the emotional debate about recombinant DNA techniques. In some countries, scientists including those in the USA who raised the question of acceptability are making significant progress with recombinant DNA techniques whereas in some other countries, including the Netherlands, expert committees and religious and political groups are still discussing whether this recent development in molecular genetics should be pursued or stopped.

Because of the ethical aspects as well as the increasing costs involved, both basic research and health care are being controlled more and more by government and society. Cost-benefit analysis has become increasingly important. The scientist applying for a grant for basic research is asked to specify the beneficial applications for the society he or she envisages before any work has been carried out! If we continue along the lines now current in many industrialized countries, I wonder whether there will be sufficient scope for creativity in the near future. Many scientists have to combine not only teaching, research, and organization, but also the handling of more and more complicated equipment. They have to write grant applications, progress reports, annual reports, and more publications than their experimental results justify. This means that all scientists have to read too many irrelevant articles, which is another loss of time. On the other hand, we cannot allow the scientists to do just what he or she wants without any control, because our modern societies ask, and rightly so, for information. If we do not provide comprehensible information about the background and purpose of our research we must not be surprised if certain developments are (temporarily) slowed down or stopped. Early communication between the basic scientist and the clinician, on the one hand, and various representatives of society, on the other, will prevent misunderstanding and promote the optimal application of new developments.

In many European countries the gap is widening between basic scientists and clinicians. Many clinicians are overloaded by routine patient care, organization of the increasingly complicated advanced patient care, and teaching. Fewer and fewer of them have time to read in fields outside their own discipline, to think, and to communicate with colleagues in basic research. The basic scientist is often too much occupied with a small area of research, national and international competition, the handling of complicated methodology, and keeping up with the ever-increasing literature. Fewer and fewer of them have time to listen to colleagues in other disciplines. Many scientists even tend to forget the initial aim of their research, which was often related to a problem that arose in patient care.

I believe that cell biology has much to offer to health care, but we must create new organizational structures that will guarantee a better understanding and collaboration between patient, clinician, and scientist. Many of our clinicians might at least partially adopt the attitude of their American colleagues, who seem to have more courage to choose and to limit their working area within a clinical discipline. The basic scientists should aim for more creativity and be less afraid of changing their subject and absorbing knowledge from other disciplines. The organizational structure should be changed in such a way that the main concern of a young scientist no longer is the acquisition of a permanent position. Less opportunity should be given to escape research by accepting all kinds of organizational tasks while still occupying a research position.

Despite all of the impressive advances made in cell biology and health care during the last decades, there still are many challenges for a young (and even an older) cell biologist or clinician. One has only to look at the data in Table 2 to realize that we still have to solve the many problems related to cancer, cardiovascular diseases, rheumatoid arthritis, and the vast majority of congenital disorders. We do not yet know the answers to such important questions as what really occurs in cell differentiation, what regulates cell proliferation, and which molecular processes are associated with the ageing of cells and intercellular structures. Even if a miracle were to occur and we could solve the main problems associated with the main diseases in the industrialized countries, we still have the enormous challenge summarized in Table 1. How can we contribute to the amelioration of the enormous suffering associated with the high rate of morbidity and mortality in the developing countries?

REFERENCES

1. McNamara RS: An address on the population problem. MIT series on World change and world security. Cambridge, MIT, 1977.
2. Greep RO, Koblinsky MA, Jaffe FS (eds): Reproduction and human welfare: a challenge to research. Cambridge, MIT, 1976.
3. Proceedings of the 6th Engineering Foundation Conference on Automated Cytology. J Histochem Cytochem 27: 1–635, 1979.
4. Stevenson AC: The load of hereditary defects in human populations. Radiat Res [Suppl] 1: 306–325, 1959.
5. Trimble BK, Doughty JH: The amount of hereditary disease in human populations. Ann Hum Genet 38: 199–223, 1974.
6. Trimble BK, Smith ME: The incidence of genetic disease and the impact on man of an altered mutation rate. Can J Genet Cytol 19: 375–385, 1977.

7. Lejeune J, Gautier M, Turpin R: Etudes des chromosomes somatiques de neuf enfants mongoliens. CR Acad Sci (Paris) 248: 1721–1722, 1959.
8. De Grouchy J, Turleau C: Atlas de Maladies Chromosomiques. Paris, Expansion Scientifique Française, 1977.
9. Boué A, Boué J: Chromosomal anomalies in early spontaneous abortion. In: Gropp A, Benirschke K (eds) Developmental biology and pathology. Berlin, Springer, 1975, pp 193–208.
10. Jacobs PA: Human cytogenetics: population aspects. In: Armendares S, Lisker R (eds) Human genetics. Proc 5th Int Congr Hum Genet Amsterdam Excerpta Medica, 1977, pp 45–52.
11. Murken JD, Stengel-Rutkowski S. Schwinger E (eds): Prenatal diagnosis. Proc 3rd European Conference on Prenatal Diagnosis of Genetic Disorders. Stuttgart, Enke, 1979.
12. Galjaard H: European experience with prenatal diagnosis of congenital disease: a survey of 6121 cases. Cytogenet Cell Genet 16: 453–467, 1976.
13. Epstein CJ, Golbus MS: Prenatal diagnosis of genetic diseases. Am Sci 65: 703–711, 1977.
14. Galjaard H: Genetic metabolic diseases; early diagnosis and prenatal analysis. Amsterdam, Elsevier Biomedical, 1980.
15. Tjio JH, Levan A: The chromosome number of man. Hereditas 42: 1–6, 1956.
16. Caspersson T, Zech L, Johansson C, Modest EJ: Identification of human chromosomes by DNA-binding fluorescent agents. Chromosoma 30: 215–227, 1970.
17. Schwarzacher HG, Wolf U (eds): Methods in human cytogenetics. Heidelberg, Springer, 1974.
18. Proceedings of the human gene mapping conferences 1–5. Bergsma D (ed): Birth Defects Orig Artic Ser. Natl Found March of Dimes, Basel, Karger, 1973–1980.
19. McKusick VA: Mendelian inheritance in man, 5th ed. Baltimore, Johns Hopkins University, 1978.
20. Stanbury JB, Wyngaarden JB, Frederickson DS (eds): The metabolic basis if inherited disease, 4th ed. New York, McGraw-Hill, 1978.
21. Levy H: Genetic screening. Pediatrics 54: 608–640, 1974.
22. Kaback MM (ed): Tay-Sachs disease: screening and prevention. Proc 1st Int Conf Tay-Sachs Disease. New York, Alan R Liss, 1977.
23. Report on genetic screening; programs, principles and research. Natl Acad Sci USA, 1975.
24. Hers HG, Hoof F van: Lysosomes and storage diseases. New York, Academic, 1973.
25. De Mars R: Some studies of enzymes in cultured human cells. Natl Cancer Inst Monogr 13: 181–191, 1964.
26. Fujimoto WY, Seegmiller JE, Uhlendorf BW, Jacobson CB: Biochemical diagnosis of an X-linked disease in utero. Lancet 2: 511–512, 1968.
27. Nadler H: Tissue culture and antenatal detection of molecular diseases. Biochimie 54: 677–681, 1972.
28. Lowry OH: The quantitative histochemistry of the brain; histological sampling. J Histochem Cytochem 1: 420–428, 1953.
29. Lowry OH, Passonneau JV: A flexible system of enzymatic analysis. New York, Academic, 1972.
30. Glick D: The contribution of microchemical methods of histochemistry to the biological sciences. J Histochem Cytochem 25: 1087–1101, 1977.
31. Galjaard H, Van Hoogstraeten JJ, De Josselin de Jong JE, Mulder MP: Methodology of the quantitative cytochemical analysis of single cells in small numbers of cultured cells. Histochem J 6: 409–429, 1974.
32. Galjaard H, Hoogeveen A, Van der Veer E, Kleijer WJ: Microtechniques in prenatal diagnosis of genetic disease. In: Armendares S, Lisker R (eds) Proc 5th Int Congr Hum Genetics. Amsterdam, Excerpta Medica, 1977, pp 194–206.
33. Orkin SH, Alter BP, Altay C, Mahoney MJ, Lazarus H, Hobbins JC, Nathan DG: Application of endonuclease mapping to the analysis and prenatal diagnosis of thalassemias caused by globin-gene deletion. N Engl J Med 299: 166–172, 1978.
34. Kan Yw, Dozy Am: Antenatal diagnosis of sickle-cell anemia by DNA analysis of amniotic fluid cells. Lancet 2: 910–912, 1978.

25. LIMITS OF OUR ABILITY TO UNDERSTAND LIVING STRUCTURES

L. VROMAN

Our senses point outward. No wonder they notice the changes around us more than they notice those inside us. They seem to mislead us into thinking that we, our true selves, are made of constant structures by which we can gauge and navigate the outer world's moving obstacles. In other words: we think ourselves able to understand at least part of the world. This understanding would involve our being able to predict all properties of the object under study. As outside conditions and influences on the object change, we must also be able to predict all possible effects of these changes; and if internal conditions in the object also may fluctuate, we must be able to predict the effects of any changing properties in the object upon all of its other properties.

Why try to understand complex structures? It seems possible that our curiosity was, long ago, limited to the areas we had to explore in order to survive, and that our efforts to understand the world of things immediately concerning us have expanded to a curiosity about things that do not affect us directly. The unlimited amount of information on the world's properties that enters our brains since our interests have expanded, must, somehow, be compressed. It must be because, since it is not consumable like food, it accumulates. We can only compress this load of information by assuming that many new observations must be covering ealier ones and deal with properties in the outside world that do not change, so that we need to store them in our memory only once. This process of compressing the accidentally accumulating by-products of our curiosity results in the product called 'knowledge.' Knowledge may then be defined as the mere ability to recognize properties, perhaps including their immediate interrelations, and implying that the laws of nature creating these properties and interrelations are as constant as what they create.

Once we would know all of the parts and laws creating an object, we would be able to say we understand that object, and we achieve this understanding by observing how the object repeats in time and/or space under various conditions. What does not repeat, and what is observed only once, must appear chaotic, and chaos eludes analysis.

Our world seems built of things that are part of bigger things, but the laws ruling any one level or arrays (of things or properties) may well differ from those ruling any other level of arrays. For example, the behavior of an

W.Th. Daems et al. (eds.), Cell Biological Aspects of Disease, 319–326. All rights reserved.

organism gives no direct information about the behavior of its organs; and observations of either organs, cells, subcellular structures, protein molecules, or atoms give no information about the substructures that each observed structured thing is made of.

As a result, every surprise is full of surprises. Digging for them, say, in a human being, we find our growing knowledge of the substructures of that person will expand exponentially as we reach the smaller and smaller sub-substructures. However, to study these, we must isolate them from the confusing influences of their fellow structures, large and small, that we had not yet analyzed. Isolated, the substructures under study will be freed, and the smaller they are, the more mobile or variable these isolated and liberated parts will be, so that our ability to understand, or even to know, the smaller things of an organism will fade as our knowledge grows.

We can also see this problem in reverse. We can, for example, imagine a free electron as a particle moving unhindered by bonds through a space containing, say, two more free electrons. The time we would need to compute its location — depending on initial location, speed, and direction as well as on collisions with those two other electrons — would be almost infinitely longer than the time consumed by the actual event. In other words, so few laws govern the motions and position of the electron that we can understand what it is doing, but not where it is doing it. Bound by several forces to the sphere of an atom, that same electron will become much easier to locate, but the laws that localize it more will be harder to understand. As the atom becomes part of a protein molecule, for example, that electron's location is even more limited but its movement will be even more complex, until, incorporated into a living body, we may know most nearly where the electron is but we will be totally unable to understand how it got there, what it is doing, and why its tiny motions, now unique for this electron, are the way they are.

To see this range of detail in perspective, imagine me touching your eye, and your eye is perfect. You will then see electrons spinning aroung the atomic nuclei of my finger tip, and farther away along my finger you will first see the atoms vibrating in their molecules, then the molecules trembling and flipping in my cell membranes, and farther away you will see my cells gently floating or crawling. Beyond you will see my blood vessels sitting quietly, and far away me, doing nothing at all (Fig. 1). But are my larger parts really doing less? How can my slowly moving body be understandable, if within me, super-human efforts are needed to understand any single one of my enzyme molecules completely? Why is an enzyme/substrate reaction in the test tube so predictable? Why can we so easily predict the half-life of a radioactive element, but not the moment when any single one of its atoms will fall apart?

Because, all we know of an apparently quiet thing is its average appearance, or to say it statistically: its mode, meaning what most of its parts are doing

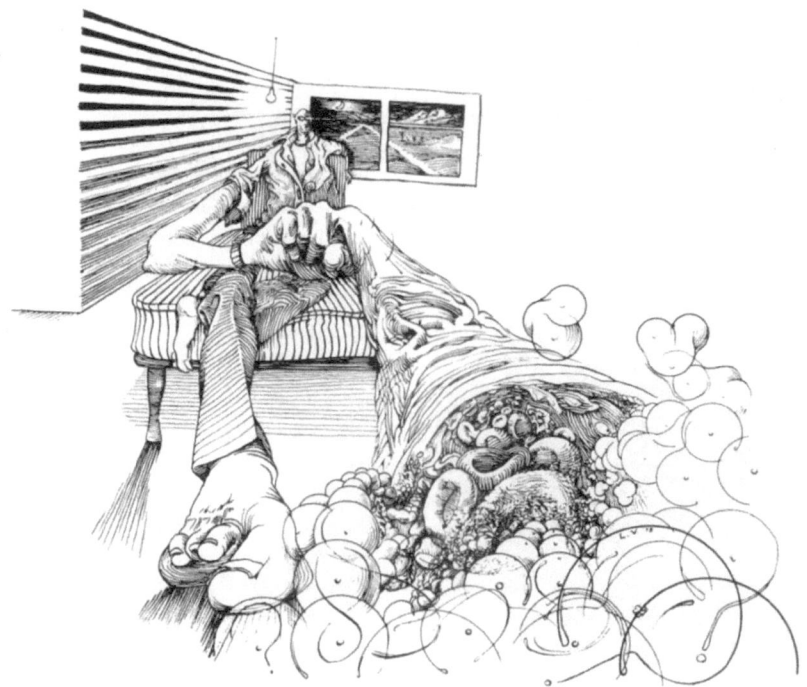

Fig. 1

most of the time. Or we know merely its overall outer mode: what it is like most of the time. Obviously, my body (Fig. 1) appears tranquil and remains predictably looking like me because its is large enough to take a distant view of it, so that we allow ourselves to be satisfied with seeing no more than my mode. We have this habit of backing away from anything, and backing away more the larger the thing is, just far enough that it neatly fills our imaging screen of our eye or our mind (see Fig. 2). The most distant object, such as the expanse of our galaxy, shrinks in our mind's eye as it responds to the word 'galaxy', until that whole section of the universe has come down to the size of an atom imagined in response to the word 'atom.' While shriveling, the giant loses all detectable variability and appears dormant.

We must not be misled. The feeling of tranquility as we gaze up to the so-called constant stars is like the joy of gazing from a mountain peak down into the valley from where we came and seeing the turmoil we just left, shrunk into a soporific blur.

Our failure to predict or understand individual things and events is most obvious when pending disasters are governed by minute substructures. The

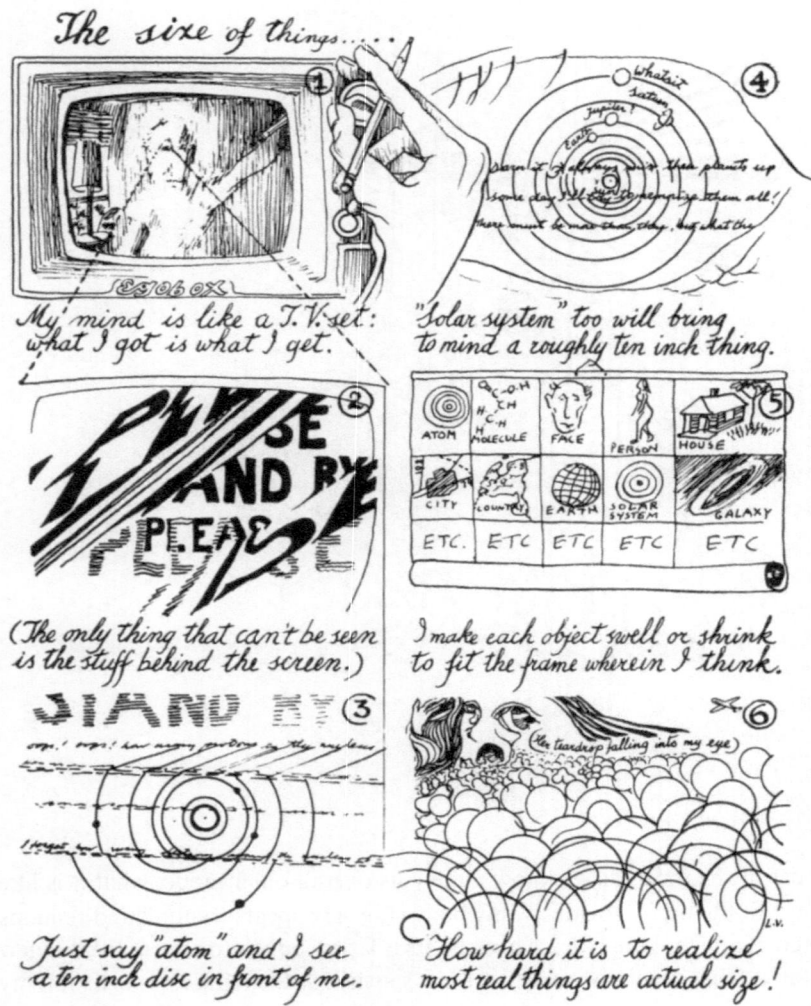

The size of things......

1. My mind is like a T.V. set: what I got is what I get.

2. (The only thing that can't be seen is the stuff behind the screen.)

3. Just say "atom" and I see a ten inch disc in front of me.

4. "Solar system" too will bring to mind a roughly ten inch thing.

5. I make each object swell or shrink to fit the frame wherein I think.

6. How hard it is to realize most real things are actual size!

Fig. 2

alertness of a mountain climber and the one pebble on which he slips over the edge of a cliff; the drunken driver or the computer error that causes death; the single new seed that starts an overgrowth; cancer — they all are events or objects governed by another, uniquely potent one. And, as I said before, uniqueness seems like chaos and defeats understanding, or even knowing. To some extent we know mitochondria, but the knowledge derived from a mostly destructive analysis of many other mitochondria represents a statistical mode that cannot be applied accurately to allow detailed predictions about any one, single, specific mitochondrion. Its exact shape can never be explained.

We can observe the shape of objects thanks only to their interfaces. Our eyes cannot help but fix on outlines, and our brain processes the information on the observed interfaces with a special appetite. Thanks to our high content of interfaces, we contain much that can be observed; but the problem with interfaces in life is that they defy accurate description: they are too mobile to sit still under any thorough probing. Besides, with their softness and mobility, our interfaces in turn induce more unpredictability in the reactions that occur on them. Even if we can predict the behavior of a dissolved enzyme molecule toward its codissolved substrate molecule, when either reacts while adsorbed onto a mobile interface the pattern of enzyme/substrate interaction is affected by spacing and orientation of the adsorbing substrate, by the microclimate and pH at the interface, and by flow. The soft substrates may adapt and reorient themselves under the influence of adhering enzyme, substrate, and reaction product.

The abundance of interfaces within us is staggering. I have tried to imagine it by thinking of stepping into a meat grinder with only a single 0.5×0.1 micron exit that will determine the cross section of the ribbon to be formed out of my entire body (see Fig. 3). Under ideal conditions, this ribbon will be long enough to encircle the earth many thousands of times. And yet, as I pas over every laboratory in the world at least once, anyone with an electron microscope can still see, anywhere in that ribbon, a wealth of interfaces in my mitochondria, microtubules, ribosomes, etcetera. To understand myself, do I have to know all aspects of and among any of these objects within me? What if we accept the following shortcut: say that the living world is a complex system of objects and events that must limit each other just enough to remain within some measurable and biologically acceptable range? If we see living things that way, they will look relaxingly soft, presenting a shimmering yet stable reality, wherein electrons are limited most strictly to their orbits to help create atoms, cells are less clearly limited to create and maintain organs, and organisms (especially humans ones) would *seem* relatively least limited, or only limited by their society. But it is difficult to say how free the organism is from the behavior of its subunits; as it chains them to each other, it is also shackling itself to them. Whereas the organism (or any living structure containing substructures) at its own level, as I said, is less free to move or change once it becomes part of a larger superstructure, it also becomes easier to find and harder to understand because of the more complex world that limits its.

In addition, the organism's behavior (or the behavior of any structured living thing) is not uniformly or predictably affected by its own substructures, which affect not only one another to maintain the superstructure, but may individually and rather directly affect it, rendering the entire organism as

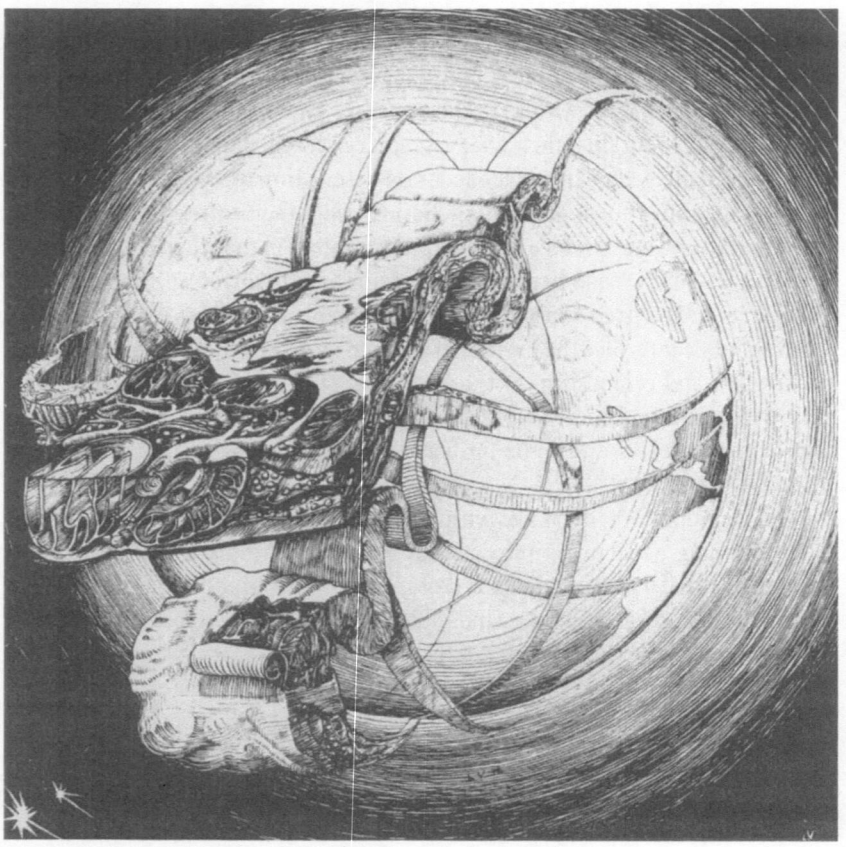

Fig. 3

unpredictable an oligarchy as any one of its dictating electrons. The behavior of the large living thing thus appears controlled by smaller and therefore less 'understandable' things, just as 'understandable' traffic may be controlled by individual and therefore less predictable or understandable collisions.

In other words: with every increase of complexity as living things evolve, the limitation they impose on their subunits become more complex, so that these subunits (1) become harder to understand, (2) change more once they are removed from their matrix (for example with the purpose of studying them in a simpler environment), and (3) can regulate the behavior of this matrix and render it less comprehensible, less significantly close to any statistical mode of behavior. Stepping back to get a reproducible image of the whole, we miss these small governing substructures entirely, and with such blurry vision we will never understand more than the modes of things. The individual human's freedom of nonessential choices — a hairdo, a new flavor of ice cream, the joy of a walk in the woods, or of music and art — all of these will remain then as much beyond understanding as the impending heart attack or traffic accident remains beyond prediction.

I think the arrogance of us, hard scientists, in ignoring so-called abnormal behavior of a few in the study of a group of many, is most obvious if we imagine ourselves being described that way. Looking down on a city as we look down on a network of blood vessels, we would ignore the collision between two cars as long as it does not happen to impede traffic drastically, or no fire breaks out. Even the drivers themselves, stepping out of their vehicles and seeing no damage, may say: 'Well... nothing happened.' It is a way of stepping back, to take an overall, statistically reassuring look at ourselves. We do the same when we study a biological event that increases in magnitude. For example, when studying the formation of a thrombus in response to some agent, we time our observations with longer and longer intervals, stepping back more and more as the thrombus gets larger and larger, and saying: 'Well, in this period less and less happens.' Seen far away, nothing does.

Now, let us discuss the digital, or True Scientific Method. Because after all, mathematics — the science that makes measurement possible — and physics, which proves measurement necessary, appear to delve down into the smallest elements of our matter and beyond, into its pure essential absence. Slowly following behind, how digital can we get? Let us start again with a single subcellular element: one mitochondrion. To express even its simplest property, its overall shape, in digital form so that we can evaluate its changes in time, we must compile very large sets of long strings of numbers that will describe, for example, the odd shapes of cross sections closely spaced from one end of the mitochondrion the the other. And we must repeat this imaginary operation as frequently as the mitochondrion's distortions with time will require. Now, to describe the distribution of one species of enzyme over this structured surface we would need an equally complex set of sets of numbers, plus two values representing the enzyme's concentration and its activity at each set of values describing its location. Any effort to define such a subcellular element would only serve to demonstrate that it cannot really be understood, and to alert us that any cell is totally beyond comprehension. Again, stepping back to avoid its annoying details, we can describe the cell as a roughly spherical object with measurable temperature, viscosity, and velocity, but in the 'noise' that a very sensitive recording of any of these overall properties would show lies the hidden music of its detailed beauty. Its protein turnover, evidence of its endearing efforts to recover from our measurements, would of course be entirely missed.

Even without this turnover and its evidence of homeostasis, negative feedback, and way for the cell to 'read itself,' we would fall behind the cell in reading its proteins. A protein molecule is like a very long word spelled with a string of amino acid residues. Knowing the sequence of these residues, we can now derive the protein molecule's overall shape from the known bond angles between each two residues. However, we will then find that it is a twisted coil, so that the residues will not spell the word as a strung-out sequence, but as a cryptogram written across a strip of paper after it had been wound around some oddly shaped thing. Subtle changes in these windings could cause drastic changes in their message, and we would have to spell each 'word' carefully even when we would think we recognized it. I once calculated from our more or less known protein turnover rates, and presuming we can read our protein molecules as rapidly as we can read simple written words, that we would need only ten million years to read one second of someone's life as long as we would not waste any time trying to understand what we were reading.

I believe many morphologists, histologists and pathologists are quite aware of the gap between quantitative information and the sensory information about the shapes to which the quantitative data must be applied. Often, the two types of data are almost incompatible, as are the scientific articles and their authors dealing with tabulated data, on the one hand, and with pictures, on the other. Understanding would require a merger of the two.

Can we unite our brains, and unite with computers, so that 'we' will be able to understand what no single person can grasp? Personally, this is a concept that is beyond my own individual ability to comprehend. The sensation of understanding, common to students of science, music, arts, and of nature itself, appears forever to be a personal one involving a feeling of totality. The idea of two people who each know half, representing together a completely understanding unit, appears to me as strange as the sum of two half-hearted listeners bursting into tears at a concert. And yet, going through a course or a textbook prepared by many only partially informed people does give us the sensation that there is a beauty hidden in the total work that no single participant could have been aware of.

INDEX

330